ERRATA

CLINICAL RADIOTHERAPY PHYSICS

Volumes I and II

The cover and title page should indicate that Subramania Jayaraman and Lawrence H. Lanzl are the sole authors of these volumes.

Clinical
Radiotherapy
Physics

Treatment Planning and Radiation Safety

Volume II

Clinical Radiotherapy Physics

Treatment Planning and Radiation Safety

Volume II

Edited by

Subramania Jayaraman, Ph.D.

Department of Radiation Oncology
Albert Einstein Medical Center
Philadelphia, Pennsylvania

Lawrence H. Lanzl, Ph.D.

Department of Medical Physics
Rush University
Chicago, Illinois

With the editorial assistance of Elisabeth F. Lanzl

CRC Press
Boca Raton   New York   London   Tokyo

Library of Congress Cataloging-in-Publication Data

Jayaraman, Subramania.

    Clinical radiotherapy physics /Subramania Jayaraman, Lawrence H.
Lanzl.
        p. cm.
    Includes bibliographical references and index.
    Contents: v. 1. Basic physics and dosimetry -- v. 2. Treatment
planning and radiation safety.
    ISBN 0-8493-6891-X (v. 1 : alk. paper). -- ISBN 0-8493-4017-9
(v. 2 : alk. paper) -- ISBN 0-8493-4018-7 (Set)
    1. Medical physics. 2. Radiotherapy. I. Lanzl, Lawrence H.
(Lawrence Herman), 1921- . II. Title.
    [DNLM: 1. Radiotherapy. 2. Physics. 3. Radiation, Ionizing.
4. Radiometry.   WN 250 J42c 1996]
R895.J39 1996
615.8′42--dc20
DNLM/DLC
for Library of Congress
                                           95-42666
                                              CIP

No claim to original U.S. Government works
International Standard Book Number 0-8493-6891-X (Volume I)
International Standard Book Number 0-8493-4017-9 (Volume II)
International Standard Book Number 0-8493-4018-7 (Set)
Library of Congress Card Number 95-42666
Printed in the United States of America 1 2 3 4 5 6 7 8 9 0
Printed on acid-free paper

PREFACE

This text is an introduction to radiotherapy physics. The emphasis in much of the work is on the clinical aspects of the field; thus, the book should be especially useful for persons who are already graduate physicists and plan for a career in clinical radiotherapy physics. At present, the treatment of cancer patients with ionizing radiation is a team effort by radiation oncologists, radiation therapists, as well as clinical physicists. The book is intended to be of use to persons in each of these areas.

Historically, clinical medical physics as a profession can be dated to the year 1913, when William Duane became the first full-time hospital-employed physicist in the United States and Sydney Russ, the first in the United Kingdom. These two physicists worked on similar problems related to the use of radium and radon for the treatment of cancer and other diseases.

Although there were no full-time clinical medical physicists before 1913, the utility of physics to the practice of medicine was recognized much earlier. For example, Galileo's work on the principle of the pendulum was used by physicians of his day for measuring the heart rate of patients. In the early 1800s, the physician Neil Arnott, in England, pioneered the idea that the curriculum of physicians in training should include the study of physics. Arnott's textbooks were translated from English into several languages. He also appears to have been the first to use the term "medical physics" in his writings (1825). To this day, the study of physics is included either in medical schools (e.g., in England, Russia, and China) or in the premedical curriculum (e.g., in the United States and Canada).

In this text we have tried to keep the treatment of a patient in perspective as much as possible, in order to keep the book clinically oriented. The sequence and depths of coverage of the different topics reflect our preference based on our own teaching experience and may be found to differ from other texts on the subject.

The text has been divided into two volumes which are to be used sequentially. We have made an attempt to have the subject develop gradually from chapter to chapter, with minimum cross-references between chapters. However, we recommend that a reader do a quick read-through of all the chapters, and then do a more thorough study of each chapter. In this way, it may be possible to appreciate best how some basic aspects that are covered in early chapters have relevance for discussions to follow in later chapters that are progressively more clinically oriented. Non-physicists can skip parts that are too mathematical, but can benefit by reading the narrative descriptions.

Volume I of the text covers basic physics and principles of radiation dosimetry. The beginning chapters cover the essentials of atomic and nuclear physics, which provide the background for the later chapters. The physics of the use of photons and electrons has been emphasized, because of their widespread use in radiotherapy clinics. The use of hadronic particles (such as neutrons, protons, pions), still being experimental, has been addressed only in minimum detail. A few paragraphs are devoted to leptons, quarks, and other recently identified fundamental particles for the purpose of completeness.

The sources of high-energy photons and electrons are particle accelerators, particularly linear accelerators. We believe that the principles of accelerators of charged particles are covered in sufficient detail for present-day medical physicists.

Radiation fields are quantified in terms of radiation units and measurements. Quantities used in clinical practice are defined and explained. The terms and definitions used in the text follow the recommendations of the appropriate international committees. However, where it was necessary, we felt the need to add a few new terms to improve the clarity of the presentations.

Volume II of the text is devoted to planning of radiation treatments and radiation safety. The text is written to include recent concepts and new refinements. Brachytherapy is an important area of present-day radiotherapy. Thus, radioactivity and the accompanying dosimetry considerations are included in the text. It should be realized that the largest exposure of man to ionizing radiations comes from deliberate irradiation in procedures of diagnostic and therapeutic radiology. Therefore, the later chapters are devoted to radiation safety and safety standards. The philosophy on which these standards are based has undergone a change in recent years, and the authors felt strongly that the changes should be included in the text.

THE AUTHORS

The two authors have been associated with each other professionally for more than 25 years. They first met in 1967, when they took on assignments in the Dosimetry Section of the International Atomic Energy Agency, Vienna, Austria.

S. Jayaraman was on leave of absence from the Bhabha Atomic Research Center, Bombay, India, and Lawrence H. Lanzl was on leave from the Argonne Cancer Research Hospital of the University of Chicago, Chicago, Illinois. For a few months in the 1970s, Lanzl spent some time at the Bhabha Atomic Research Center. Next, in the 1980s, both Jayaraman and Lanzl worked in the Departments of Medical Physics and Therapeutic Radiology at Rush-Presbyterian-St. Luke's Medical Center, Chicago. It was then that the idea of writing this book crystallized.

At present, S. Jayaraman is Staff Medical Physicist in the Department of Radiation Oncology, Albert Einstein Medical Center, Philadelphia, and L.H. Lanzl is Professor of Medical Physics, Department of Medical Physics, Rush University, Chicago.

ACKNOWLEDGMENTS

When writing a book, one calls on past experiences and insights from one's teachers, associates, students, both past and present, as well as previous writers. I would like to acknowledge my debt to all of these. The authors thank Elisabeth F. Lanzl, who has helped to make the volumes readable by her expertise in editing.

Lawrence H. Lanzl

First I wish to thank my father, Ayakarambulam Rajagopalan Subramanian, and my mother, Saraswathi Subramanian, for showering their love and affection on me, as they believed in me and encouraged me since childhood toward accomplishment. So also I acknowledge the special love and affection of my wife Syamala and my daughters, Saramati and Sahana.

My career in medical physics developed largely due to the opportunities of associations with several eminent physicists in the field. Among them I wish especially to recognize and thank Professor Lawrence H. Lanzl, Professor Nagalingam Suntharalingam (of Thomas Jefferson University, Philadelphia), Dr. R. Chidambaram (Chairman, Atomic Energy Commission, India), and S. Somasundaram (Bhabha Atomic Research Center, India). Their expressions of faith in me at different phases in my career made my progress possible.

I also find it appropriate to mention the extraordinary resilience of my coauthor, Lawrence H. Lanzl, who worked with me to see this text to its completion amidst several difficult health challenges. He has been an inspiration to me in many ways ever since I first met him in 1967.

I am thankful for the philosophy of the Albert Einstein Medical Center, Philadelphia, Pennsylvania, which encourages academic achievement by its staff, and for the active endorsement of that objective by Dr. Sucha O. Asbell, Chairman, Department of Radiation Oncology, where I have worked during the last seven years. The encouraging words and appreciation from all staff members of my Department were of great help. Especially I express my thanks to my coworkers in the physics laboratory, including physicist Alan S. Baker, and dosimetrists Shirley A. Johnston and Lori M. Lichtman, for their keen interest in the completion of this text. Our thanks are also owed to Marsha Baker and Renee Taub of CRC Press, Inc. for steering this book through its publication.

Subramania Jayaraman

TABLE OF CONTENTS

VOLUME I

Chapter 1
Scope of Clinical Radiotherapy Physics 1
  1.1 A Physicist in a Clinic? 1
  1.2 Physical Concepts and Radiotherapy 1
  1.3 Cooperation between Physicist and Physician 1
  1.4 Scope of This Book 2

Chapter 2
Atoms, Molecules, and Matter 3
  2.1 Historical Origin of Atomic Physics 3
  2.2 Formation of Atoms and Elements 3
  2.3 Atomic Electron Configuration 7
      2.3.1 Electron Orbits and Energy Levels 7
      2.3.2 Ionization and Excitation of Atoms 9
      2.3.3 Characteristic X-Rays and Auger Electrons 10
  2.4 Definition of an Electron Volt (eV) 10
  2.5 Atomic Mass, Molecular Mass, and Atomic Mass Unit 11
  2.6 Avogadro's Number (N_{Av}) 11
  2.7 Periodic Table of Elements 12
  2.8 Molecular Bonds 12
      2.8.1 Ionic Bonds 12
      2.8.2 Covalent Bonds 12
      2.8.3 Hydrogen Bonds 14
  2.9 Elementary Particles 15
  2.10 Outer Space and Particle Research 18

Chapter 3
Propagation of Energy by Electromagnetic Waves 21
  3.1 Radio Waves, Heat Waves, and Light Waves 21
  3.2 Wave Propagation 21
  3.3 Photons, Quanta, and the Electromagnetic Spectrum 23
  3.4 Louis de Broglie's Matter Waves 24

Chapter 4
Nuclear Transitions and Radioactive Decay 25
  4.1 Discovery of Natural Radioactivity 25
  4.2 Nuclear Forces and Energy Levels 25
  4.3 Nuclear Decay Schemes 26
  4.4 Alpha Decay 27
  4.5 Beta Decay 27
      4.5.1 Neutron-Proton Imbalance 27
      4.5.2 Beta-Minus (β^-) Decay 28
      4.5.3 Beta-Plus (β^+) Decay 29
      4.5.4 Electron Capture (EC) 30
  4.6 Internal Conversion (IC) 31
  4.7 Isomeric Transition 32
  4.8 Nuclear Fission 33
  4.9 Nuclear Fusion 34

4.10 Induced Nuclear Transformations..35

Chapter 5
Radioactive Decay Calculations 37
5.1   Introduction..37
5.2   Decay of a Single Isotope...37
      5.2.1 Observing an Instant...37
      5.2.2 Observing Decay Over Lengthy Periods...37
      5.2.3 Half Life (T_h) 39
      5.2.4 Mean Life (T_M) 40
5.3   Radioactive Decay Chains..41
      5.3.1 Daughter Product Buildup and Decay...41
      5.3.2 Secular Equilibrium..43
      5.3.3 Transient Equilibrium...44
5.4   Neutron Activation...45

Chapter 6
Collision and Radiation Loss in Charged-Particle Interactions......................49
6.1   Slowing Down of Charged Particles 49
6.2   Collision Loss...49
      6.2.1 Collision Energy Loss Formula 49
      6.2.2 Bragg Ionization Curve...51
6.3   Radiative Loss..52
      6.3.1 Bremsstrahlung...52
      6.3.2 Radiative Stopping Power...53
      6.3.3 Angular Distribution of Bremsstrahlung X-Rays...............................53
      6.3.4 Energy Distribution of Bremsstrahlung Radiation 53
      6.3.5 Linear Energy Transfer 56

Chapter 7
Photon Interactions..59
7.1   Nature of the Interactions...59
7.2   Attenuation Coefficient..59
      7.2.1 Diminution of Photon Flux..59
      7.2.2 Linear Attenuation Coefficient..60
      7.2.3 Mass Attenuation Coefficient..61
      7.2.4 Atomic Attenuation Coefficient 61
      7.2.5 Electronic Attenuation Coefficient..61
7.3   Coherent Thompson Scattering 62
7.4   Photoelectric Absorption 62
      7.4.1 Early Photoelectron Experiment 62
      7.4.2 Photon Energy and Photoelectric Interaction.....................................65
      7.4.3 Atomic Number and Photoelectric Interaction...................................65
      7.4.4 Local Energy Absorption in Photoelectric Interaction........................66
      7.4.5 Angular Emission of Photoelectrons 66
      7.4.6 Photoelectric Cross Section...66
7.5   Incoherent Compton Scattering...66
      7.5.1 Kinematics of Compton Scattering...66
      7.5.2 Angular Distribution of Scattered Photons...68
      7.5.3 Scattered Energy at Specific Angles 68
      7.5.4 Compton Cross Section..68
      7.5.5 Energy and Atomic Number vs. Compton Cross Section.....................70

7.6   Negatron-Positron Pair Production 71
       7.6.1 Threshold Energy for Pair Production 71
       7.6.2 Electron-Positron Annihilation 72
       7.6.3 Pair Production Cross Section 72
       7.6.4 Photon Energy and Atomic Number vs. π 72
       7.6.5 Local Energy Absorption and Pair Production 73
7.7   Summing up the Local Energy Absorbed 73
7.8   Components of μ at Different Energies 74
7.9   Attenuation Coefficients for Mixtures and Compounds 75
       7.9.1   Weighted Addition of μ/ρ Values 75
       7.9.2   Effective Z for Mixtures and Compounds 75
7.10   Broad- and Narrow-Beam Attenuation Geometries 76
       7.10.1 Primary and Scatter Fluence 76
       7.10.2 Scatter Build-Up Factor 77
7.11   Photonuclear Reactions 78

Chapter 8
Conventional X-Ray Machines 81
8.1   Discovery of X-Rays 81
8.2   Gas-Discharge X-Ray Tube 81
8.3   Features of Modern X-Ray Tubes 81
       8.3.1   Coolidge's X-Ray Tube 81
       8.3.2   Heat Generation 82
       8.3.3   Line Focus Principle 83
       8.3.4   Heel Effect 84
       8.3.5   Rotating Anode 84
       8.3.6   Avoidance of Overheating 84
8.4   High-Voltage Supply and Rectification 85
       8.4.1   Stepping up the AC Supply 85
       8.4.2   Self-Rectified X-Ray Tube 85
       8.4.3   Half-Wave Rectification 85
       8.4.4   Full-Wave Rectification 86
       8.4.5   Three-Phase Power Supply and Full-Wave Rectification.........87
8.5   A Typical X-Ray Circuit 88
8.6   X-Ray Spectra and Quality 88
       8.6.1   X-Ray Spectra in Practice 88
       8.6.2   Beam Quality and Half-Value Thickness 90
       8.6.3   Homogeneity Index 91

Chapter 9
Equipment for Radioisotope Teletherapy 93
9.1   Concept of Teletherapy 93
9.2   Radioisotope Sources 93
       9.2.1   Requirements for the Source 93
       9.2.2   Some Radioisotopes to be Considered for Teletherapy 93
9.3 ^{60}Co Teletherapy Machines 95
       9.3.1   The Source Head 95
       9.3.2   Light Beam Localizer 96
       9.3.3   Source on-off Mechanism 96
       9.3.4   Source Capsule 96
       9.3.5   Geometric Penumbra 96
       9.3.6   Transmission Penumbra 98

        9.3.7   Designs of Adjustable Diaphragms...98
  9.4   Miscellaneous Features and Accessories...98
        9.4.1   Movement of Treatment Head and Patient Support 98
        9.4.2   Optical Distance Indicator...98
        9.4.3   Back-Pointing Device..100
  9.5   Closing Remarks..100

Chapter 10
Particle Accelerators...103
10.1   Three Categories of Accelerators 103
10.2   Direct-Voltage, Electrostatic Accelerators...103
        10.2.1 Tube for Acceleration..103
        10.2.2 Cockcroft-Walton Voltage Multiplier 103
        10.2.3 Van de Graaff Electrostatic Generator 104
10.3   Linear Accelerators 105
        10.3.1 Principle of Linacs 105
        10.3.2 Phase Stability in Linacs 106
        10.3.3 Wave Guides...107
        10.3.4 Standing Wave and Traveling Wave...107
        10.3.5 Clinical Linear Accelerator 108
10.4   Betatron...110
10.5   Cyclotron...112
10.6   Microtron 114

Chapter 11
Quantification of Radiation Field: Radiation Units and Measurements...........117
11.1   Radiation Field..117
11.2   Some Theoretical Concepts 117
        11.2.1 Fluence...117
        11.2.2 Energy Fluence 117
        11.2.3 Fluence Rate 118
        11.2.4 Energy Fluence Rate 118
        11.2.5 Energy Transferred and Kerma (k_{med})...119
        11.2.6 Energy Absorbed and Dose (D_{med})..119
        11.2.7 Charged-Particle Equilibrium 120
        11.2.8 Relationship between Kerma and Dose 121
11.3   Dose and Kerma Profiles — An Interface Example 121
11.4   Air Kerma (k_{air}) and Water Kerma (k_{water})..123
11.5   Exposure..123
        11.5.1 Concept of Exposure 123
        11.5.2 Relationship among Exposure, Air Kerma, and Dose to Air 124
        11.5.3 Relationship of Dose in Medium to Air Kerma and Exposure.............125
11.6   Measurement of Exposure 127
        11.6.1 Free-Air Ionization Chamber 127
        11.6.2 Cavity Chambers 128
        11.6.3 Exposure Calibration Factor...130
11.7   Use of Calibrated Ion Chamber in Therapy Beams 131
        11.7.1 Need for Calibration of Beams 131
        11.7.2 "Dose to Tissue in Air" for a Cobalt-60 Beam.....................................131
        11.7.3 Dose in Water for a Cobalt-60 Beam 132
        11.7.4 Ideal Bragg-Gray Cavity 133
        11.7.5 Less than Ideal (Larger) Cavity 134

11.7.6 Walled Chamber in a Medium 134
11.7.7 Determining N_{gas} from $N_{X,co}$ 135
11.7.8 Dose Delivered by Electron Beams 136
11.7.9 Dose to Water 137
11.8 Air-Kerma Rate Constant for Radionuclide Sources 137

Chapter 12
Instruments for Radiation Detection 143
12.1 Introduction 143
12.2 Ionization Detectors 143
    12.2.1 Role of Applied Potential 143
    12.2.2 Condenser Chamber 144
    12.2.3 Cylindrical (Thimble) Chamber 145
    12.2.4 Parallel-Plate (Pancake) Chamber 146
    12.2.5 Extrapolation Chamber 146
12.3 Photographic Film Detector 146
    12.3.1 Photographic Process 146
    12.3.2 Optical Density 147
    12.3.3 Calibration of a Film 147
    12.3.4 Film Response Curves 147
    12.3.5 Intensifying Screens and Grids 148
    12.3.6 High-Energy Port Films 149
12.4 Scintillation Detector 149
12.5 Semiconductor Diodes 150
12.6 Thermoluminescent Dosimeters (TLDs) 150
    12.6.1 Thermoluminescence 150
    12.6.2 TLD Instrumentation 151
    12.6.3 Measuring an Unknown Dose by TLD 151
12.7 Chemical Dosimeters 152
12.8 Calorimetry 153

Chapter 13
Basic Ratios and Factors for the Dosimetry of External Beams 155
13.1 Introduction 155
13.2 Defining the Beam Geometry 155
13.3 Quality of Beams 157
13.4 Central-Axis Dose Profile 157
13.5 Calculation of Dose in the Depth: General Approach 159
13.6 Dose to Tissue in Air 159
13.7 Inverse-Square Fall-Off 160
13.8 Irradiation Parameters 161
13.9 Tissue–Air Ratio (TAR) 163
13.10 Peak Scatter Factor (PSF) 163
13.11 Normalized PSF (NPSF) 165
13.12 Percent Depth Dose (PDD) 165
13.13 Tissue Maximum Ratio (TMR) 166
13.14 Tissue–Phantom Ratio 170
13.15 Dose Output Factors 173
    13.15.1 Calibrated Dose Output 173
    13.15.2 In-Air Output and Peak Output 173
13.16 Gathering Depth-Dose Data 175
13.17 Methods of Deriving the Dose Rate $\dot{D}_P$ at Point P 175

13.18 Calculation of Treatment Duration 177
13.19 Equivalent Squares and Circles 177
13.20 Relationship of TAR and TMR to PDD..178
13.21 Converting PDD for One SSD to that for Another...180

Chapter 14
Beam Dosimetry
Additional Corrections — Special Situations 193
14.1 Introduction 193
14.2 Scatter Considerations 193
    14.2.1 Scatter in Blocked Fields 193
    14.2.2 Effective Rectangular Field...193
    14.2.3 Scatter–Air Ratio, SAR(d, A_d) 196
    14.2.4 Scatter-Radius Integration 197
    14.2.5 Day's Method..199
14.3 General Approach for Off-Central Axis Points..200
    14.3.1 Surface Curvature, Distance, and Depth...200
    14.3.2 Off-Center Ratios in Air, OCR_{air} 200
    14.3.3 Dose Rate at Off-Center Point Q...201
14.4 Correction for Body Inhomogeneities...202
    14.4.1 Inhomogeneities..202
    14.4.2 Inhomogeneity Correction Factor (ICF) 202
    14.4.3 Lung and Bone..202
    14.4.4 Lung Phantom Geometry 203
    14.4.5 Effective Depth (d_{eff}) 203
    14.4.6 ICF Based on Accounting for d_{eff}..204
    14.4.7 Effective Field Size (A_{eff})...204
    14.4.8 ICF Based on Equivalent TAR, with d_{eff} and A_{eff}...........................204
    14.4.9 ICF by Batho's Method 204
    14.4.10 Comparison of ICF Obtained by Different Methods 206
    14.4.11 Lung Density and Lateral Electronic Equilibrium 208
14.5 Bone Attenuation and Absorption 208
14.6 Advanced Methods and Future Trends..209

Appendix A
Electron Mass Stopping Power (in MeV cm² g⁻¹) for Various Materials 215

Appendix B
Mass Attenuation Coefficients, Mass Energy Transfer Coefficients, and
Mass Energy Absorption Coefficients (in cm² g⁻¹) for
Various Materials 225

INDEXES 233
Subject Index (Volume I) 233
Author Index (Volume I)..245
Subject Index (Volume II)..249
Author Index (Volume II) 259

Chapter 15
Treatment Dose Distribution Planning: Photon Beams 1
15.1   Introduction 1
15.2   Isodose Surfaces and Curves 1
15.3   Single-Beam Isodose Curves 1
        15.3.1 General Features...1
        15.3.2 Low-Energy Kilovoltage X-ray Beam 2
        15.3.3 Co^{60} Beam...4
        15.3.4 Megavoltage X-rays 4
15.4   Concept of Combining Beams..7
15.5   Derivation of Dose Distribution 7
        15.5.1 General Approach 7
        15.5.2 Dose at P_i for Fixed SSD Technique 9
        15.5.3 Dose at P_i for Isocentric Technique 9
        15.5.4 Correction for Contour Shape 10
                Ratio-of-TAR Correction Method...11
                Isodose Shift and Effective SSD Correction Method 11
                Partial Isodose Shift Correction Method...11
        15.5.5 Influence of Obliquity on Dose Build-Up 12
15.6   Planning of Dose Distributions 13
        15.6.1 Zones to be Considered 13
        15.6.2 Examining a Dose Distribution 14
15.7   Principles of the Use of Wedge Filters 17
        15.7.1 Wedge Angle..17
        15.7.2 Wedged Oblique Pair 17
        15.7.3 Three-Field Techniques with Wedges..17
15.8   Irradiations with Parallel Opposed Beams 21
        15.8.1 On a Body Section of Medium Thickness 21
        15.8.2 On a Thin Body Section 22
        15.8.3 On a Thick Body Section 23
        15.8.4 In a Four-Field Box Geometry 24
        15.8.5 On a Section of Uneven Body Thickness 24
15.9   Other Common Techniques 26
15.10   Treatment Planning: A Practical Case..35
        15.10.1 Therapy Simulator..35
        15.10.2 Localization for Treatment of the Esophagus 35
        15.10.3 Case-Specific Isodose Planning...38
        15.10.4 Comparative Evaluation of the Plans 38
        15.10.5 Use of Dose-Volume Plots...40
        15.10.6 Integral Dose (Σ)...40
        15.10.7 Simulating the Accepted Plan..42
15.11   Use of CT Data..43
        15.11.1 CT Transverse Cuts..43
        15.11.2 CT for Field Shaping..44
15.12   Treatment of Adjacent Sites 46
        15.12.1 Problem of Concern..46
        15.12.2 Both Sites Treated from One Direction..48
        15.12.3 Adjacent Parallel Opposed Fields..49
        15.12.4 Matching Opposed Beams with a Single Beam 50
        15.12.5 Angle Match Between Orthogonal Beams..50

Chapter 16
Physical Aspects of Electron Beam Therapy 55

16.1   Electron Transport...55
16.2   Electron Beam from Machine to Patient...55
16.3   Electron Beam After Entering the Patient...56
16.4   Electron Beam Depth Dose Data 61
16.5   Planning a Simple Electron Beam Treatment 62
16.6   Electron Beam Depth Dose and Field Size..62
16.7   Electron Pencil Beam 63
16.8   Oblique Incidence and Depth Dose...63
16.9   Electron Beams: Some Practical Considerations 65
        16.9.1   Electron Beam Output Factors 65
        16.9.2   Output Factors for Non-Square Fields 67
        16.9.3   Field Shaping and Selective Shielding..68
        16.9.4   Effective SSD 70
        16.9.5   Agreement of Light Field and Radiation Field.......................................71
16.10   Influence of Inhomogeneities 72
16.11   Comparison of Kilovoltage X-ray and Electron Beams 74
16.12   Total-Skin Electron Treatment...75
16.13   Intraoperative Electron Therapy 76
16.14   Electron Arc Therapy..77
16.15   Adjacent Electron Fields...79

Chapter 17
Physics of the Use of Small Sealed Sources in Brachytherapy 85

17.1   Brachytherapy 85
17.2   Categories of Applications..85
17.3   Source Strength of Brachytherapy Sources...88
        17.3.1   Need for Specification of Source Strength...88
        17.3.2   Specification by Radium-Equivalent Mass..89
        17.3.3   Specification by Activity..90
        17.3.4   Specification by Air-Kerma Rate Yield 90
        17.3.5   Specification by Water-Kerma Rate Yield 91
17.4   Source Strength and Time Product..91
        17.4.1   Significance..91
        17.4.2   Milligram Hour of Treatment 91
        17.4.3   Air-Kerma Yield of Treatment 92
17.5   Dosimetry of a Point Source in Water 93
        17.5.1   Theoretical Approach...93
        17.5.2   AAPM and ICWG Empirical Approach for
                 Dosimetry of Radioactive Seeds...95
17.6   Dosimetry of a Linear Source 97
        17.6.1   Encapsulated Source in Air 97
        17.6.2   Unencapsulated Source in Air 99
        17.6.3   Linear Source in Water 100
        17.6.4   Dose Distribution for Linear Sources...101
        17.6.5   AAPM and ICWG Approach for Linear Source Dosimetry 101
17.7   A Simple Line Source Treatment..103
17.8   Forming Multiple Source Arrays...105
        17.8.1   Sources as Dose Building Blocks..105
        17.8.2   Uniform vs. Differentially Distributed Arrays 105

17.9   Systems for Brachytherapy 111
         17.9.1   What Are Systems or Approaches? 111
         17.9.2   Quimby Approach 112
         17.9.3   Paris Approach 113
         17.9.4   Approach of Memorial Hospital in New York 114
         17.9.5   Manchester Approach of Paterson and Parker 115
         17.9.6   Pitfalls of Mixing Systems or Approaches................................117
17.10   Manchester (Paterson and Parker) Distribution Rules 119
         17.10.1 Surface Applications 119
                  Circular Areas: Distribution Rules 119
                  Rectangular Areas: Distribution Rules 120
                  Areas of Irregular Shape: Distribution Rules..........................120
         17.10.2 Single-Plane Implants 120
         17.10.3 Two-Plane Implants 121
         17.10.4 Volume Implants 122
17.11   Planning and Implementing a Practical Case..125
         17.11.1 A Sample Target Volume 125
         17.11.2 Planning the Geometry of the Array 125
         17.11.3 Determining the Source Strengths...125
         17.11.4 Procuring the Sources 127
         17.11.5 Implanting the Sources 127
         17.11.6 Radiographic Localization of Sources...127
                  Tube Shift Radiographic Localization 128
                  Orthogonal Radiographic Localization 129
         17.11.7 Orthogonal Reconstruction — A Practical Case.......................130
         17.11.8 Dosimetry Using Computer and Interpretation 132
17.12   Permanent Implants 134
17.13   Intracavitary Irradiation 134
         17.13.1 Vaginal Cylinder 134
         17.13.2 Pairs of Colpostats 135
         17.13.3 Irradiations of Uterine Cervix 136

Chapter 18
Radiation Safety Standards 143
18.1   Introduction 143
18.2   Harmful Effects of Radiation 143
         18.2.1   Acute Radiation Syndrome..143
         18.2.2   Stochastic Effects and Deterministic Effects 144
         18.2.3   Somatic and Genetic Effects..144
18.3   Evaluation of Dose for Radiation Protection 144
         18.3.1   Inadequacy of Dose as an Index of Harm..................................144
         18.3.2   Microscopic Energy Deposition 145
         18.3.3   Relative Biological Effectiveness (RBE)....................................145
         18.3.4   Quality Factor and Dose Equivalent..146
         18.3.5   Weighting Factors for Different Radiations 147
         18.3.6   Equivalent Dose 147
         18.3.7   Weighting Factors for Different Body Tissues...........................149
         18.3.8   Effective Dose 149
18.4   Uncertainties in Radiation Risk Assessment...150
         18.4.1   Problem of Sample Size 150
         18.4.2   Imperfect Knowledge of Radiation Dose 151
         18.4.3   Dose-Response Projection 151

	18.4.4	Lifetime Risk Projection	151
	18.4.5	Dose and Dose Rate Effectiveness Factor (DDREF)	153
	18.4.6	Assessed Radiation Risk	153
18.5	Radiation Safety Philosophy		154
	18.5.1	Natural Background Radiation	154
	18.5.2	Medical Exposures	154
	18.5.3	Risk vs. Benefit Philosophy	154
18.6	Safety of Radiation Workers		155
	18.6.1	Limits for Adult Workers	155
	18.6.2	Limits for Embryo or Fetus	156
	18.6.3	Limits for Workers under Age 18	156
	18.6.4	Personnel Monitoring	157
18.7	Safety of the General Public		158

Chapter 19
Radiation Safety in External-Beam Therapy 161

19.1	Introduction		161
19.2	Time, Distance, and Shielding		161
19.3	Approach to Shielding Design of a Beam-Therapy Facility		162
	19.3.1	Selection of Acceptable Weekly Equivalent Dose Limits (P)	162
	19.3.2	Radiation Components	162
	19.3.3	Recommended Leakage Levels	162
	19.3.4	Shielding Data	164
	19.3.5	Architectural and Equipment Data	166
	19.3.6	Workload (W)	166
	19.3.7	Use Factor (U)	167
	19.3.8	Occupancy Factor (T)	167
19.4	Estimating the Allowable Barrier Transmission		168
	19.4.1	Primary Shielding Barrier	168
	19.4.2	Secondary Protective Barrier	169
		Leakage Radiation	169
		Scattered Radiation	169
	19.4.3	Entrance Door Barrier	170
	19.4.4	Roof Protection and Skyshine	172
19.5	High-Energy X-rays and Neutron Production		173
	19.5.1	Neutron Shielding at the Door	173
	19.5.2	Neutron Capture Gamma Rays	175
	19.5.3	Induced Radioactivity	175
19.6	An Example of Shielding Calculations for a Facility		175
	19.6.1	Basic Data and Assumptions	175
	19.6.2	Side Walls	177
	19.6.3	Entrance Door Shield	177
	19.6.4	Skyshine Shielding	178
19.7	Ozone Production		181
19.8	Miscellaneous Aspects of Planning a Facility		182

Chapter 20
Radiation Safety in Brachytherapy 195

20.1	Introduction	195
20.2	Role of Time and Afterloading	195
20.3	Role of Distance	196
20.4	Role of Shielding	196

20.5   Monitoring Instruments 197
20.6   Source Storage and Preparation...197
20.7   Source Inventory 198
20.8   Source Wipe Tests..198
20.9   Source Transport 199
20.10   Safety of Nurses and Visitors during Treatment 199
20.11   Procedure After Treatment...200
20.12   Permanent Implants 200
20.13   Personnel Monitoring...202
20.14   Conclusion...202

INDEXES 205
Subject Index (Volume I) 205
Author Index (Volume I)..217
Subject Index (Volume II)..221
Author Index (Volume II) 231

Chapter 15

TREATMENT DOSE DISTRIBUTION PLANNING: PHOTON BEAMS

15.1 INTRODUCTION

Before a patient is treated with radiation, the target volume for delivery of the radiation dose is delineated by the physician, who takes into account the stage and extent of the tumor and the clinical objective of palliation or cure. The methods and processes available for delivery of radiation, as well as the mechanisms of radiation interaction, are such that we cannot restrict the dose delivery strictly to the target volume alone, with no incidental irradiation elsewhere.

After a target volume is decided upon and designated to receive a prescribed dose, an acceptable or optimum treatment strategy needs to be worked out. The treatment should be planned in such a way that (i) the designated target volume, which includes the tumor, is given a uniform dose; (ii) incidental irradiation of the surrounding normal structures is minimal; and (iii) the dose to any vital body organ does not exceed its tolerance level. The entire dose distribution pattern made possible by a particular treatment plan should be evaluated carefully before the plan is accepted for implementation on a patient. Several different treatment strategies can be compared and the optimum one selected.

In this chapter, we restrict the subject of dose distribution planning to the use of photon beams. Planning for the use of electron beams and discrete sealed radioactive sources in the brachytherapy mode will be covered in the two chapters that follow.

15.2 ISODOSE SURFACES AND CURVES

When a beam passes through a patient, different points within the patient will receive different doses; that is, there will be a spatial dose distribution. Because it is convenient to think in terms of relative rather than absolute doses, it is usual to select a particular point in the irradiated field as a reference point and to designate the dose it receives as 100%. Let us say that a particular point in the field receives a dose of p% (relative to 100%). Then there may be several other points in the field that receive a dose of p%. The surface formed when all of these points are connected is referred to as an isodose surface for p%. Isodose surfaces are three-dimensional (3D) constant-value surfaces, just like isotherms and isobars in weather maps. The line or curve obtained at the intersection of a plane with an isodose surface is an isodose curve. Isodose curves are two-dimensional (2D) entities because they lie in a plane intersecting the 3D dose distribution. Because of the fact that the isodose surfaces or curves represent a specific dose value, the isodose surfaces or curves for two different dose levels cannot cross one another. Isodose curves have been used more commonly than isodose surfaces for analysis of dose distributions, because the fact that they are 2D allows them to be displayed on paper. Three-dimensional displays and surface representations are becoming feasible with the use of computed tomography (CT) and graphic work stations.[1-9] However, they are still in the development stage. Their full practical import for routine clinical treatment planning will be realized in the future.

15.3 SINGLE-BEAM ISODOSE CURVES

15.3.1 GENERAL FEATURES

In Chapters 13 and 14 (Volume I), we discussed the dose calculation at points on and away from the central axis. Calculation of the dose received at many points in the beam can reveal the geometric dose distribution pattern for any radiotherapy beam. The dose distribution obtained for any beam will depend on its geometric divergence, energy and depth-dose characteristics, off-central-axis fall-off of intensity and penumbra, and the influence of any beam-modifying filters such as wedge filters or beam-flattening filters inserted in the beam.

Figure 15.1a is a 3D view of a radiation beam of rectangular cross section. Figures 15.1b and c represent two mutually perpendicular planes through this beam — a plane perpendicular to the central axis of the beam, and the plane that contains the central axis and a major axis of the rectangular cross section, respectively. The lines marked G on both of these diagrams are the geometric edges of the beam (see Section 9.3.5).

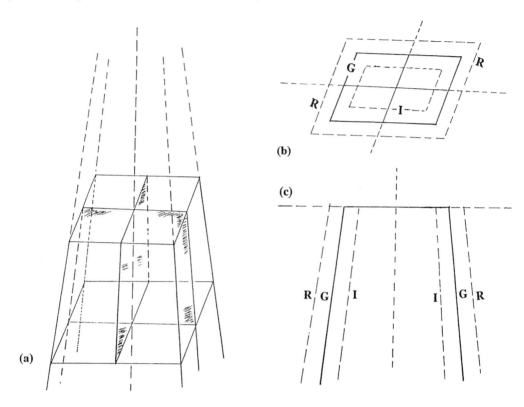

FIGURE 15.1   (a) Three-dimensional view of a beam of rectangular cross section. (b) View of a plane perpendicular to the central axis of the beam. (c) View of a plane containing the central axis of the beam and a principal axis of the rectangle. G is the geometric edge. Lines I and R are drawn to define the inner region (within I) and the remote region (beyond R), respectively.

For the purpose of understanding and analyzing the dose distribution, any single radiation beam can be visualized as consisting of three zones. These are (i) the useful inner region lying between lines I, covering up to 80 or 90% of the geometric width of the beam; (ii) a penumbra or fall-off region lying between lines I and R on either side of the geometric edge; and (iii) a distal or remote region that lies well beyond lines R, where most of the dose is contributed by radiation leaking through the diaphragms and by scattered radiation. The ideal would be to have a cross-beam radiation intensity profile that is highly uniform in the inner region, with a rapid and abrupt fall-off in the penumbra and a negligible magnitude in the remote regions. In practice, beams are not so perfect, as our further discussion will reveal. Single-beam isodose curves have been published in the form of atlases for academic study.[10,11]

15.3.2 LOW-ENERGY KILOVOLTAGE X-RAY BEAM
Figure 15.2a is a schematic diagram of the source and diaphragm geometry for a low-energy X-ray beam. A small X-ray focal spot gives a near-point source of radiation emission. The beam size is limited by thin diaphragms made of lead, which need to be only a few millimeters thick

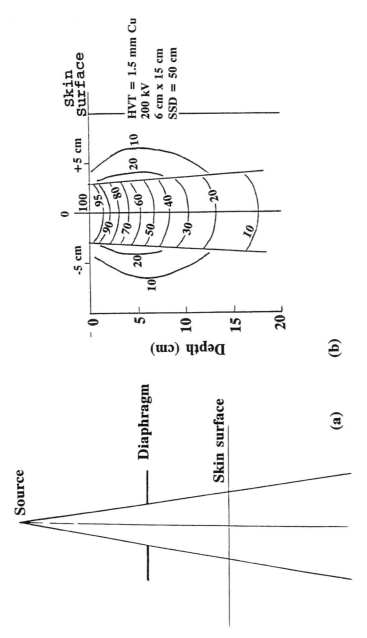

FIGURE 15.2 (a) Schematic diagram of a low-energy X-ray beam emerging from a near-point source through a thin beam-limiting diaphragm. (b) Isodose curves for a 200-kV X-ray beam.

because of the high efficiency of absorption in lead at low energies. Figure 15.2b presents the isodose curves for such a beam. The peak dose at the surface on the central axis has been designated as 100% for normalization.

The isodose curves are concave upward in the central region of the beam. This indicates a reduction in the dose from the central axis outward, because the amount of scattered radiation falls off from the central axis toward off-axis points. As we know, the scatter dose at any point depends on the location of the point in the irradiated field and on the geometry of the scattering volume. The central-axis point at a given depth receives more scatter than does an off-central-axis point. The scattered dose component for low-energy X-rays is considerably greater than that at megavoltage energies.

Looking at the penumbral region in Figure 15.2b, we notice that the isodose curves have a sharp cut-off at the geometric edge of the beam. In low-energy X-ray beams, the combination of a near-point source and thin collimating diaphragms produces such sharp beam edges, with almost no penumbra.

At low energies, outside the geometric beam edge, the primary radiation levels are reduced to negligible amounts by the beam-limiting diaphragms. However, in Figure 15.2b we observe 20% and 10% isodose curves in the regions outside the edges. This dose comes from the photons scattered sideways from the beam. At such low energies Compton-scattered photons spread over a wide angle and make the lateral scatter prominent. These isodose curves are concave toward the central axis, giving an appearance of a beam that is being propagated laterally outward from the central axis and perpendicular to it.

15.3.3 Co^{60} BEAM

Figure 15.3a is a schematic diagram of a beam produced by a ^{60}Co teletherapy machine. The source has a finite size, often in the range of 1.0 to 2.0 cm in diameter. Collimating a beam of high-energy photons (1.17 MeV and 1.33 MeV) requires thick diaphragms made of several centimeters of a heavy metal such as lead, tungsten, or uranium. The overall geometry is such that (i) a geometric penumbra is caused by the finite size of the source, and (ii) the partial transmission of some oblique rays from the source through the corners of the diaphragms adds a transmission penumbra (see also Section 9.3.6).

Figure 15.3b presents a typical isodose pattern for a ^{60}Co beam. The isodose curves are normalized to 100% at the peak dose on the central axis. In the inner regions, the curves are flat and perpendicular to the central axis. Near the beam edge the curves are parallel to the edge and go all the way up to the surface. The dose fall-off is gradual across the edge. This is in contrast to the discontinuity that we observed at the beam edge for the low-energy X-rays in Figure 15.2b. The isodose curves outside the field edges are not as prominent as are those for low-energy X-rays because, at this energy, there is no significant lateral scatter. Outside the beam edges, some dose is contributed by direct transmission of photons through the collimator diaphragms. Such leakage through the collimator diaphragms usually amounts to about 0.5 to 3% of the peak dose on the central axis.

15.3.4 MEGAVOLTAGE X-RAYS

In Sections 6.3 and 10.3.5, we discussed the fact that the high-energy X-ray emission has a forward peak and that the X-ray intensity needs to be flattened by an interposed beam-flattening filter. Figure 15.4a is a schematic diagram of the geometric features of a megavoltage photon beam. The isodose curves for an 8-MV X-ray beam are shown in Figure 15.4b. The 100% dose has been taken to be the peak dose on the central axis.

As illustrated in Figure 15.4a, the focal spots (sources) in megavoltage X-ray machines are smaller than the size of the sources in ^{60}Co machines.[12] This helps to reduce the geometric penumbra. However, the diaphragms have to be thick, as with ^{60}Co, and hence, a transmission penumbra cannot be avoided. In addition, at high energies the range of the secondary electrons increases. Although the secondary electrons travel mostly in the forward direction, they can spill over the geometric

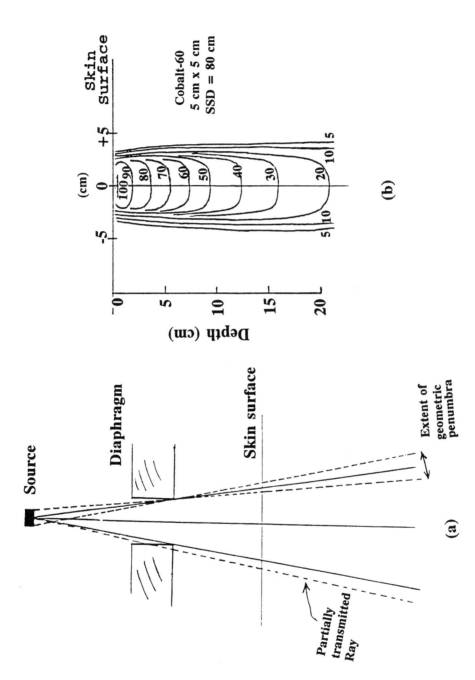

FIGURE 15.3 (a) Schematic diagram of a cobalt-60 beam emerging from a source of finite size through a thick beam-limiting diaphragm. The geometric penumbra and a partially transmitted ray are shown on the right and left edges of the beam, respectively. (b) Isodose curves for a cobalt-60 beam.

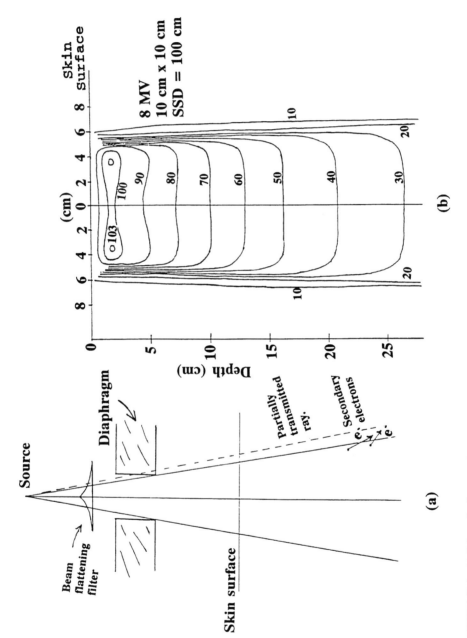

FIGURE 15.4 (a) Schematic diagram of a megavoltage X-ray beam showing the source of emission, the beam flattening filter, the thick beam-limiting diagram, a partially transmitted ray through the diaphragm, and secondary electron spill over the beam edge. (b) Isodose curves for an 8-MV X-ray beam.

edge of the beam and blur the edge. Most high-energy beams have less penumbra than does a ^{60}Co beam, but exceptions cannot be ruled out.

In the design of the beam-flattening filter, the presence of scatter fluence in an irradiated medium is also taken into account. The flattening filter is usually optimized to give a flatness of ±3% in the inner region covering about 80% of the geometric field width at a depth of about 10 cm in water. This depth is chosen with the understanding that the target volume is usually located at about that depth in patients. Because scatter accumulates with depth, its contribution to the total dose is low at the surface and increases with depth. The scatter aids in beam flattening because it tends to disperse the fluence. A beam-flattening filter that is designed to give beam flatness at 10 cm depth, taking into account the scatter at that depth, can produce a beam with horns or humps on either side of the central axis at shallow depths, where the scatter is less. This is why, in Figure 15.4b, the dips in the 90% isodose curve and the hot spots of 103% near the surface occur. The humps may be particularly prominent in beams of large width.

15.4 CONCEPT OF COMBINING BEAMS

The tolerance of sensitive tissues through which a beam may pass from its entrance to its exit in the patient can limit the total tumor dose that can be delivered by that beam. When a beam is directed to irradiate a tumor located in the depth, the entrance region (just beyond the build-up) will receive a much higher dose than does the tumor. A beam in transit will give a higher dose on the entrance side of the target than on the exit side. (Some exceptions occur in rare contexts when photon beams of very high energies, 40 MV and above, are used.) Often, the higher dose received by the subcutaneous tissues near the entrance surface limits the total tumor dose that can be delivered by a single beam. By using more than one beam focused and directed toward the tumor, one can distribute the doses along multiple entrance and exit paths around the target volume and concentrate the dose at the tumor. The positions and paths of the beams can be planned so as not to exceed the tolerance dose of normal tissues that lie around the target volume and are irradiated incidentally. Multiple beams can be combined with the added objective of molding the dose distribution to conform to the shape of the volume to be treated and to make the dose uniform within the target. The aim should be to create an optimum or at least an acceptable dose distribution in the patient.

15.5 DERIVATION OF DOSE DISTRIBUTION

15.5.1 GENERAL APPROACH

Single-beam isodose curves are the basis for inferring the dose distribution for a combination of beams. In the early days of the practice of external-beam therapy, physicists added the dose distributions of single beams manually to obtain the composite dose distribution for multiple-beam arrangements. In the modern practice of radiation oncology, dose distribution calculations and plotting of isodose curves are done by computerized treatment-planning systems, and the arduous and time-consuming manual calculations have mostly been dispensed with. Although computers speed up the process, manual methods form the basis of computer calculations. Hence, we cover these methods here next.

The dose distribution in a patient is a 3D entity. 3D dose calculations and 3D display of dose distributions are rather voluminous and complex. In many situations, for practical purposes, a simpler dose distribution plotted in a 2D mid-transverse section of the patient provides useful insight for dose distribution planning. Figure 15.5a shows a transverse contour of a patient. A total of M beams, 1, 2, 3, . . ., M, are set up to converge at a point T inside the patient. Let us assume that all are beams of rectangular cross section. It is common to refer to the field dimension in the direction of the long axis of the patient as "field length" and to that in the transverse plane of the contour as "field width." To find the dose distribution, we set up a rectangular grid of points P_1, P_2, P_3, . . . to cover the region of interest (Figure 15.5a). Our approach is to determine the doses received at the individual grid points for each individual beam and to add them to obtain the total

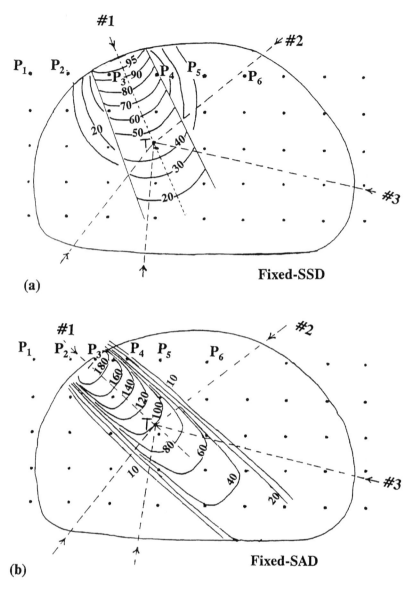

FIGURE 15.5 A patient's transverse contour with the grid of points chosen for dose estimation and an isodose curve placed at the position of a beam. (a) Use of isodose charts with 100% at the peak dose, as applicable for a fixed-SSD-type setup. (b) Use of isodose charts that have 100% at the depth of the isocenter, as applicable to an isocentric setup.

dose for the beam combination. From knowing the doses at the grid points, it should be possible to designate a particular dose level as 100% and to plot the isodose curves for the combination of beams. Usually, the 100% level is selected to be the dose at the center of the target volume to be treated. Many times it may be the dose at point T, where the beam axes converge.

The field widths, W_1, W_2, ...,W_M, of the individual beams are generally planned to cover the width of the target volume as seen from the direction of the beam. After other aspects of the plan (the beam angles, widths, treatment times, etc.) have been accepted in a review of the 2D plan, the field lengths (which may have the same value, L, for all beams) can be selected to cover the length of the target volume. It is worth reiterating that the dose distribution in this central 2D transverse plane need not necessarily represent the dose distribution obtainable in other transverse sections along the length of the patient. However, this information, when used with caution, has proved to be useful in the practice of radiotherapy.

15.5.2 DOSE AT P_i FOR FIXED-SSD TECHNIQUE

For the fixed source-to-skin distance (SSD) technique, we set up all of the beams to have a constant, preselected SSD. The set of isodose curves appropriate for the chosen SSD for a field width W_1 and length L is placed on the patient contour to provide the dose distribution from beam 1, as shown in Figure 15.5a. The percentage (depth) dose $PDD_{i,1}$ as shown by the isodose curve at point P_i is read with the 100% being the peak dose. If the treatment duration for beam 1 is such that the 100% dose (also called the "given dose") is G_1, then the dose $D_{i,1}$ at P_i due to beam 1 is given by

$$D_{i,1} = PDD_{i,1} \frac{G_1}{100}$$

The procedure can be carried out first for beam 1 for all grid points and then for all M beams. The total dose D_i at point P_i is

$$D_i = \sum_{j=1}^{j=M} PDD_{i,j} \cdot \frac{G_j}{100}$$

15.5.3 DOSE AT P_i FOR ISOCENTRIC TECHNIQUE

For treatment with a machine that is capable of isocentric rotation, the central point T can be chosen to be at the isocenter for all of the M beams. During treatment, the patient needs to be positioned only once for the first beam to have T at the isocenter. Subsequently, a mere rotation of the gantry of the machine can give the other beam locations without any need for moving the patient. (This is not possible for the fixed-SSD technique, which requires a movement of the patient for each individual beam so that the chosen SSD is obtained.)

To infer the dose distribution for isocentric situations, we need to use special isodose curves that are normalized to have the 100% dose level at the depth of the isocenter (Figure 15.5b). This means that, for a given field width, we will need many different isodose patterns with 100% chosen to be at various depths of normalization. In theory, all depths of normalization are possible. Although this implies that innumerable isodose charts covering every possible depth of normalization should be available, this is not so in practice. Fortunately, percent depth doses read from isodose charts normalized at a particular depth are not too sensitive to the depth of the normalization (i.e., the position of the surface). This is because the different points in the beam remain at the identical distances from the source, irrespective of the depth of normalization. The isodose curves merely reflect the differences in dose caused by attenuation and scatter. Hence, it is possible to do the treatment planning with a limited number of isodose charts for a few discrete depths of normalization without losing much accuracy. The percent (depth) dose at point P_i can be read to be $PDD_{i,1}$ for beam 1. The absolute value of the 100% dose is a function of the time of irradiation with beam 1. If the 100% dose (or given dose) for beam 1 is G_1, the dose $D_{i,1}$ at point p_1 from beam 1 is

$$D_{i,1} = G_1 \cdot \left(PDD_{i,1}/100 \right)$$

G_1 is given by the product of the dose to tissue in air, $(D_{air})_1$, and the tissue–air ratio TAR_1 for beam 1. Thus,

$$D_{i,1} = \left(D_{air} \right)_1 \cdot TAR_1 \cdot \left(PDD_{i,1}/100 \right)$$

The evaluation can be carried out first for beam 1 for all of the grid points and then for the rest of the M beams. The total dose D_i at point p_i then is

$$D_i = \sum_{j=1}^{j=M} \left(D_{air}\right)_j \cdot TAR_j \cdot \left(PDD_{i,j}/100\right)$$

15.5.4 CORRECTION FOR CONTOUR SHAPE

The isodose charts that we used in the previous examples are for beams incident on a flat surface. In practice, the patient's contour may be curved, or the beam may be incident obliquely on the surface, as shown in Figure 15.6. The data read from the standard isodose curves need to be modified for nonstandard situations. This is also referred to as the "missing tissue" problem. A solution can be to flatten the surface by filling the "missing tissue" with a tissue-equivalent material or bolus. However, this will have the negative effect of producing a build-up of secondary electrons on the patient's surface, and of enhancing the skin dose, with the resulting loss of skin sparing. Here we present different methods of correcting the standard isodose curves for incidence on a flat surface to allow for the presence of body curvature.[13]

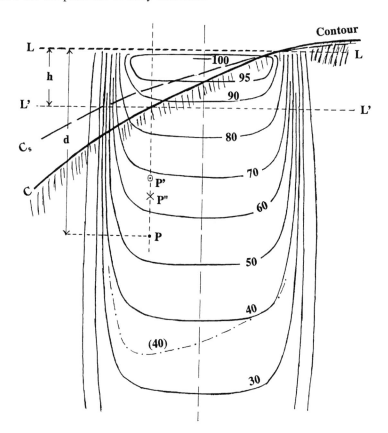

FIGURE 15.6 A beam incident on a curved contour C. P is the point where the dose is estimated. Line L is at the level of the SSD. Line L′ is at the level of the surface point directly above P. The depth of P is d, and h is the thickness of the "missing" tissue. C_s is the effective contour obtained by the 2/3 shift method. P′ and P″ are effective positions of point P in two different interpretations.

The diagram in Figure 15.6 shows a standard set of isodose curves positioned as if the body surface were flat and located at the level of line L. Let us say that we desire to know the percent depth dose (PDD) at point P, which is at depth d below line L. Line L′ is drawn through the actual point on the surface (on contour C) directly above P. The thickness of "missing tissue" is h, and the actual depth of P is (d − h). (The "missing tissue" problem discussed here is only a part of the overall problem of off-central-axis and inhomogeneity corrections discussed in Sections 14.3 and 14.4.)

Ratio-of-TAR Correction Method

If A_d is the field size at the level of point P in Figure 15.6, a correction factor CF for the value of PDD as read from the normal isodose chart can be worked out from the ratio of TARs as follows:

$$CF = \frac{\text{TAR for the effective depth } (d-h)}{\text{TAR for depth d implied in the isodose curve}}$$

$$= \frac{\text{TAR}(d-h, A_d)}{\text{TAR}(d, A_d)}$$

PDD actual = PDD read from isodose chart $\times$ CF

Isodose Shift and Effective SSD Correction Method

We could slide the isodose chart down so that its surface matches the line L′ and read a PDD value at P. Then the PDD value read will correspond to that for the point P′. Although this value is for the true depth (d – h), the distance of the 100% reference value in the isodose curve has changed from (SSD + d_m) to (SSD + h + d_m). Because this change of distance is not really true for point P, we obtain the PDD at P by applying an inverse square distance correction to the PDD read at P′, as follows:

$$\frac{\text{PDD at P}}{(\text{Surface L}')} = \frac{\text{PDD read at P}'}{(\text{Surface L})} \times \left[\frac{(\text{SSD}+d_m)}{(\text{SSD}+h+d_m)} \right]^2$$

The above method, although it uses a different route, is the same in principle as the ratio-of-TAR method discussed previously.

Partial Isodose Shift Correction Method

In this method also, the isodose chart is shifted down, not through the entire distance h to the level of line L′, but through a fractional distance $k \times h$. Table 15.1 gives the values of k recommended for different energies in ICRU Report 24.[13] These values of k are empirical and are designed to allow for the net effect of primary, scatter, and inverse-square fall-off, as observed in practical cases. For Co^{60}, k can be taken as 2/3, and hence this method is also referred to as the "2/3 shift method." A 2/3 shift will move point P to P″ in the dose distribution of Figure 15.6.

TABLE 15.1
Isodose Shift Factors, k, for Different Beam Qualities

X-Ray Quality	150 kV to 1 MV	1 MV to 5 MV	5 MV to 15 MV	15 MV to 30 MV	30 MV and Above
k	0.8	0.7	0.6	0.5	0.4

From ICRU-24.[13]

This method can be used easily for generating an entire isodose distribution for a change in contour shape. In Figure 15.6, the 40% isodose curve has been redrawn based on this method. The 2/3 shifts for the missing tissue result in an effective contour C_S in Figure 15.6.

Example 15.1

Derive the percent depth dose at point P in Figure 15.6 by the three methods of correction discussed above. The beam is from Co^{60}. Point P is at 10 cm depth from line L, but is at an actual depth of 7 cm. The SSD = 90 cm and the field size is 9 cm × 9 cm at SSD.

Ratio of TAR:

In this example, d = 10 cm, the field size at depth d is A_d = 10 cm × 10 cm, h = 3 cm, and the beam is from ^{60}Co.

The PDD read from the isodose curves at P is 55%.

$$\text{TAR}\left(d, A_d\right) = \text{TAR}\left(d = 10 \text{ cm}, A_d = 10 \text{ cm} \times 10 \text{ cm}\right) = 0.718 \qquad \text{(Table 13.2)}$$

$$\text{TAR}\left(d - h, A_d\right) = \text{TAR}\left(d = 10 - 3 \text{ cm}, A_d = 10 \text{ cm} \times 10 \text{ cm}\right)$$
$$= \text{TAR}(7, 10 \times 10) = 0.830 \qquad \text{(Table 13.2)}$$

Correction factor, CF = 0.830/0.718 = 1.156

Corrected PDD = PDD read × CF

$$= 55 \times 1.156 = 63.6\%$$

Isodose Shift and Effective SSD:

After the isodose chart is shifted down by h = 3 cm, the position of P will move up to P′.

PDD read at P′ = 68%

SSD = 90 cm, $\text{SSD} + d_m = 90 + 0.5 = 90.5$ cm

$\text{SSD} + d_m + h = 90 + 0.5 + 3.0 = 93.5$ cm

$$\left[\left(\text{SSD} + d_m\right) / \left(\text{SSD} + d_m + h\right)\right]^2 = \left[90.5/93.5\right]^2 = 0.937$$

PDD actual = PDD read × 0.937 = 68.0 × 0.937 = 63.7%

Partial (2/3) Shift Method:

For h = 3 cm, 2/3 of h is 2 cm. The isodose chart shifted by 2 cm places the point P at P″ (Figure 15.6). A vertical interpolation between the 60 and 70% isodose curves gives a PDD at point P″ of 64%. In this example, the three methods give nearly the same result.

15.5.5 INFLUENCE OF OBLIQUITY ON DOSE BUILD-UP

The corrections for contour shape and obliquity of the surface that we discussed above are applicable at points that lie beyond the depth of the peak dose. At depths closer to the surface, where full secondary electron build-up has not been attained, the dose estimation becomes more complex. The secondary-electron build-up and the depth at which the peak dose occurs are influenced by the obliquity of the surface with respect to the direction of incidence of the beam.[14-18] In Figure 15.7, a beam is incident on an oblique surface S. The dashed line S′ indicates a flat surface perpendicular to the direction of the beam. We know from Chapter 7 that secondary electrons from Compton scatter can emerge up to a maximum angle of 90° with respect to the direction of an incident photon. Points P′ and P have been chosen on a vertical ray below each other on surfaces S′ and S, respectively. Points Q′ and Q have also been chosen on these surfaces, on a vertical ray displaced laterally, but within a secondary-electron range. If the surface is S, P can receive secondary electrons from several points between Q and Q′, but if it is S′, P′ can receive secondary electrons only from Q′. Thus, the secondary electron fluence at P on surface S can be greater than that at point P′ on surface S′. Thus, the obliquity of the surface can cause an enhancement of the skin

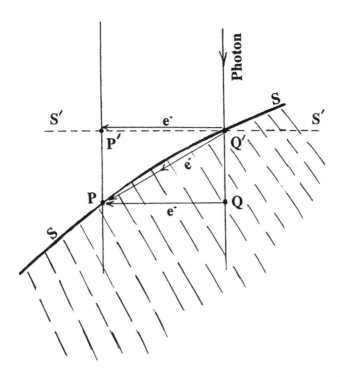

FIGURE 15.7 Diagram to explain the enhancement of skin dose caused by obliquity of incidence of a high-energy photon beam. Lines marked e⁻ define the path of the secondary electrons produced by photon interactions.

dose because of partial secondary-electron build-up. The additional build-up caused by obliquity moves the depth of the peak dose closer to the skin. Proper assessment of the dose in the build-up region remains a challenging problem,[19] because it is subject not only to the partial build-up effects that we just discussed, but also to the influence of secondary electrons from the beam-limiting diaphragms, trays, shielding blocks, and other accessories in the path of the beam.[20-25] A note of caution should be sounded that many computer algorithms used for dose distribution calculations do not allow for these effects in sufficient detail to give an accurate dose assessment in the build-up regions.

15.6 PLANNING OF DOSE DISTRIBUTIONS

15.6.1 ZONES TO BE CONSIDERED

In every beam of a multiple-beam arrangement, the following zones can be identified (see Figure 15.8):

A build-up zone (BZ) at the skin entrance
An entrance zone (ENZ) after the initial build-up, but prior to intersection with other beams
A target zone (TZ), where the beam crosses the target volume treated and where it may overlap
  with other beams
The exit zone (EXZ) beyond the target volume and before the beam exits from the patient
The penumbra zone (PZ) at the beam edges
The annular zones (AZ) that form the regions not directly irradiated by any beam

These various zones have been identified in Figure 15.8 for a simple case of a combination of two oblique beams. During the planning of multiple-beam treatments, it is necessary to determine where the various zones will fall in relation to the tissues to be treated or protected. The direction

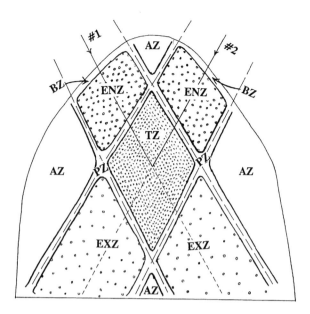

FIGURE 15.8   A combination of two oblique beams. BZ, ENZ, TZ, EXZ, PZ, and AZ identify build-up zone, entrance zone, target zone, exit zone, penumbra zone, and annular zone, respectively.

of a beam should be such that the entrance and exit paths minimize the dose to normal tissues that have critical or limited tolerance. Short entrance and exit routes are preferable to long ones. After it has passed through the build-up zone, any beam delivers a gradually decreasing dose as it goes from its entrance zone through its target zone to its exit zone. Multiple beams should divide the entrance and exit doses suitably and ensure that the tolerance doses of normal tissues along the paths of the beams are not exceeded. The combined beams should give a concentrated, uniform dose to the target volume. Ideally, the beams should be located so that any highly radiosensitive organ will fall in an annular zone.

15.6.2 EXAMINING A DOSE DISTRIBUTION

The dose distribution for the arrangement of two oblique beams is shown in Figure 15.9a for X-ray beams of 4 MV energy. The entrance zones and exit zones receive about 70% and 40% of the target dose, respectively. This may or may not satisfy the requirement of not exceeding the tolerance of tissues in the entrance and exit zones in a specific clinical situation. However, in the target zone (i.e., the zone where the beams overlap), an uneven dose distribution is observed, with the dose received ranging from 110% on one side to 70–80% on the opposite side. This may not be acceptable if we desire that the target dose should be uniform within ±10%. The reason for this nonuniformity can be understood if it is realized that the part of the target zone receiving the higher dose of 110% is at a shallow depth for both beams, and that the zone receiving 70 to 80% in the target volume is at a greater depth for both beams. The uniformity can be improved if the photon fluence reaching the region of 110% is reduced and that in the region of 70% is increased. The use of wedge-shaped, beam-modifying filters, called "wedge filters," in the manner illustrated in Figure 15.9b can help. Figures 15.10a and b show dose distributions for the same beam arrangement for Co^{60} beams. Wedge filters of different designs and performance are usually available in a clinic for various treatment situations.

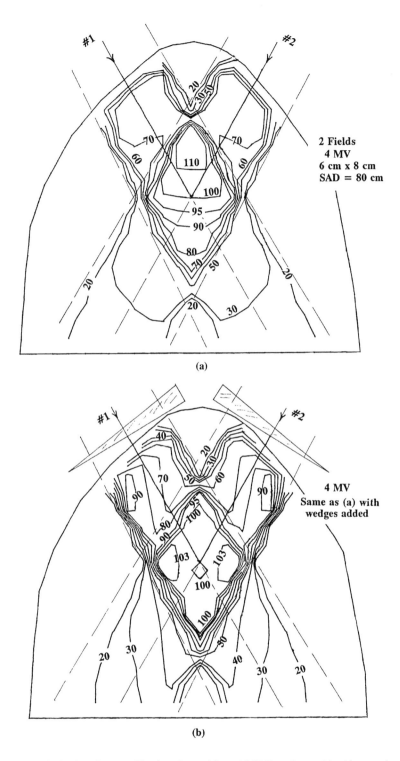

FIGURE 15.9 Dose distributions for a combination of two oblique 4-MV X-ray beams (a) without wedges and (b) with wedges.

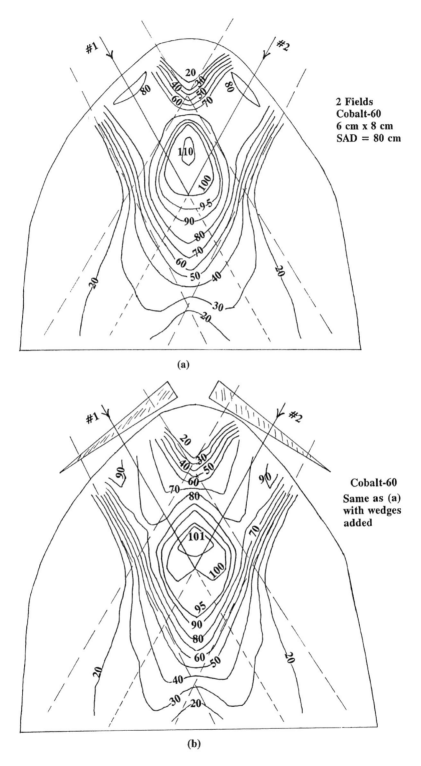

(a)

(b)

FIGURE 15.10 Dose distribution for a combination of two oblique cobalt-60 beams (a) without wedges and (b) with wedges.

15.7 PRINCIPLES OF THE USE OF WEDGE FILTERS

15.7.1 WEDGE ANGLE

Figure 15.11 shows a single-beam dose distribution with a wedge filter. The isodose curves are inclined with respect to the central axis. The 50% isodose curve forms an angle θ with respect to the perpendicular to the central axis. The angle θ, which is called the "wedge angle," is a measure of the tilt of the isodose line from its normal horizontal course (i.e., when there is no wedge). There have been various definitions of the wedge angle. This angle can be defined in terms of the tilt of an isodose curve at a particular dose level (say, 50%) or at a specified depth (such as 10 cm). The wedge angle is a characteristic of the dose distribution that results when the wedge is inserted in the beam.

It will be noticed from Figure 15.11 that the angles of higher-percentage isodose curves are more than θ. On the other hand the angles of the lower-percentage isodose curves are less than θ. Thus, the value of θ stated for any wedge is merely a value that indicates the differences among the many wedges that a clinic has on hand. Wedge filters for wedge angles of 15°, 30°, 45°, and 60° are common. The design and use of wedge filters have been discussed in the literature.[26-30] It is important to note that the wedge angle is not the physical measure of the angle of the narrow end of the wedge itself. The wedge is usually placed at a distance of 15 to 30 cm above the skin to reduce electron contamination (see Sections 9.3.5, 11.3, and 13.4).

15.7.2 WEDGED OBLIQUE PAIR

Figures 15.12a and b illustrate a wedged beam of wedge angle θ and the "hinge angle" φ at which two wedged beams with angle θ have been combined, with the thick ends of the wedges facing toward the junction. When φ is selected to be equal to (180° − 2θ), the isodose curves for the two wedge beams tend to run parallel to the vertical line AC that bisects the angle φ, and a near-uniform dose can result in the region of overlap of the two beams. This is seen in Figure 15.13, in which two wedged beams are combined at a hinge angle of (180° − 2θ) and overlap over the diamond-shaped area ABCD. The line AC falls on an isodose curve. Along diagonal BD, in the direction from B to D, the dose falls off for one beam, but increases for the other. The decrease and increase can compensate each other to improve the uniformity of the dose along line BD. In an ideal situation, in which the isodose curves are equally spaced and parallel, the entire area ABCD can receive a uniform dose. The hinge angle of (180 − 2θ) is the appropriate one for wedge angle θ.

Because the ideal of equally spaced and parallel isodose curves does not occur in reality, it is difficult to achieve perfect uniformity. In addition, the dose fall-off in the penumbral zones of the beams cannot be avoided. Figures 15.14a, b, and c show 30°, 45°, and 60° wedge pairs combined at their respective appropriate (i.e., 180 − 2θ) hinge angles of 120°, 90°, and 60°, respectively. It is to be noted that, in the entrance zone, the wedge fields may produce hot spots toward the thin end of the wedge, as can be seen in Figures 15.9b and 15.10b.

15.7.3 THREE-FIELD TECHNIQUES WITH WEDGES

Apart from being used in wedge-pair geometries, wedges can be used in certain three-beam geometries. Figure 15.15a shows two 30° wedged fields, 1 and 2, combined at a hinge angle of 140°, which is larger than the hinge angle of 120° (i.e., 180° − 2θ) that is appropriate for using two 30° wedged beams. A dose gradient is observed along a line bisecting the hinge angle in the target zone. The delivery of a part of the dose by a third beam, 3 in Figure 15.15b, removes this gradient and makes for better dose uniformity.

Figure 15.16a shows a combination of two parallel opposed beams and a third beam normal to them. Beams 2 and 3 are lateral beams from the left and right sides of the patient, and beam 1 is incident from the front. The dose distribution is uniform within the target volume along the axes

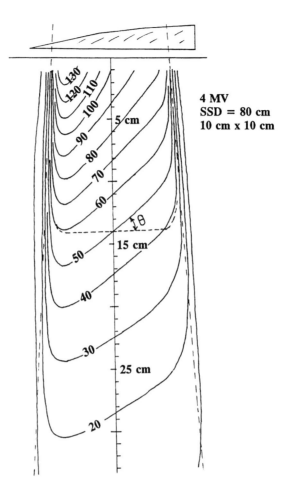

**4 MV
SSD = 80 cm
10 cm x 10 cm**

FIGURE 15.11 Single-beam dose distribution with a wedge. Angle θ is defined as the wedge angle.

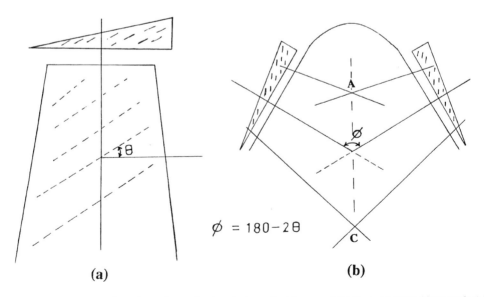

$$\phi = 180 - 2\theta$$

(a)   **(b)**

FIGURE 15.12 Illustration of (a) the wedge angle of a single wedged beam and (b) the appropriate hinge angle ϕ for combining two wedge fields with thick ends of the wedges toward the beam-bisecting line.

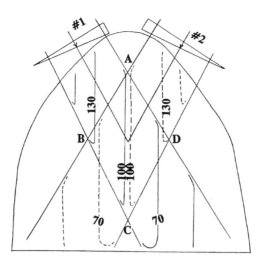

FIGURE 15.13 Composite dose distribution at the region of overlap of two wedged beams with the thick ends of the wedges adjacent to each other. Compensating field gradients occur between points B and D when the beams are combined at the appropriate hinge angle. Then bisector AC falls on an isodose curve.

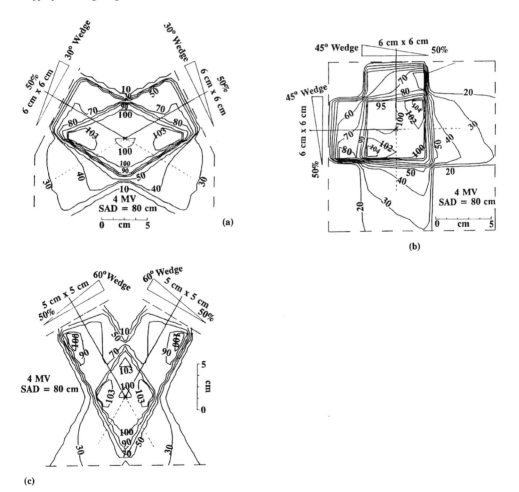

FIGURE 15.14 Isodose curves for pairs of wedged beams combined at their appropriate hinge angles (a) 30° wedges, (b) 45° wedges, (c) 60° wedges.

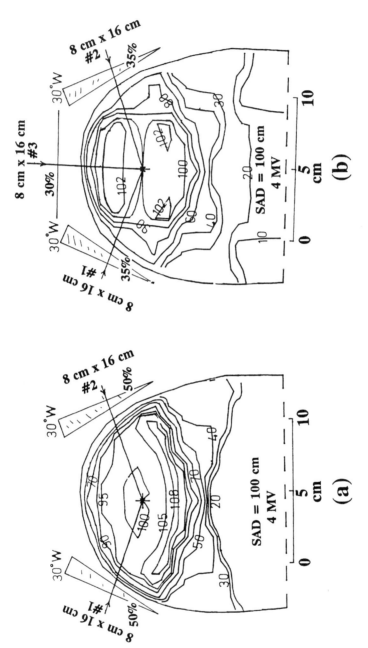

FIGURE 15.15 (a) Two 30° wedges combined at a hinge angle of 140°; (b) the same, with a normally incident beam added along the bisecting line.

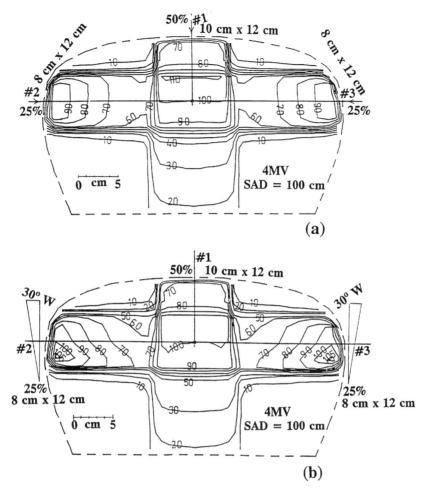

FIGURE 15.16 (a) A three-field technique with bilateral opposing beams and an anterior beam perpendicular to them. (b) The same technique, with wedges added in the lateral beams as shown.

of beams 2 and 3. This is because beams 1 and 2 oppose each other and their gradients balance each other. However, the fall-off of dose along the axis of beam 1 causes a dose gradient from 110% to 90% across the target volume in the direction perpendicular to the central axis of beams 2 and 3. The inclusion of wedge filters in beams 2 and 3 (Figure 15.16b) compensates for the gradient caused by beam 1. It will be noticed that hot spots of 105% appear toward the thin end of the wedge in the entrance zones of beams 2 and 3.

This technique, sometimes referred to as "three-field box," requires optimization of the dose that is administered by each beam and of the wedges to be used.

15.8 IRRADIATIONS WITH PARALLEL OPPOSED BEAMS

15.8.1 ON A BODY SECTION OF MEDIUM THICKNESS

A combination of two opposing beams is a very simple and commonly used technique in radiation oncology. Figure 15.17 shows the central-axis dose profile for one set of opposing beams for different beam energies and a body thickness of 20 cm. Equal doses are delivered by the two beams at the patient's midline; hence, we refer to these as "equally weighted." In a clinical context, this resembles the treatment of a body section by an anterior (i.e., from the front) beam and an opposing posterior (i.e., from the back) beam. Figure 15.18 illustrates the isodose distributions

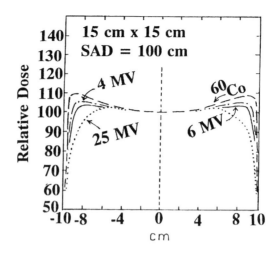

FIGURE 15.17 Central-axis depth-dose profiles for parallel opposed beams in a patient of body thickness 20 cm.

obtained with opposing beams for different energies and treatment SADs. With such a technique, one can deliver a nearly uniform dose in the central region of the patient, with the falling dose gradient of one beam compensating for the rising gradient of the opposing beam. However, the phenomena of exponential attenuation and inverse-square fall-off of photon fluence are such that exact compensation cannot occur over an extended region. Therefore, high doses can result at points close to the beam entry. For example, in Figure 15.17, the profile for cobalt-60 shows high doses or "horns" at points far removed from the patient's midline and close to the entry of the beams. The uniformity improves for higher energies because of the reduced attenuation and less rapid depth-dose fall-off.

An initial dose increase with depth is noticeable in the profiles of the high-energy beams (Figure 15.17). This is caused by the secondary-electron build-up. As we discussed in Section 13.12, the treatment distance also can influence the depth-dose fall-off, although less dramatically than does the energy. Figures 15.18a and b are both for cobalt-60, but are for two different SADs. Figures 15.18c and d are comparisons for two SADs at 4 MV. Figure 15.18e is for a 25-MV beam for a SSD of 100 cm.

The technique in which two beams in a parallel opposed beam arrangement deliver unequal doses at the patient's midline is given the name "unequally weighted parallel opposed beams." In the example shown in Figure 15.19, the beams are weighted 80%:20% in favor of beam 1. The target volume is located off-center and closer to the entrance surface of beam 1. The weighting has been planned so that a minimum dose of 90% will be delivered to the designated target volume.

15.8.2 ON A THIN BODY SECTION

Figure 15.20 addresses a situation in which equally weighted opposing beams irradiate a thin body section measuring 10 cm. The build-up region of the high-energy beams results in underdosing of a major part of the body section. Figure 15.21 represents a clinical parallel to this, with equally weighted bilateral fields used for treatment of the whole brain with ^{60}Co, 4-MV and 25-MV beams. In such treatments, if it becomes necessary to ensure adequate dose delivery even at shallow depths, the large build-up zone of very high-energy beams can become a disadvantage. One approach with a high-energy beam could be to place a layer of tissue-equivalent "bolus" materials near or on the patient's skin and to provide secondary-electron build-up to the superficial regions.[31,32] However, this procedure, called "bolusing," will increase the skin dose, and the skin-sparing advantage of high-energy beams will be compromised. Overall, lower-energy beams, such as Co^{60} beams, are preferable for such situations.

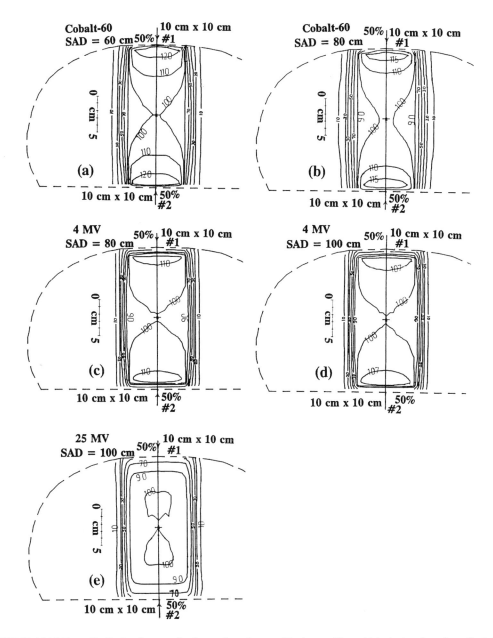

FIGURE 15.18 Dose distribution for opposing beams from front and back on a 20 cm thick chest region of a patient: (a) and (b), for cobalt-60; (c) and (d) for 4 MV; and (e) for 25 MV.

15.8.3 ON A THICK BODY SECTION

Figure 15.22 addresses the use of equally weighted opposing beams on a large body section of 50 cm thickness. The difference between high and low energies is very significant for this thickness. Thicknesses of such magnitude may be encountered when opposing lateral beams (from the right and left sides) are used on a very thick body section. Figure 15.23 presents the isodose curves for equally weighted bilateral beams of different energies and SADs, incident on a patient with an average body thickness of 34 cm. The lateral subcutaneous doses are reduced from 220% in Figure 15.23a to 112% in Figure 15.23e by gradual improvement of the depth-dose fall-off with the use of increasing SAD and energy.

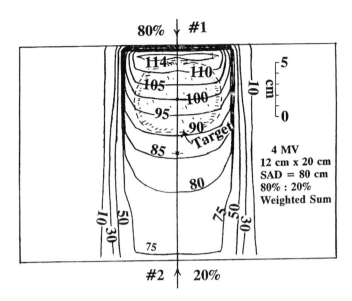

FIGURE 15.19 Unequally weighted opposing beams for treatment of a target volume located anteriorly. The anterior beam delivers 80% of the target dose.

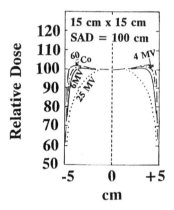

FIGURE 15.20 Central-axis depth-dose profiles for parallel opposed beams in a body section of thickness 10 cm.

15.8.4 IN A FOUR-FIELD BOX GEOMETRY

Using lateral beams alone to deliver a high target dose is rarely done in practice. It is more common to use lateral beams in combination with anterior and posterior beams. Thus, the isodose patterns shown in Figure 15.24 for four-beam combinations (also called "four-field box") reflect the relative merits of increasing the SAD or the energy, or both, in a way that more accurately reflects actual practice.

15.8.5 ON A SECTION OF UNEVEN BODY THICKNESS

In situations where the thickness of the patient changes significantly within the field, parallel opposed beams can give a dose gradient along the patient's midline. Figure 15.25a illustrates this for parallel opposed 6-MV beams irradiating the neck and chest region of a patient. The dose is seen to vary from 109% to 90% along the patient's midline from the thin side to the thick side. In Figure 15.25b, the uniformity is improved when a bolus or wax is used on the patient's surface to fill the thickness deficits and level the surface. Such bolusing on the skin is a disadvantage, as the secondary electrons from the bolus will enhance the skin dose and eliminate the build-up and skin-sparing advantage of high-energy photon beams. In an alternative approach, which is shown in

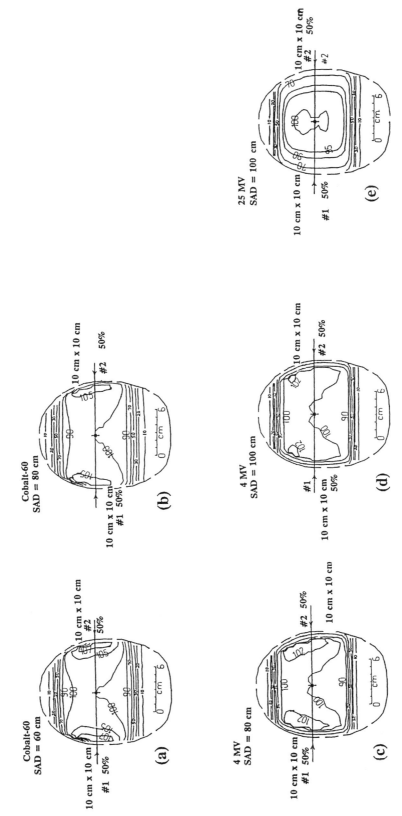

FIGURE 15.21 Dose distribution for opposing beams irradiating a 14 cm thick section of the head of a patient: (a) and (b), for cobalt-60; (c) and (d) for 4 MV; and (e) for 25 MV.

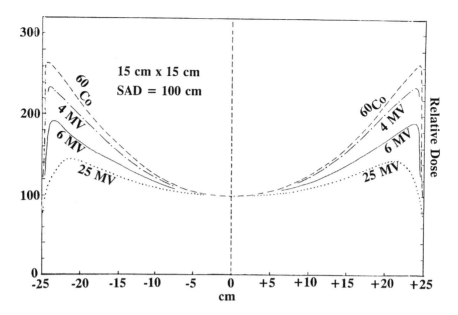

FIGURE 15.22 Central-axis depth-dose profiles for parallel opposed beams in a body section of thickness 50 cm.

Figure 15.25c, a specially designed filter called a "tissue compensating filter" is placed at a distance above the surface to filter the radiation in such a way as to improve the dose uniformity. One can specially design the shape of the compensating filter by exactly taking into account the variation in the patient thickness across the field.[33-37] The compensating filter can be placed at a large distance (20 cm or more) from the skin, so that the fluence of secondary electrons from the filter does not contribute significantly to the skin dose and thereby spoil the dose build-up and skin-sparing effect.

In situations where the change in patient thickness within the field is gradual, wedge filters can be used as compensating filters. Figures 15.26a and b illustrate the dose distributions without and with wedge compensation in a case of irradiation of the breast and chest wall by tangentially opposing beams.

15.9 OTHER COMMON TECHNIQUES

Figures 15.27 to 15.31 present the isodose distributions for some commonly employed techniques of irradiation. The techniques covered are

"Three-field-obliques," with three beams in an oblique geometry (Figure 15.27)
"Four-field-obliques," with four beams in an oblique combination (Figure 15.28)
"Full 360° rotation," which uses an isocentric beam that makes a complete circle around the patient (Figure 15.29)
"Posterior skip arc," with a moving beam that rotates around an isocenter, but skips an 80° arc segment at the posterior side of the patient (Figure 15.30)
"Bilateral arcs," that is, two arcs on either side of the patient (Figure 15.31)

Each illustration provides four isodose patterns covering the following energies and SADs:

(a)   Cobalt-60, SAD = 60 cm
(b)   Cobalt-60, SAD = 80 cm
(c)   4-MV X-rays, SAD = 100 cm
(d)   25-MV X-rays, SAD = 100 cm

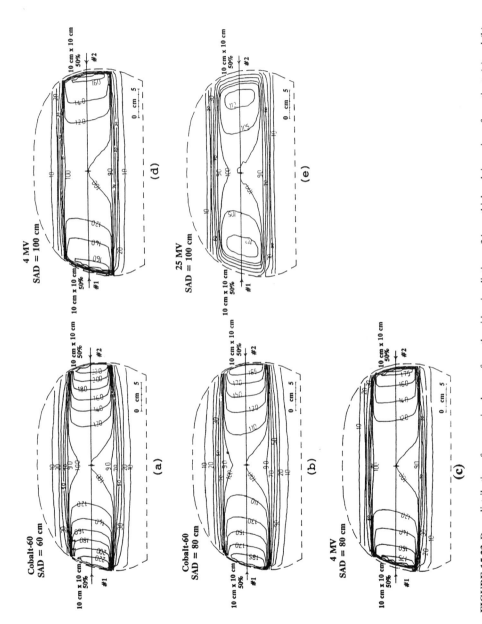

FIGURE 15.23 Dose distributions for opposing beams from the sides, irradiating a 34 cm thick pelvic region of a patient: (a) and (b), for cobalt-60; (c) and (d) for 4 MV; and (e) for 25 MV.

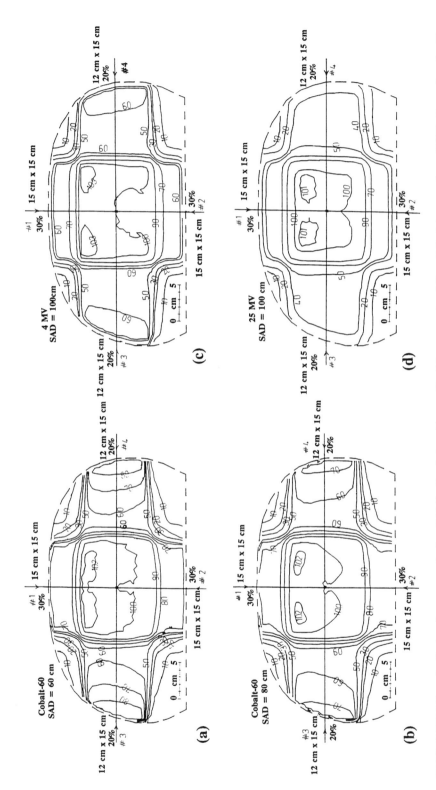

FIGURE 15.24 Dose distributions for a rectangular four-field "box" technique. Front and back beams together deliver 60% of the target dose of 100%. Beams from the sides deliver the remaining 40%. (a) Cobalt-60, SAD 60 cm; (b) cobalt-60, SAD 80 cm; (c) 4-MV X-rays, SAD 100 cm; (d) 25-MV X-rays, SAD 100 cm.

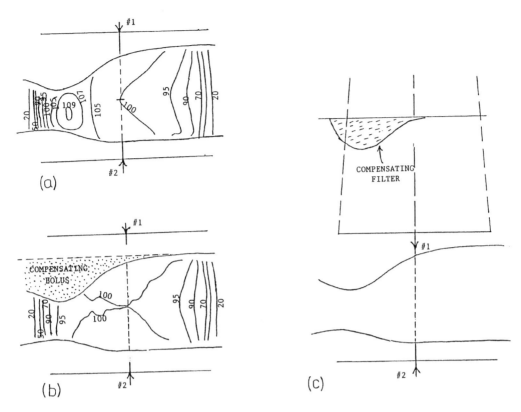

FIGURE 15.25 (a) A pair of 6-MV parallel opposed beams irradiating the neck and chest regions of a patient, resulting in nonuniform delivery of dose along the patient's midline. (b) A compensating bolus has been placed on the patient's skin to level the surface and improve the dose uniformity. (c) A compensating filter is inserted in the beam.

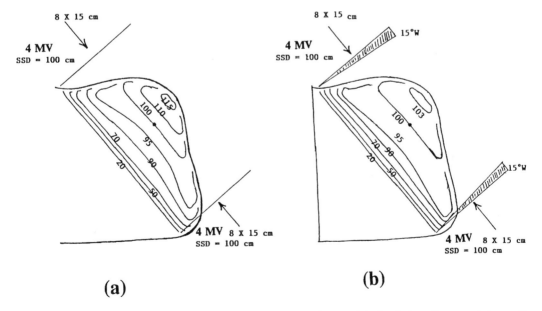

FIGURE 15.26 Dose distributions obtained for tangentially opposing fields used for irradiation of breast and chest wall. (a) Without tissue compensation wedges, (b) with wedges used for tissue compensation.

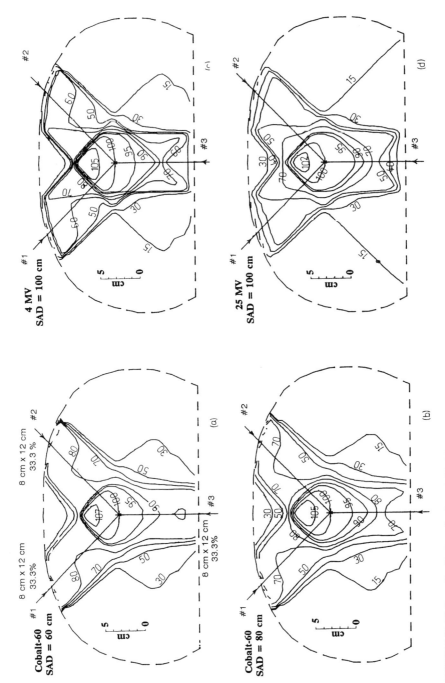

FIGURE 15.27 Dose distributions for three-field oblique technique with an equal part of the 100% target dose delivered by each beam. (a) Cobalt-60, SAD 60 cm; (b) cobalt-60, SAD 80 cm; (c) 4-MV X-rays, SAD 100 cm; (d) 25-MV X-rays, SAD 100 cm.

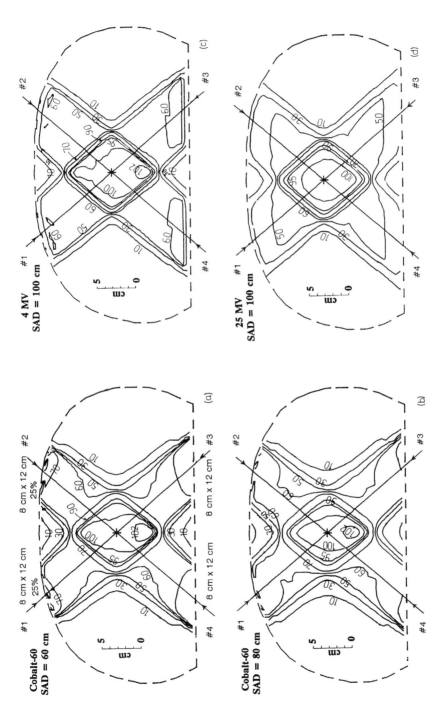

FIGURE 15.28 Dose distributions for a combination of four oblique fields with equal amount of 100% target dose delivered by each beam. (a) Cobalt-60, SAD 60 cm; (b) cobalt-60, SAD 80 cm; (c) 4-MV X-rays, SAD 100 cm; (d) 25-MV X-rays, SAD 100 cm.

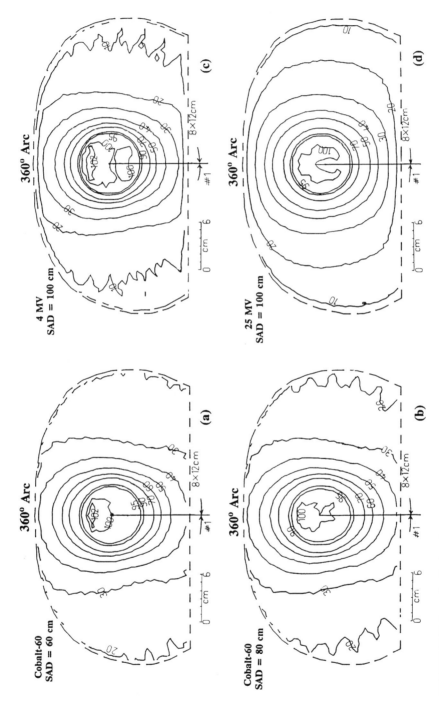

FIGURE 15.29 Dose distributions for 360° rotation. (a) Cobalt-60, SAD 60 cm; (b) cobalt-60, SAD 80 cm; (c) 4-MV X-rays, SAD 100 cm; (d) 25-MV X-rays, SAD 100 cm.

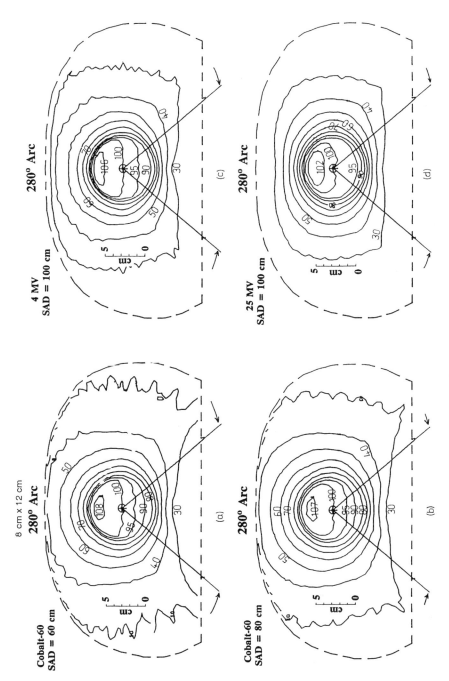

FIGURE 15.30 Dose distribution for "posterior skip arc" with a 280° moving beam. (a) Cobalt-60, SAD 60 cm; (b) cobalt-60, SAD 80 cm; (c) 4-MV X-rays, SAD 100 cm; (d) 25-MV X-rays, SAD 100 cm.

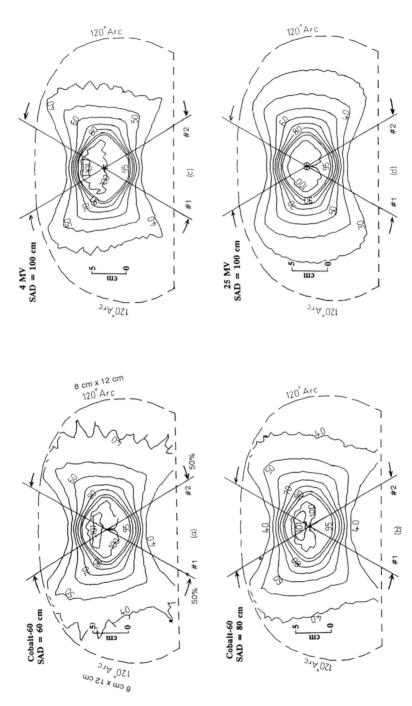

FIGURE 15.31 Dose distribution for bilateral 120° arcs. (a) Cobalt-60, SAD 60 cm; (b) cobalt-60, SAD 80 cm; (c) 4-MV X-rays, SAD 100 cm; (d) 25-MV X-rays, SAD 100 cm.

From (a) to (d), the above sequence upgrades the machine from an early cobalt machine to a high-energy accelerator through two interim stages. The reader is advised to observe the isodose patterns to discern (i) the shape of the target zones covered, (ii) the hot spots and cold spots in the target zone, (iii) the doses at the entrance and exit zones, (iv) the location of the annular zones, (v) the fall-off in the penumbral zones, and (vi) the dose increase in the build-up zones. In a given clinical situation, the selection or suitability of one dose distribution over another can be guided by the above factors. Atlases of multiple-beam and moving-beam dose distributions have been published for study and teaching purposes.[38,39]

15.10 TREATMENT PLANNING: A PRACTICAL CASE

15.10.1 THERAPY SIMULATOR

A radiotherapy simulator is a machine that uses a diagnostic X-ray tube as a radiation source and mimics, in all of its adjustments and motions, the radiotherapy machine to be used for the actual treatment.[40-42] Simulation is a process of developing, evaluating, and accepting a treatment strategy for a given patient situation. The planning phase of the treatment of a patient can require a considerable amount of time, and it is therefore not wise to use a treatment machine for planning purposes. The treatment machine is best utilized for treating as many patients as possible with strategies that are already finalized. A part of the planning and of accepting the treatment strategy is to take projection radiographs for particular beam conditions. The radiotherapy simulator is a major tool for this purpose. The image contrast obtainable in the film with the diagnostic X-ray beam from the simulator is different from that obtainable in a "port film" obtained with the high-energy therapy beam.

Figures 15.32a and b show a simulation film of a field irradiating the vocal cord and the corresponding port film. The bony shadows are seen in better contrast in the simulation film, whereas the soft-tissue outlines are clearer in the high-energy therapy beam image. The kilovoltage X-ray beam of the simulator can be used for localizing the bony structures for dose distribution planning. It is prudent to verify whether the location of the different beams and the coverage provided by them conform to the plan chosen. Injection of contrast medium into the body cavities can aid in the localizing and verification process where appropriate. The simulated radiographic image in Figure 15.32a includes the images of horizontal and vertical pairs of wires which delineate the geometric edges of a rectangular field intended for treatment. The X-ray beam used for radiographing can be larger than the intended field of treatment to show a broader background. The radiograph also shows the image of a graduated cross hair at the two principal axes of the rectangular field. These gradations, which signify 1-cm spacings at the distance of the isocenter, are helpful in the evaluation or in suggesting changes.

Simulation radiographs involve much less exposure to the patient than does imaging with the therapy beam itself. Changes can be made in successive steps until the optimum beam coverage is achieved. With modern simulators, the beam delineation and orientation and patient positioning can be done under fluoroscopic observation. Any treatment beam should also be verified with a port film radiograph taken with the therapy beam, as illustrated in Figure 15.32b. A port film can combine two images on one film — the first obtained with a therapy beam of a size identical to that of the intended treatment beam and the second obtained with a larger beam covering the surrounding body structures as well.

15.10.2 LOCALIZATION FOR TREATMENT OF THE ESOPHAGUS

We now discuss the specific case of a patient with cancer of the esophagus. Figures 15.33a and b are AP (i.e., front to back) and lateral (i.e., side view) radiographic projections of a section of the patient taken with barium contrast medium in the esophagus. The contrast medium outlines the organ and helps the physician to identify the target volume of treatment which includes subclinical disease and the surrounding routes of spread. (The target volume for dose delivery may often include more than the known tumor volume.) Figures 15.34a and b are line drawings of the visible

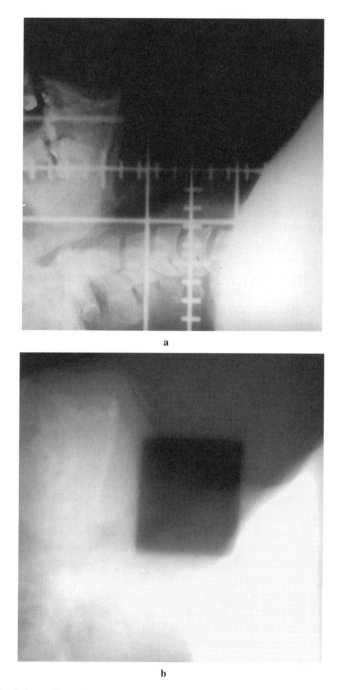

a

b

FIGURE 15.32 (a) Simulation radiograph obtained with 80-kV X-rays. (b) A therapy port radiograph obained with 4-MV X-rays.

outlines from the radiographs in Figures 15.33a and b. In Figure 15.34a, the marks (A_R, A_L), (B_R, B_L), and (C_R, C_L) indicate the right and left extents of the target volume at three levels in the patient as indicated by the physician. Likewise, in Figure 15.34b, at the same three levels, the upper and lower (i.e., anterior and posterior) limits of the target volume have been identified as (A_U, A_D), (B_U, B_D), (C_U, C_D). The course of the spinal cord is also seen and is observed in both projections.

We would like to have available a transverse contour of the patient through point M_0 (Figure 15.34b), where M_0 is the center of the field on the body surface. The contour can usually be obtained

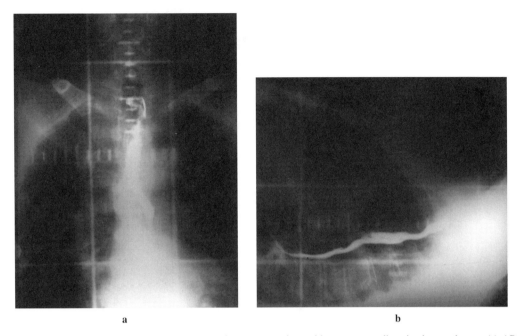

FIGURE 15.33 The first simulation radiographs of a cancer patient with contrast medium in the esophagus. (a) AP projection, (b) lateral projection.

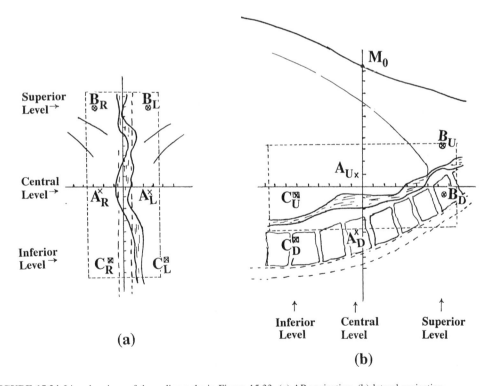

FIGURE 15.34 Line drawings of the radiographs in Figure 15.33. (a) AP projection, (b) lateral projection.

by placing of a moldable plaster-of-paris cast on the patient's surface and waiting for it to harden. Then the cast is removed and placed on a sheet of paper (Figure 15.35). When the cast is on the patient, marks (e.g., M_0, M_1, and M_2 as shown in Figure 15.35) are made on it to identify the points of entry of the AP beam and the entrance and exit points of the lateral beam as simulated. The

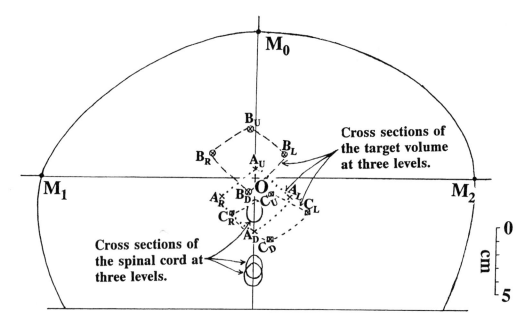

FIGURE 15.35 Patient contour drawn with skin marks M, M_1, and M_2, and localization of the front-to-back (i.e., AP–PA) and left-to-right (i.e., lateral) extents of the target volume and spinal cord, as interpreted from Figure 15.32. x, $\otimes$ and $\boxtimes$, refer to A points, B points, and C points, respectively.

measured lateral and front-to-back thicknesses of the patient between these (and any other) fiducial marks are used for appropriate placement of the plaster-of-paris cast on a sheet of paper for tracing of the contour, as shown in Figure 15.35. The vertical line through M_0 and the horizontal line M_1M_2 intersect at O. The point O, which is the location of the isocenter at simulation, can be used as the origin of a rectangular (x,y) coordinate system.

As a next step, the positions of points (A_R, A_L) and (A_U, A_D) (from Figures 13.34a and b) should be localized with respect to the origin O in Figure 15.35. In the absence of full information (such as a CT scan may provide) in the transverse plane, the points A_R, A_L, A_U, and A_D have been localized in Figure 15.35 with the assumption that the lines A_RA_L and A_UA_D bisect one another. In the same manner, the points (B_R, B_L, B_U, B_D) and (C_R, C_L, C_U, C_D) have been localized. These give a perspective of the progression of the target volume along the length of the patient. In Figure 15.35, the points have been connected to indicate the areas to be covered in the irradiation. By a similar approach, the sections of spinal cord have been drawn at the three levels, because it is a critical organ with limited radiation tolerance.

15.10.3 CASE-SPECIFIC ISODOSE PLANNING

Let us say that the physician desires to deliver a dose of 60 Gy to the target volume. He would like to use a technique that would (i) keep the dose to the spinal cord below 45 Gy and (ii) minimize the dose to the lungs. Figures 15.36, 15.37, and 15.38 illustrate the design of three different treatment plans, assuming that a 4-MV X-ray machine is available in the clinic. The first plan, in Figure 15.36, is a four-field box technique that delivers 66% of the target dose by AP–PA fields 1 and 2 and the remaining 34% by lateral fields 3 and 4. The second plan, in Figure 15.37, uses front-to-back fields 1 and 2 to deliver 66% of the target dose and employs opposing oblique fields 3 and 4 for the remaining 34%. The third plan, in Figure 15.38, uses front-to-back fields 1 and 2 to deliver 60% of the total dose and a 240° arc to add the remaining 40%.

15.10.4 COMPARATIVE EVALUATION OF THE PLANS

Uniformity of dose within the target volume is accomplished in all three plans. This is to be expected, because they were designed to achieve this as a minimum objective. The total dose

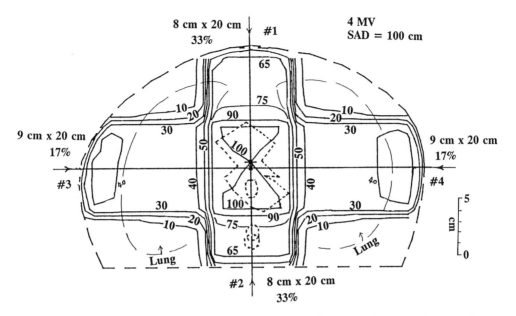

FIGURE 15.36 A rectangular four-field box technique for treating the esophagus case of Figure 15.32. Front-to-back beam delivers 66% of the target dose and lateral opposing beams deliver the remaining 34%.

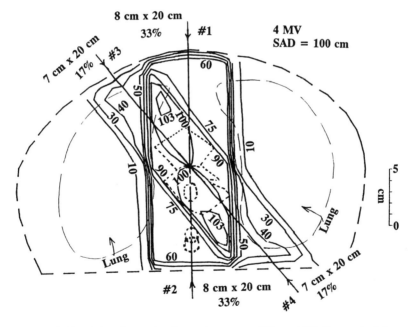

FIGURE 15.37 A four-field technique for treating the esophagus case of Figure 15.32. Front-to-back beams deliver 66% of the target dose, and oblique opposing beams deliver the remaining 34%.

delivered with any plan, however, can be limited by the tolerance dose of the other organs that are irradiated incidentally. Therefore, let us first look at the plans from the point of view of the spinal cord tolerance. All three plans have been designed so as to deliver not more than 75% of the prescribed target dose of 60 Gy to the mid- and lower segments of the spinal cord. However, the upper segment of the spinal cord is much closer to the isocenter and is seen to receive the same dose as the target dose. Here, we need to remember that the plan we see is two-dimensional and

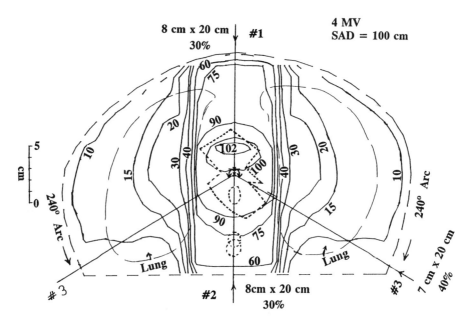

FIGURE 15.38 A technique that combines front-to-back beams for delivery of 60% of the dose, with a 240° arc technique to deliver the remaining 40%, for treating the esophagus case of Figure 15.33.

does not display all of the details along the length of the patient. At simulation, we can observe the fields along their lengths. The protection of the upper spinal cord can be taken care of by shaping of the field with blocks during the stages of simulation and verification of the beams.

The three plans differ with regard to protecting the lungs and minimizing pulmonary damage. The plans of Figures 15.36 and 15.38 are both poor in this respect compared to that in Figure 15.37. It appears that the plan of Figure 15.37 is the most acceptable overall. A more quantitative comparison for this purpose can be made with the use of dose-volume plots.

15.10.5 USE OF DOSE-VOLUME PLOTS

A graphic plot of the fraction of any organ (or volume) that receives more than various assigned dose levels is a useful tool for evaluating the performance of different dose distributions. Such plots are called dose-volume plots. A typical dose-volume plot for a target volume to be irradiated may have an appearance as shown in Figure 15.39, for any plan designed to give a uniform dose. The figure compares the plot for ideal dose uniformity within the target volume with what can be obtained in real situations. For any critically sensitive organ, different treatment plans will give different dose-volume plots. For example, an evaluation of the dose distribution in the lungs in Figures 15.36, 15.37, and 15.38 resulted in the dose-volume plots shown in Figure 15.40. Thus, the relative merits of these three plans from the point of view of sparing the lung volume are compared side by side. If a cut-off level of 20% dose is used for lung tolerance, the plot labeled B, applicable to the plan in Figure 15.37, is seen to irradiate a minimum lung volume above this dose, compared to the two others labeled A and C. This again affirms the selection of the plan of Figure 15.37.

15.10.6 INTEGRAL DOSE (Σ)

Ideally, one would like to irradiate the target volume only, with no dose delivered elsewhere. After assuring that the target dose is uniform, we can look among several techniques for one that results in minimum energy absorbed in the whole body. Integral dose (Σ) was defined as an index by Mayneord[43] for such a comparative evaluation. If a volume of tissue having mass M receives an average dose D_{Av}, Σ is given by

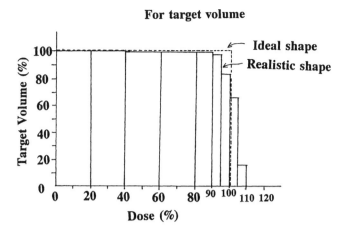

FIGURE 15.39   A typical dose-volume plot for a target volume.

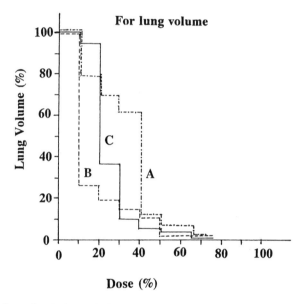

FIGURE 15.40 Dose-volume plots for lung. The three curves labeled A, B, and C are for the plans of Figures 15.36, 15.37, and 15.38, respectively.

$$\Sigma = \text{mass} \times \text{average dose} = M \times D_{Av}$$

Example 15.2

A cylindrical body section has a diameter of 20 cm and a length of 15 cm. The density of tissue is 1.0 g cm^{-3}. In a treatment plan adopted for irradiation, the average dose to the volume is assessed to be 1200 cGy. Calculate the integral dose.

Radius of cylinder (r) = 20/2 = 10 cm; Length (L) = 15 cm; volume (V) = $\pi r^2 L$ = 3.1416 $\times$ $10^2 \times 15$ = 4712 cm^3

$$\text{Mass of volume} = 4712 \text{ cm}^3 \times 1.0 \text{ g cm}^{-3} = 4.712 \text{ kg}$$

$$\text{Integral dose} = \text{average dose} \times \text{mass receiving the dose}$$

$$= 1200 \text{ cGy} \times 4.712 \text{ kg} = 4.712 \text{ kg} \times 1200 \times 10^{-2} \text{ J kg}^{-1}$$

$$= 56.5 \text{ J}$$

In general, different volumes may be enclosed between different isodose surfaces plotted in a plan. If so, Σ is given by the following sum:

$$\Sigma = {}_i\Sigma\rho\left|V_{i+1} - V_i\right|\left(D_{i+1} + D_i\right)/2$$

where V_i = volume enclosed within isodose level i; D_i = dose corresponding to isodose level i; and ρ = density of the medium.

From the two-dimensional isodose curves, it is possible only to obtain area A_i enclosed by an isodose curve for dose D_i. In a simplistic way, if the same distribution is assumed to be valid in all transverse planes along the field length L, the following approximation results:

$$V_i = A_i \times L$$

and

$$\Sigma = {}_i\Sigma\rho L\left|A_{i+1} - A_i\right|\left(D_{i+1} + D_i\right)/2$$

$$= {}_i\Sigma\rho L\,\Delta A_i\left(D_{i+1} + D_i\right)/2$$

where ΔA_i is the annular area enclosed between isodose levels i and i + 1. Figures 15.41a, b, and c are plots of the annular areas between different isodose curves of Figures 15.36, 15.37, and 15.38. The average doses estimated for the three planes are 21%, 17%, and 16%, respectively. These numbers are directly proportional to the Σ values for the three plans. However, these diagrams and numbers are not particularly useful for making any decision. This is because Σ is a sum that does not distinguish between different organs and their individual tolerances. Σ increases with the thickness of the patient through which the beam passes. For example, in the case of a centrally located target site, Σ will be larger for a technique that uses lateral beams than for another technique that employs AP–PA beams. However, the overall dose distribution, rather than Σ, should influence how much dose can be given in each beam orientation. As in our example in Section 15.10.3, the tolerance of an organ (such as the spinal cord) can be a more significant factor for limiting the AP–PA component than is any fear of a possible increase in Σ by use of any other beam directions.

15.10.7 SIMULATING THE ACCEPTED PLAN

The geometric aspects of the paper plan of Figure 15.37 should now be implemented on the patient. Beams 1 and 2 have the isocenter at O, which is the same isocenter that was used during the first simulation. This isocenter can be identified within the patient by means of the skin marks M_0, M_1, and M_2 (see Figure 15.35), which are retained by the patient. To implement the treatment plan in which the two oblique beams 3 and 4 are used, we need to simulate these beams. In general, these beams may have their isocenter at a point I different from O. Setting the isocenter at I can be done through the following steps:

(i)   Identify the offsets a and b (Figure 15.42a) from isocenter I with respect to O.
(ii)   Set up beam 1 with the isocenter at O, as was done during the initial localizing simulation.
(iii)   The patient is moved in the left–right direction through a distance **a** to have the beam axis go through the isocenter I (see Figure 15.42b).
(iv)   The patient is then moved in the front–back direction through a distance **b** so that the isocenter coincides with I.
(v)   The beam is swung to assume the oblique direction of beam 3 (Figure 15.42c), and a simulation radiograph is obtained.
(vi)   The same procedure is repeated for beam 4.

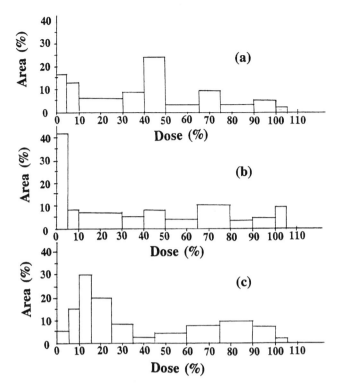

FIGURE 15.41 Plots of the percent area of the patient's cross section enclosed between different isodose levels. Diagrams (a), (b), and (c) are for the dose distributions in Figures 15.36, 15.37, and 15.38, respectively.

Figure 15.43 shows the simulation radiographs for oblique beam 3. Figure 15.44 is a line drawing of the contents of Figure 15.43. In the plan of Figure 15.37, the oblique beams were designed to treat the target volume without irradiating the spinal cord in the midtransverse section of the fields. In Figures 15.43 and 15.44, it is seen that the field edges (as indicated by the shadow of field-delineating wires) fall far from the spinal cord in the lower sections of the field. However, the spinal cord courses within the field at one corner. For protection of this part of the spinal cord, a shielding block is added. With the block included, the entire field length of beam 3 conforms to the geometric criteria (concerning the field edge) that made the paper plan of Figure 15.37 acceptable. A similar block can be designed for oblique field 4 after that field is simulated. With such specially shaped oblique fields the patient can be treated.

We refer the reader to References 44, 45, and 46 for several other practical aspects of photon beam treatment planning.

15.11 USE OF CT DATA

15.11.1 CT TRANSVERSE CUTS

Computed-tomography (CT) scanners provide detailed anatomic and diagnostic information in successive transverse sections of the patient. The CT images can be used directly for treatment planning, provided the CT scan is made with the patient placed in a position identical to the treatment position. In the positioning, one should use similar patient supports with the same positions of arm, shoulder, neck, etc. With any change of position, the organ delineations can differ between the CT and the treatment position of the patient.

Many advances arc being made in the transfer and processing of CT images for direct 3D planning in radiotherapy.[1-9] It is not within the scope of this text to discuss this subject in detail. We will merely illustrate how CT data can be used for field shaping, using just one example.

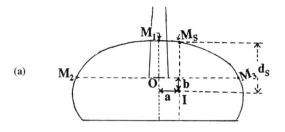

(a)

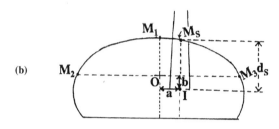

(b)

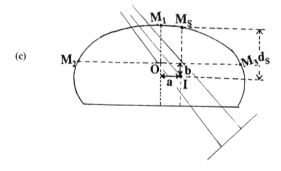

(c)

FIGURE 15.42 Diagrams (a), (b), and (c) show the steps by which the isocenter is placed at point I of the plan in Figure 15.36. In (a), the patient is set up so as to have the isocenter at point O used during initial simulation. The patient is then moved by offset distances a and b in (b) and (c).

15.11.2 CT FOR FIELD SHAPING

We use the example of a lung tumor for which the physician has already simulated an anterior field, as shown in Figure 15.45. This radiograph does reveal the presence of the tumor, but not in the same detail and clarity as provided by a CT scan. Figure 15.46 shows some examples of CT images of the patient. We can interpret the CT tumor outlines and project them on the simulation radiograph. The tumor outline in Figure 15.45 has been drawn based on the CT images by a projection procedure that is described next. Figure 15.47 gives the line drawing representation of the same CT images. These drawings highlight the tumor, the vertebral body, the sternum, and the outer body contour in each section. A minified line drawing of the film view is shown in Figure 15.47e which shows the apex of the lung, the bronchial carina, and the diaphragm, along with bony structures. The scale in the middle marks the levels of the different CT images from 3 to 21. These have been localized by identification of the levels of a few salient anatomic landmarks, such as the apex of the lung, the bronchial carina, and the diaphragm. In Figures 15.47a to d, rays through the edges of the tumor have been drawn that project points AA, BB, CC, and DD at the level of the

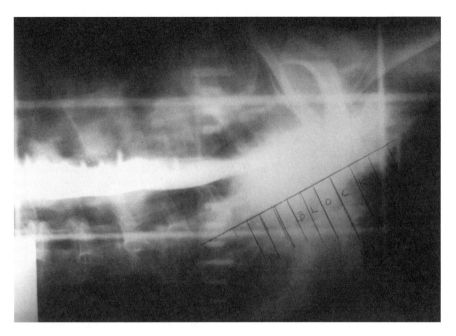

FIGURE 15.43 Simulation radiograph of oblique field no. 3 of Figure 15.36. A block is shown shielding the cord where it falls within the collimated rectangular field.

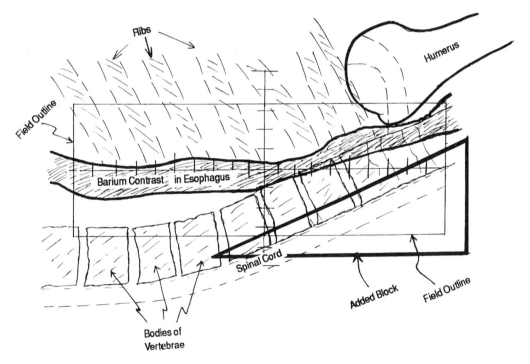

FIGURE 15.44 Line drawing of the radiograph in Figure 15.43.

film. The distance of these points from the midline M of the patient is first measured on the CT image. Then these points are relocated in the film, as illustrated in Figure 15.47e. The scale of the CT image is usually small compared to the scale of the actual patient. On the other hand, because of the beam divergence, the simulation radiograph shows the patient anatomy on a magnified scale. Thus, both the scale of the CT image and that of the simulation radiograph should be taken into

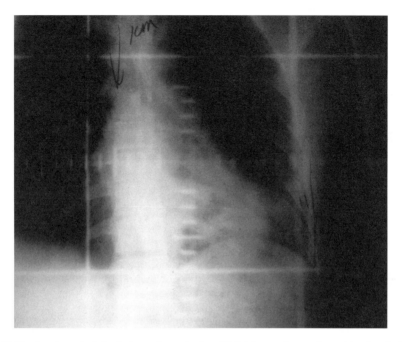

FIGURE 15.45 The first (tentative) simulation radiograph of an AP field setup for a patient with a lung lesion.

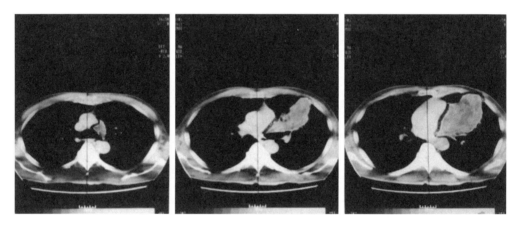

FIGURE 15.46 Examples of CT images of the patient with a lung lesion. The tumor outlines have been drawn.

account in the projection of the extent of the CT image of the tumor on the simulation radiograph. Such a "beam's-eye" projection of any structure seen in CT on the film plane is very useful for shaping the treatment field. Figure 15.48 is a port film of the field showing the tumor volume projected from CT and a block placed to shape the field accepted for treatment.

Here we have dealt with a simple situation of projecting a tumor volume from CT for a vertical beam of simple geometry irradiating a patient from front to back. With the use of computers and complex coordinate transformation algorithms, one can project the beam's-eye view of a tumor or any other organ from CT for any arbitrary beam orientation.[1-9]

15.12 TREATMENT OF ADJACENT SITES

15.12.1 PROBLEM OF CONCERN

In radiotherapy practice, situations may be encountered in which it becomes necessary to treat a site adjacent to a site either treated previously or under current treatment. If both sites are being

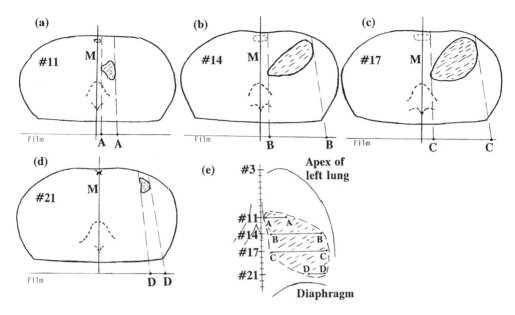

FIGURE 15.47 (a) to (d) Line drawings of the CT images of Figure 15.46, showing the salient structures. The rays projecting the right-left extent of the tumor onto the plane of the simulation radiograph are also illustrated schematically. (e) Line drawing of the AP radiograph of Figure 15.45, including the projection of the tumor volume from CT images.

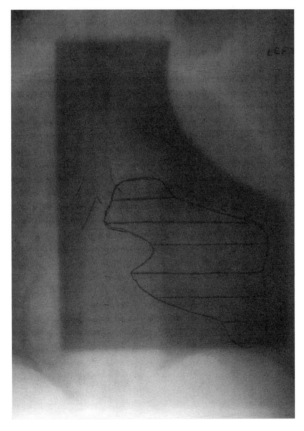

FIGURE 15.48 Port film image of a shaped field including a block and the tumor volume projected from CT.

treated concurrently, the reason for the split may be that the maximum field size provided by the treatment machine is inadequate to include both sites in a single beam. When separate fields are used, it is important to take into account the overlap or gaps between the edges of the adjacent fields. Ignoring this can result in overdosage because of superposition of the beam edges or underdosage because of gaps between them at the interface.[47,48] The gradual fall-off of dose caused by a beam with a penumbra is a blessing in these situations, as it can diffuse the severity of the effects of mismatches, gaps, or overlaps.

The junction problem has been studied and reported for various situations. Different approaches have been used for overcoming the problem. These include the use of a separation between the adjacent beam edges on the skin, angular rotation of the beam to orient its edges, adopting half-beam blocking and using the nondiverging central axis of the adjacent beams to coincide, using penumbra spreaders, and moving the junction during phases of treatment, etc.[48-59] In the next sections, we discuss the general aspects of this problem.

15.12.2 BOTH SITES TREATED FROM ONE DIRECTION

A very simple situation is shown in Figure 15.49a, where two beams irradiate adjacent sites. Fields 1 and 2 have their field lengths L_1 and L_2 specified at their respective SAD_1 and SAD_2 of treatment. The skin is at level d above the junction between the two fields. The divergences of the beams are such that a separation (or skin gap) S between the edges of the fields is needed at the skin level so that the edges intersect at the depth d. The field lengths L_1' and L_2' of the two fields at the skin surface are

$$L_1' = L_1 \times \frac{(SAD_1 - d)}{SAD_1} = L_1 - L_1 \times \frac{d}{SAD_1}$$

$$L_2' = L_2 \times \frac{(SAD_2 - d)}{SAD_2} = L_2 - L_2 \times \frac{d}{SAD_2}$$

The skin gap S is related to L_1, L_2, L_1', and L_2' by

$$2S = (L_1 + L_2) - (L_1' + L_2') = \left[\frac{L_1}{SAD_1} + \frac{L_2}{SAD_2}\right]d$$

Hence, the skin gap

$$S = \frac{1}{2}\left[\frac{L_1}{SAD_1} + \frac{L_2}{SAD_2}\right]d$$

If $SAD_1 = SAD_2 = SAD$,

$$S = \frac{d(L_1 + L_2)}{2 \times SAD}$$

Example 15.3

Two adjacent fields have lengths of 17 cm and 20 cm as specified at an SAD of 80 cm. Calculate the skin gap needed for matching of the field edges at 5 cm depth.

In this example,

$$L_1 = 17 \text{ cm}; \ L_2 = 20 \text{ cm}, \ SAD = 80 \text{ cm}; \ d = 5 \text{ cm}$$

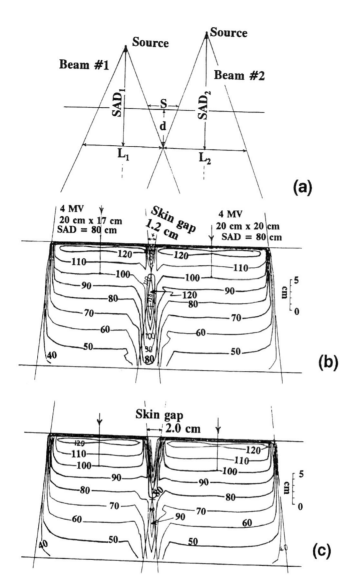

FIGURE 15.49 (a) Diverging edges of two adjacent fields of lengths L_1 and L_2 set up at distances SAD_1 and SAD_2. (b) The dose distribution for two adjacent beams with 4-MV X-rays positioned for a skin gap of 1.2 cm to match the diverging edges at 5 cm depth. (c) Dose distribution for the same beams when the skin gap is increased to 2 cm.

$$S = \frac{d(L_1 + L_2)}{2 \times SAD} = \frac{5(17 + 20)}{2 \times 80} = 1.2 \text{ cm}$$

Figure 15.49b shows the isodose curves for this example for 4 MV beams. The prescription dose of 100% has been taken at a depth of 5 cm for both sites. It is seen that, at the overlap between the fields, the dose rises to 120%. An increase of the skin gap to 2.0 cm (see Figure 15.49c) reduces the dose at the overlap to 90%, but at the cost of underdosing the tissue just below the skin gap.

15.12.3 ADJACENT PARALLEL OPPOSED FIELDS

The beam divergence calculation that gave the skin gap S is equally applicable to situations in which adjacent sites are treated by parallel opposed beams. For such beams, the dose prescription is usually made at the midplane of the patient. The beam edges can also be matched at the patient's midplane.

Figures 15.50a to d consider the use of different skin gaps for two adjacent sites treated by fields of lengths 12 cm and 15 cm at an SAD of 80 cm. In Figure 15.50a, no skin gap is used, and the field edges are matched on the skin. It is seen that an overdose of up to 170% occurs at the junction. The skin gap which would match the field edges at the midplane without overlap is calculated in the next example.

Example 15.4

The patient's thickness at the junction is 18 cm.

$$L_1 = 12 \text{ cm}, \ L_2 = 15 \text{ cm}, \ d = 18/2 = 9 \text{ cm}, \ SAD = 80 \text{ cm}$$

$$\text{Skin gap } S = \frac{d(L_1 + L_2)}{2 \times SAD} = \frac{9(12+15)}{2 \times 80} \approx 1.5 \text{ cm}$$

The dose distribution obtained with the above 1.5-cm skin gap is shown in Figure 15.50b. There are cold spots at shallow depths under the skin gap. Figure 15.50c uses a more generous skin gap of 2.0 cm, which results in a 60% cold spot at the junction. On occasion, it is not enough merely to use a skin gap and accept the cold spots. A method that one can use to remove the extent of underdosing below the skin gap is to change the lengths of the adjacent fields and to move or "feather" the junction during the course of treatment. This can be done only when both sites are treated concurrently. The result of feathering is illustrated in Figure 15.50d, where the position of the beam edges changes from a–a′ to b–b′ and to c–c′ during three successive segments of the treatment. The greater the number of segments, the less can be the inadequacy of any cold spot or the severity of a resulting hot spot. Feathering once a week can be a clinically practicable procedure. Feathering can also diffuse the consequence of any random errors in daily positioning and setup.

15.12.4 MATCHING OPPOSED BEAMS WITH A SINGLE BEAM

In Figures 15.50e and f, we consider a site previously treated by parallel opposed beams, with the dose prescribed to the midline. Let us say that an adjacent site is now to be treated by a beam from only one side of the patient and that the dose is prescribed at a depth of 5 cm. We assume that the dose prescribed for the current treatment is the same as that delivered at the previously treated site. First, let us match the new field edge at 5 cm depth with the previously treated beam from its own side only (i.e., ignoring the second beam that irradiated the patient from the opposite side). This suggests a skin gap of 1.0 cm. Figure 15.50e shows the resulting dose distribution. There is a considerable overlap with the (ignored) beam from the opposite side at the junction, resulting in hot spots of up to 140%. If the opposing beam is not to be ignored, the matching should be done at the patient's midline. This needs a larger skin gap of 1.5-cm. Figure 15.50f shows the dose distribution with the 1.5-cm skin gap. This avoids the overlap and the high doses, but regions under the skin gap at shallow depths become underdosed. Such trade-offs of hot spots and cold spots are unavoidable when adjacent sites are treated with different fields. The physician's clinical insight and discretion should govern how much dose to prescribe, where to position the junction, what level of a high or low dose to accept, and what skin gap to use.

15.12.5 ANGLE MATCH BETWEEN ORTHOGONAL BEAMS

In Figure 15.51, beam no. 1 treats the spinal column at the back of a patient. Beams 2 and 3 are laterally incident, parallel opposed beams that treat the patient's brain from the sides. The continuous edges of beams 2 and 3 represent the beam outlines in the patient's lateral midplane. The outlines shown by dashed lines are the field outlines at the level of the surface of head where the beams enter. These are smaller because they are at a distance closer to the source. The diverging angle of the edge of beam 1 is given by

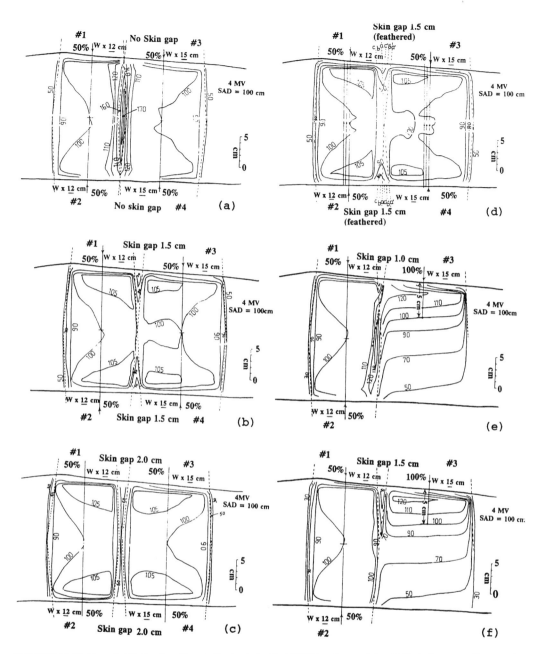

FIGURE 15.50 Dose distribution for adjacent sites treated with 4-MV X-ray beams. (a) to (d) Both sites treated by opposing beams: (a) with edges matched on the skin, leaving no skin gap; (b) with a calculated 1.5-cm skin gap to match the edges of the beams at the patient's midline; (c) with a 2-cm skin gap; (d) with a 1.5-cm calculated gap and "feathering" in three steps, with moving of the junction from a–a′ to b–b′ to c–c′. (e) and (f) The left site is treated by opposing beams with 100% dose at the midline. The right site is treated by a beam from one side only, with 100% dose at 5 cm depth. (e) A calculated skin gap of 1.0 cm is used which matches the edges of the new beam with the previously treated beam at 5 cm depth. (f) A skin gap of 1.5 cm to match the edges of all three beams at the midline.

$$\tan\theta = \frac{0.5 \times L}{SAD}$$

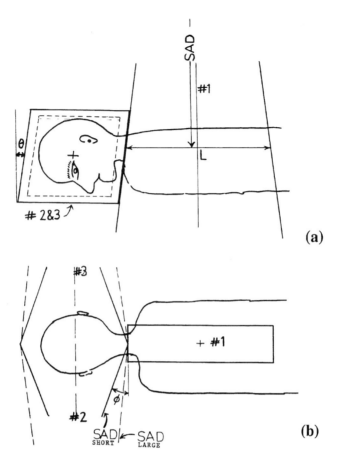

(a)

(b)

FIGURE 15.51 Angular matching of orthogonal beams. Beam no. 1 treats the patient from the back. Fields 2 and 3 treat the patient from the sides. (a) Outlines of beams 2 and 3 are rotated to match the diverging edge of beam 1 at the patient's lateral midline. (b) The diverging edges of beams 2 and 3 are shown in the plane perpendicular to the central axis of beam 1. Angle ϕ can be compensated for by a couch rotation.

where L is the field length of beam 1 at the SAD. A rotation of the collimator by θ, for beams 2 and 3, will match their field outline at the midplane with the edge of beam 1. The dashed edge (at the surface of entrance) also can next be matched by a rotation of the patient's couch around a vertical axis through an angle ϕ. In clinical practice, the light-beam localizer can be used for verifying that the calculated angles do give the expected matches between the adjacent field edges on the surface of the patient.

REFERENCES

1. Tepper, J.E., and Chaney, E.C. (Eds.), Three-Dimensional Treatment Planning, Seminars in Oncology, Vol 2 (No. 4), W.B. Saunders, Philadelphia, 1992.
2. Goitein, M., and Mark, A., Multi-dimensional treatment planning. I. Delineation of anatomy, Int. J. Radiat. Oncol. Biol. Phys., Vol 9, p777-787, 1983.
3. Goitein, M., Abrams, D., Rowell, H., Pollari, H., and Wiles, J., Multi-dimensional treatment planning. II. Beam's-eye-view, back projection, and projection through CT sections, Int. J. Radiat. Oncol. Biol. Phys., Vol 9, p789-797.
4. Mohan, R., Barest, G., Brewster, L.J., Chui, C.S., Kutcher, G.J., Laughlin, J.S., and Fuks, Z., A comprehensive three-dimensional radiation treatment planning system, Int. J. Radiat. Oncol. Biol. Phys., Vol 15, p481-495, 1988.

5. Rosenman, J., Sherouse, G.W., Fuchs, H., Pizer, S.M., Skinner, A.L., Mosher, C., Novins, K., and Tepper, J.E., Three-dimensional display techniques in radiation therapy treatment planning, Int. J. Radiat. Oncol. Biol. Phys., Vol 16, p263-269, 1989.

6. Jacky, J., 3-D radiation therapy treatment planning: Overview and assessment, Am. J. Clin. Oncol., Vol 13, p331-343, 1990.

7. Nishida, T., Nagata, Y., Takahashi, M., Abe, M., Yamaoka, N., Ishihara, H., Kubo, Y., Ohta, H., and Kazusa, C., CT simulator, a new 3-D planning simulating system for radiotherapy: I. Description of system, Int. J. Radiat. Oncol. Biol. Phys., Vol 18, p499-504, 1990.

8. McShan, D.L., Frass, B.A., and Lichter, A.S., Full integration of the beam's eye view concept into computerized treatment planning, Int. J. Radiat. Oncol. Biol. Phys., Vol 18, p1485-1494, 1990.

9. Ling, C.L., Rodgers, C.C., and Morton, R.J. (Eds.), Computed Tomography in Radiotherapy, Raven Press, Washington, D.C., 1982.

10. Tsien, K.C., and Cohen, M., Isodose Charts and Tables for Medium Energy X-Rays, Butterworths, London, 1962.

11. Webster, E.W., and Tsien, K.C., Atlas of Dose Distributions, Vol I, Single-field Isodose Charts, International Atomic Energy Agency, Vienna, Austria, 1965.

12. Munro, P., Rawlinson, J.A., and Fenster, A., Therapy imaging: Source sizes of radiotherapy beams, Med. Phys., Vol 15, p517-524, 1988.

13. ICRU, International Commission on Radiological Units and Measurements, Determination of absorbed dose in a patient irradiated by beams of x or gamma rays in radiotherapy procedures, ICRU Report 24, International Commission on Radiological Units and Measurements, Washington, D.C., 1976.

14. Bush, R.S., and Johns, H.E., The measurement of build-up on curved surfaces exposed to cobalt-60 and cesium-137 beams, Am. J. Roentgenol., Vol 87, p89-93, 1962.

15. Jackson, W., Surface effects of high-energy X-rays at oblique incidence, Br. J. Radiol., Vol 44, p109-115, 1971.

16. Orton, C.G., and Seibert, J.B., Depth dose in skin for obliquely incident cobalt-60 radiation, Br. J. Radiol., Vol 45, p271-275, 1972.

17. Hughes, H.A., Measurements of superficial absorbed dose with 2 MV X-rays used at glancing angles, Br. J. Radiol., Vol 32, p255-258, 1959.

18. Gagnon, W.F., and Peterson, M.D., Comparison of skin doses to large fields using tangential beams from cobalt-60 gamma rays and 4 MV X-rays, Radiology, Vol 127, p785-788, 1978.

19. Klein, E.C., and Purdy, J.A., Entrance and exit dose regions for a Clinac-2100, Int. J. Radiat. Oncol. Biol. Phys., Vol 27, p429-435, 1993.

20. Khan, F.M., Use of electron filter to reduce skin dose in cobalt-60 teletherapy, Am. J. Roentgenol., Vol 111, p180-181, 1971.

21. Saylor, W.L., and Quillin, R.M., Methods for enhancement of skin sparing in cobalt-60 teletherapy, Am. J. Roentgenol., Vol 111, p174-179, 1971.

22. Khan, F.M., Moore, V.C., and Levitt, S.H., Effect of various atomic number absorbers on skin dose for 10 MV X-rays, Radiology, Vol 109, p209-212, 1973.

23. Rao, P.S., Pillai, K., and Gregg, E.C., Effect of shadow trays on surface dose and build-up for megavoltage radiation, Am. J. Roentgenol., Vol 117, p168-174, 1973.

24. Leung, P.M.K., and Johns, H.E., Use of electron filters to improve the build-up characteristics of large fields from cobalt-60, Med. Phys., Vol 4, p441-444, 1977.

25. Gagnon, W.F., and Horton, W.L., Physical factors affecting absorbed dose to the skin from cobalt-60 gamma rays and 25 MV X-rays, Med. Phys., Vol 6, p285-290, 1979.

26. Tranter, F.W., Design of wedge filters for use with 4 MeV linear accelerator, Br. J. Radiol., Vol 30, p329-330, 1957.

27. Cohen, M., Burns, J.E., and Sear, R., Physical aspects of cobalt-60 therapy using wedge filters. I. Physical investigation, Acta Radiol., Vol 53, p401-413, 1960.

28. Cohen, M., Burns, J.E., and Sear, R., Physical aspects of cobalt-60 therapy using wedge filters. II. Dosimetric considerations, Acta Radiol., Vol 53, p486-504, 1960.

29. van de Geijn, J.A., A simple wedge filter technique for cobalt 60 teletherapy, Br. J. Radiol., Vol 35, p710-712, 1962.

30. Aron, B.S., and Scappicchio, M., Design of universal wedge filter system for a cobalt 60 unit, Am. J. Roentgenol., Vol 96, p70-74, 1966.

31. Doppke, K., Novack, D.H., and Wang, C.C., Physical considerations in the treatment of advanced carcinomas of the larynx and pyriform sinuses using 10 MV X-rays, Int. J. Radiat. Oncol. Biol. Phys., Vol 6, p1251-1255, 1980.

32. Binder, W., and Karcher, K.H., "Super-stuff" als Bolus in der Strahlentherapie, Strahlentherapie, Vol 153, p754-757, 1977.

33. Ellis, F., Hall, E.J., and Oliver, R., A compensator for variations in tissue thickness for high energy beam, Br. J. Radiol., Vol 32, p421-422, 1959.

34. Khan, F.M., Moore, V.C., and Burns, D.J., The construction of compensators for cobalt teletherapy, Radiology, Vol 96, pp187-192, 1970.

35. Sewchand, W., Bautro, N., and Scott, R.M., Basic data of tissue equivalent compensators for 4 MV X-rays, Int. J. Radiat. Oncol. Biol. Phys., Vol 6, p327-332, 1980.

36. Khan, F.M., Williamson, J.F., Sewchand, W., and Kim, T.H., Basic data for dosage calculation and compensation, Int. J. Radiat. Oncol. Biol. Phys., Vol 6, p745-751, 1980.

37. Leung, P.M.K., Van Dyk, J., and Robins, J., A method for large irregular field compensation, Br. J. Radiol., Vol 47, p805-810, 1974.

38. Cohen, M., and Martin, S.J., Atlas of Dose Distributions, Vol II, Multiple-Field Isodose Charts, International Atomic Energy Agency, Vienna, Austria, 1966.

39. Tsien, K.C., Cunningham, J.R., Wright, D.J., Jones, D.E.A., and Pfalzner, P.F., Atlas of Dose Distributions, Vol III, Moving-Field Isodose Charts, International Atomic Energy Agency, Vienna, Austria, 1967.

40. Bomford, C.K., Dawes, P.J.D.K., Lillicrap, S.C., and Young, D.J., Treatment Simulators, Brit. J. Radiol. Supplement 23, British Inst. of Radiology, London, 1989.

41. McCullough, E.C., and Earl, J.D., The selection, acceptance testing, and quality control of radiotherapy treatment simulators, Radiology, Vol 131, p221-230, 1979.

42. Karzmark, C.J., and Rust, D.C., Radiotherapy simulators and automation, Radiology, Vol 105, p157-161, 1972.

43. Mayneord, W.V., The measurement of radiation for medical purposes, Nature, Vol 149, p600-601, 1942.

44. Rozenfeld, M., Treatment planning with external beams. Introduction and historical overview, Radiographics, Vol 8, p557-571, 1988.

45. Hendrickson, F.R., Radiation treatment planning. The physician's role, Radiographics, Vol 8, p987-991, 1988.

46. Jayaraman, S., Pathways and pitfalls in treatment planning with external beams: The role of the clinical physicist, Radiographics, Vol 8, p1147-1170, 1988.

47. Hopfan, S., Reid, A., Simpson, L., and Ager, P.J., Clinical complications arising from overlapping of adjacent radiation fields, Int. J. Radiat. Oncol. Biol. Phys., Vol 2, p801-808, 1977.

48. Agarwal, S.K., Marks, R.D., and Constable, W.C., Adjacent field separation for homogeneous dosage at a given depth for the 8 MV (Mevatron 8) linear accelerator, Am. J. Roentgenol., Vol 114, p623-630, 1972.

49. Armstrong, D.J., The matching of adjacent fields in radiotherapy, Radiology, Vol 108, p419-422, 1973.

50. Williamson, T.J., A technique for matching orthogonal megavoltage fields, Int. J. Radiat. Oncol. Biol. Phys., Vol 5, p111-116, 1979.

51. Hale, J., Davis, L.W., and Bloch, P., Portal separation for pairs of parallel opposed portals at 2 MV and 6 MV, Am. J. Roentgenol., Vol 114, p172-175, 1972.

52. Frass, B.A., Tepper, J.E., Glatstein, E. et al., Clinical use of a match line wedge for adjacent megavoltage radiation field matching, Int. J. Radiat. Oncol. Biol. Phys., Vol 9, p209-216, 1983.

53. Svensson, G.K., Bjarngard, B.E., Chen, G.T.Y. et al., Superficial doses in treatment of breast with tangential fields using 4 MV X-rays, Int. J. Radiat. Oncol. Biol. Phys., Vol 2, p705-710, 1977.

54. Burkoritz, A., Deutsch, M., and Slayton, R., Orthogonal fields, Variation in dose vs. gap size for treatment of the central nervous system, Radiology, Vol 126, p795-798, 1978.

55. Gillin, M.T., and Kline, R.W., Field separation between lateral and anterior fields on a 6 MV linear accelerator, Int. J. Radiat. Oncol. Biol. Phys., Vol 6, p233-237, 1980.

56. Dupont, J.C., Rosenwald, J.C., and Beauvais, H., Convolution calculations of dose in the build-up regions of high energy photon beams obliquely incident, Med. Phys., Vol 21, p1391-1400, 1994.

57. Siddon, R.L., Tonnesen, G.L., and Svensson, G.K., Three field techniques for breast treatment using a rotatable half-beam block, Int. J. Radiat. Oncol. Biol. Phys., Vol 7, p1473-1477, 1981.

58. Johnson, P.M., and Kepka, A., A double junction technique for total central nervous system irradiation with a 4 MV accelerator, Radiology, Vol 145, p467-471, 1982.

59. Van Dyk, J., Jenkins, R.D.T., Leung, P.M.K. et al., Medulloblastoma treatment technique and irradiation dosimetry, Int. J. Radiat. Oncol. Biol. Phys., Vol 2, p993-1005, 1977.

Chapter 16

PHYSICAL ASPECTS OF ELECTRON BEAM THERAPY

16.1 ELECTRON TRANSPORT

For the clinical applications of electron beams, the physical behavior of electrons has to be well understood. In this chapter, we discuss the fundamental features of electron transport and the ways in which they influence the dose distribution patterns. Electrons are more complex than photons in their transport behavior. The dose distribution for electron beams can be well documented for standard conditions of a beam incident on a unit-density medium with a flat surface. For nonstandard situations that may be encountered in actual clinical contexts, the interpretation and prediction of electron beam dose distributions pose many challenges.

In Chapter 4, we discussed the collision and radiation energy losses suffered by charged particles. The electrons in a clinical electron beam also undergo such energy losses. Apart from losing their energies, the electrons change their direction of motion in the electric fields of the nucleus and of the atomic orbital electrons in the target material.[1-5] These changes are caused by electron-nuclear scattering and electron-electron scattering. In electron-nuclear scattering with a high-Z nucleus, the large charge of the nucleus deflects the electron trajectory considerably. However, the energy loss suffered is negligible because the mass of the nucleus is much greater than that of the electron. The electron-nuclear scattering probability is proportional to Z^2/E, where E is the electron energy and Z is the nuclear charge.

Electron-electron scattering contributes not only to deflection of the path of the electron, but also to energy loss. The electron-electron scattering probability for any atom is approximately proportional to Z, which equals the number of electrons per atom. In high-Z materials, nuclear scattering predominates over scattering by electrons. The details of the scattering of electrons are explained well only by relativistic wave mechanics. Explanations based on principles of classical mechanics fail in the range of nuclear dimensions, which are of the order of 10^{-13} cm. In electron beam therapy, there are two regions in which an understanding of multiple scattering of electrons is of importance. One of these is the region between the electron source and the surface of the patient's body, and the other is the region within the body.

16.2 ELECTRON BEAM FROM MACHINE TO PATIENT

The energetic electron beam emerging through the vacuum window of an accelerator is a very thin pencil beam and is not suitable for use on a patient. There are two established methods by which the electron fluence of the pencil beam can be spread over a larger area. In one approach (illustrated in Figure 16.1a), an electromagnetic steering device is used which scans the pencil beam over a large area.[6] In the other approach (illustrated in Figure 16.1b), the electrons are spread over a large area by multiple scattering in foils made of a high-Z material that is interposed in the pencil beam.[5,7] The thickness of the foils and the Z of its material together influence the number of multiple scattering events that can occur within it and the extent of spread of the beam. The foil also produces bremsstrahlung and contributes a photon component to the electron beam. The foil can be optimized to produce the desired angular spread with a very low bremsstrahlung component. Most commercially available electron beam machines are designed to give a choice of preselectable electron energies and at least one photon energy. Different scattering foils may be used for different electron energies.

Figure 16.2 illustrates an electron beam delivery system that incorporates two scattering foils: a primary scattering foil that spreads the electron beam and a secondary scattering foil that functions as a beam-flattening filter.[7] The broadened electron beam needs first to pass through the primary

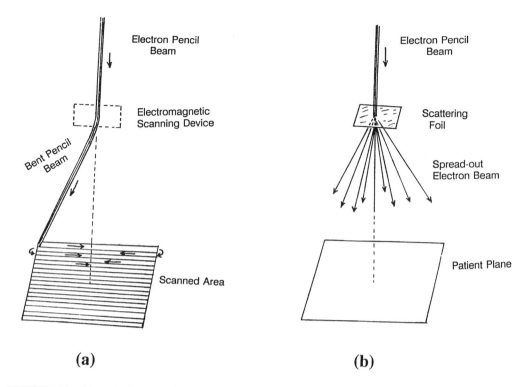

FIGURE 16.1 Schematic diagrams of spreading of an electron pencil beam to cover a clinically useful area. (a) Use of electromagnetically steered scanning. (b) Use of a scattering foil.

collimator, which is used for photons and electrons. The primary collimator is usually placed well above the level of the skin of the patient because it is a part of the treatment head. Because the electrons that strike the primary collimator are scattered further, a rather diffuse beam edge results. The electron beam edges can be sharply defined only if the collimation is extended toward the skin of the patient by attachment of trimmers, as shown in Figure 16.2. Without trimmers, the field projected by the light beam localizer through the primary photon (variable) collimator will give a very misleading impression of the true electron field.[8] Usually, the primary collimating aperture and the trimmers for the electron beams are optimally designed to give an electron beam of uniform fluence, conforming to the light beam indication at the level of the patient's skin. The reflecting mirror shown in Figure 16.2 is retracted away from the beam during patient irradiation.

16.3 ELECTRON BEAM AFTER ENTERING THE PATIENT

Figure 16.3 is a photographic image of an electron beam of 22 MeV energy, alongside a 25-MV X-ray beam, as they enter and penetrate the body. The images were obtained by sandwiching of a film between polystyrene blocks and irradiation of the film. It will be observed that the electron beam penetrates to a finite depth with a clear-cut range. The photon beam, on the other hand, proceeds with no indication of any finite range. The range of penetration of the electron beam is a function of the electron energy. Figure 16.4 shows the film blackening for electron beams of different energies.

The dose distribution in an electron beam is influenced by the following:

(a)   The energy loss interactions suffered by the incident primary electrons
(b)   The extent of production of secondary electrons
(c)   The change in direction and the dispersion of the electrons
(d)   The bremsstrahlung contamination in the beam
(e)   The beam divergence contributing to the inverse-square fall-off of the electron fluence

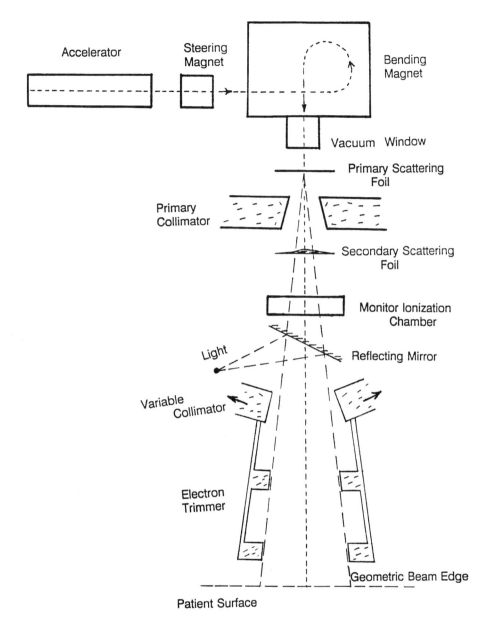

FIGURE 16.2 Components of a typical electron beam delivery port.

The characteristics of the electrons, which undergo changes in their directions of travel and lose energy along their paths by ionization and excitation until all their energies are spent, influence the dose distributions resulting from electron beams.

The central-axis dose profile of a typical electron beam of 21 MeV energy is shown in Figure 16.5. The curve is made up of three segments: an initial increase, a fall-off, and a flat tail. The dose is D_S at the surface and increases to a peak value D_m at the depth d_m. The convention for normalization is to take this peak dose as 100%. Beyond depth d_m, the dose falls off slowly at first, then quite rapidly in a straight line. Extrapolation of the straight-line segment to zero dose defines the maximum electron range R_p. This is referred to as the extrapolated range. The relatively flat tail in the depth-dose curve that is beyond the extrapolated range is attributable to the bremsstrahlung component in the beam.

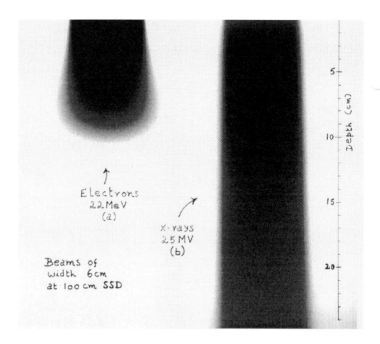

FIGURE 16.3   Photographic images of depth dose for a 22-MeV electron beam (left) and a 25-MV X-ray beam (right). (From Jayaraman, S., Radiographics, 8, 1147–1170, 1988. With permission.)

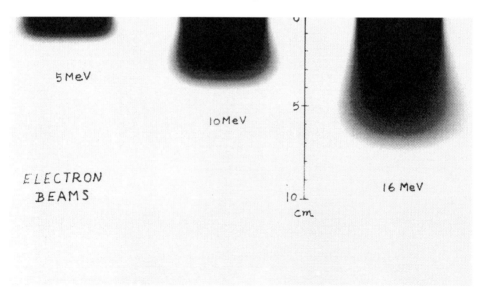

FIGURE 16.4   Photographic images of penetration of electron beams of different energies. (From Jayaraman, S., Radiographics, 8, 1147–1170, 1988. With permission.)

The reason for the surface dose build-up of a photon beam was discussed in Section 11.3. It is caused by the build-up of the secondary-electron fluence. We explained that the dose delivered to a layer is approximately proportional to the number of electrons crossing that layer. In the case of electron beams also, secondary electrons are set in motion by the primary electrons. However, the dose build-up due to the increase in the number of secondary-electron tracks is marginal and is dominant only in the initial shallow depths.

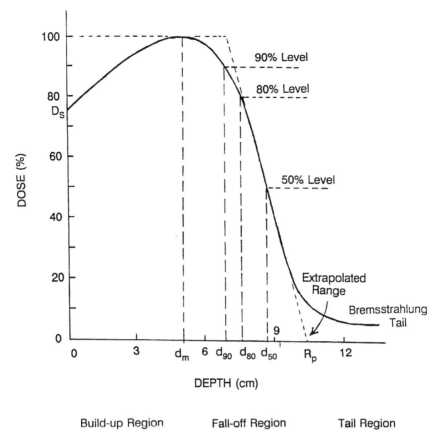

Build-up Region   Fall-off Region   Tail Region

FIGURE 16.5 Shape of the central-axis depth dose curve for an electron beam.

A more significant effect than this is a dose build-up that occurs in electron beams as a direct result of their angular scattering and dispersion. This is illustrated in Figures 16.6a to c. The electrons, as they enter the patient, are essentially parallel and normal to the body surface. Figure 16.6a shows an electron beam incident on an area A, and deflected through an angle θ, which then passes through an area A′. The fact that A′ is smaller than A, but the number of electron tracks has remained the same, means that the fluence and the dose have increased. This same phenomenon is illustrated in a different way in Figure 16.6b, where a series of electron tracks are deflected through an angle θ. Volumes V_1 and V_2 are identical in size. Being crossed by the inclined tracks, V_2 sees more fluence than does V_1, which is in the initial beam. The dose to V_2, thus, will be greater than that to V_1.

In the above discussion, the assumption that all electrons are deflected through the same angle θ with respect to the incident direction and travel parallel to each other does not correspond to reality. We made such a simple assumption merely to explain how angular deflection can contribute to a build-up of fluence and dose. In reality, neither do all electrons undergo the same angle of deflection, nor do they continue to travel parallel to each other.

To add just one further degree of complexity, in Figure 16.6c, we consider two possible directions of deflection for the electrons, to the left as well as to the right, with the same probability. The number of incident electrons has been doubled (compared to that in Figure 16.6b). The fluence in V_2 is greater than that in V_1. A lateral electronic equilibrium is created because, whereas some electrons are deflected away from reaching V_2, some others come into V_2 from the opposite side and compensate for the loss. (Overall, the flux in V_2 in Figure 16.6c is twice that in Figure 16.6b,

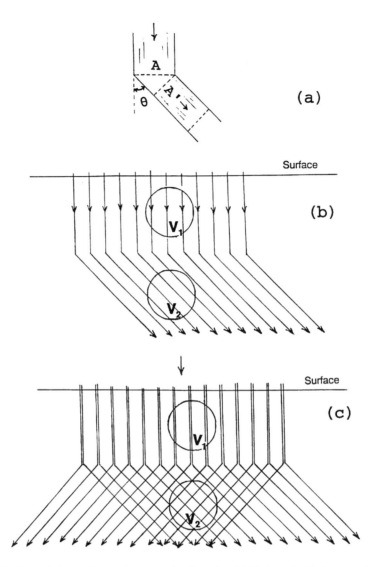

FIGURE 16.6   Build-up of electron fluence due to angular dispersion. (a) Electrons incident on area A are deflected by angle θ to go through area A′ = A cos θ, which is smaller than A. (b) Multiple electron tracks deflected by angle θ pass through volumes V_1 and V_2 of identical dimensions. (c) Electrons are shown deflected to the right and left with equal probability.

because of the twofold increase in the number of incident electrons.) Figure 16.6c also shows how the beam broadens with depth due to angular dispersion.

   With increasing depth, the electron-electron and electron-nuclear scattering cause the moving electrons to have progressively larger angles with the initial beam direction. The extent of the surface dose build-up changes as a function of the electron energy. Low-energy electrons undergo deflections by larger angles, and thus the surface dose build-up is greater at lower than at higher energies. One typical accelerator gave skin doses of 74%, 82%, and 93% of the peak dose for electron beams of 5 MeV, 10 MeV, and 16 MeV with a field of 10 cm × 10 cm cross section.

   The fall-off part of the electron beam depth dose curve is caused by the finite range of travel of the primary electrons. The fall-off is steep, but gradual, indicating that different electrons penetrate to different depths. This is called "range straggling." An electron that suffers minimum angular scattering and travels mostly in a straight line will have the maximum depth of penetration.

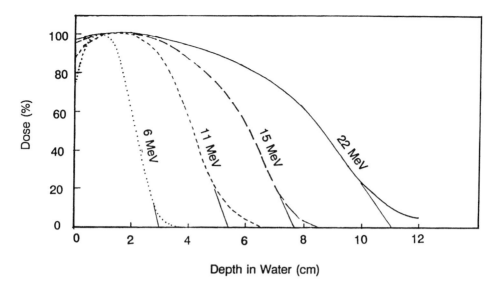

FIGURE 16.7 Central-axis depth dose curves for broad electron beams of different energies.

At any chosen depth, there will be a distribution of electron energies. This is because, even if all of the electrons incident on a material have the same initial energy, their energy losses occur in individual interactions. The statistical variations in the number of these interactions and the energy losses that occur in them cause a spread in electron energies. This is referred to as "energy straggling." The extrapolated range R_p is also called the "practical range" of the electrons (Figure 16.5). The depth d_{50}, where the dose is 50% of the maximum dose, is the "50% range."

We pointed out that the tail part of the depth dose curve is due to the bremsstrahlung component in the beam. The bremsstrahlung yield (see Chapter 4) increases with the energy of the electrons and the Z of the scattering foils. In practical situations, the bremsstrahlung tail may contribute a dose that is 0.5 to 5% of the maximum dose.

Because electrons are indistinguishable from one another, in an electron-electron interaction the electron with the higher energy is considered to be the primary electron and the lower-energy electron is regarded as the secondary electron.

16.4 ELECTRON BEAM DEPTH DOSE DATA

Central-axis depth dose curves for broad (compared to the range of the electrons) electron beams of different energies are shown in Figure 16.7. For routine clinical selection of electron beam energies, it is useful to have the depth dose features presented in the form shown in Table 16.1. "Gradient" refers to the decrease in dose per unit depth. The features listed are strongly machine-dependent because the electron energy spectrum incident on the patient is greatly influenced by the design of the machine. The stated initial energy is a typical value specified by the manufacturer. The values of the characteristics as tabulated converge and become stable for broad beams. However, for narrow beams of dimensions comparable to the electron range, the absence of lateral electronic equilibrium can cause a considerable reduction in the depth dose values (see Sections 16.5 and 16.8). For any given electron beam, the depth dose characteristics tend to stabilize and become unique for large fields. Stated in terms of the extrapolated range R_p, the stability occurs for field diameters of 1.5 R_p at 3.2 MeV, 1.0 R_p at 8 MeV, and 0.6 R_p at 15 MeV and above.[9] For broad beams in water, the following approximations hold, when the electron beam energy E is expressed in MeV:

TABLE 16.1
Typical Electron Beam Data for Broad Beams

Beam Energy (MeV)	Surface Dose (% of Peak Dose)	d_m	d_{90}	d_{80}	d_{50}	d_{10}	Practical Range (cm) R_p
5	74	0.9	1.2	1.4	1.7	2.2	2.3
7	76	1.6	2.0	2.2	2.7	3.3	3.4
10	82	2.4	3.1	3.4	3.9	4.8	4.9
13	88	3.2	4.0	4.3	5.1	6.1	6.4
16	93	3.4	5.1	5.6	6.5	8.0	8.0
19	94	2.6–3.6	5.9	6.7	7.8	9.5	9.5
22	96	2.6–3.6	6.5	7.6	9.3	11.3	11.4
25	96	2.6–3.6	6.5	8.0	10.1	12.4	12.4

The "Depth (cm)" heading spans columns d_m, d_{90}, d_{80}, d_{50}, d_{10}.

$$R_p \approx E/2 \text{ cm}$$

$$d_{80\%} \approx E/3 \text{ cm}$$

These expressions are not exact, but can provide some guidelines for treatment planning.

16.5 PLANNING A SIMPLE ELECTRON BEAM TREATMENT

Electron beam treatments are generally designed for irradiation of the superficial regions of tissue up to a chosen depth. For example, let us say that the superficial lymph nodes in a patient's neck extend to an assessed maximum depth of 3 cm. It is decided to treat them with electrons in such a way that the deepest aspect of the nodes receives at least 90% of the peak dose. From Table 16.1, it can be seen that a 10-MeV electron beam can achieve this objective. The surface dose will be 82% of the peak dose, which helps to assure some degree of skin sparing. The skin sparing can be improved, when needed, by delivery of a part of the dose by a photon beam of 4 MV or from cobalt-60. At lower electron energies, the surface dose falls and a nonuniform dose distribution results from the surface to the depth of the peak dose. For this reason also, a part of the total dose might preferably be delivered by a photon beam. For very high-energy electron beams, the surface dose is nearly the same as the peak dose, and there is practically no advantage of a dose build-up. The difference between the depth of the 80% dose and that of the 10% dose is an indication of the excess tissue irradiated on the exit side of the beam. This difference increases from 1.4 cm at 10 MeV to 4.4 cm at 25 MeV. This, together with the fact that there is very little skin sparing at higher electron energies, makes energies above 16 MeV less useful clinically than lower energies.

16.6 ELECTRON BEAM DEPTH DOSE AND FIELD SIZE

When the field sizes are large compared to the range of the electrons and the distance of their lateral spread, the depth dose characteristics stabilize and become unique for a given energy. The data given in Table 16.1 are limiting values for such large or "infinite" beam sizes. For small field sizes, the depth dose values drop off considerably. Figure 16.8 shows the depth dose for 10-MeV electrons for a small field of 1 cm × 1 cm and for a larger field of 5 cm × 5 cm. The superficial dose build-up is reduced for small fields, because of the lack of lateral scatter. Such a deficiency of laterally scattered electrons occurs at the field edges even for large fields and has to be allowed for in planning of the field dimensions to cover the target volume. To ensure that the deeper aspects of the edges of the target volume are within the 90% isodose curve, the field size at the surface should be more generous than a size that will merely include the target cross section at the surface inside 90%. This is particularly important at high electron energies. Figures 16.9a and b illustrate

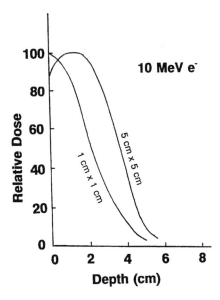

FIGURE 16.8 Dependence of depth dose on field size for two narrow electron beams.

this. Thus, very small electron fields may not be suitable with regard to both depth dose and lateral dose.

16.7 ELECTRON PENCIL BEAM

Figure 16.10 shows the dispersion of electrons in an incident pencil beam. The figure is a cloud chamber image of a finite number of electrons. There are sparse and dense regions, which will become more alike when the number of electrons becomes very large and the pencil beam disperses into a balloon-shaped volume. In general, the behavior of electron beams can be understood if one thinks of the beam as consisting of several narrow pencil beams that are dispersed in the shape of a balloon.

Many successful theoretical calculation models for predicting the dose distribution in electron beams rely on the dispersion and diffusion of thin electron pencil beams by multiple scattering. Many articles have been published on this subject; a few[10-27] are listed at the end of this chapter for interested readers. Some of these models allow for the scattering effect of edges and inhomogeneities. It is advisable to validate the dose distributions predicted by any model for specific experimental situations before it is adopted for clinical decision making.[28] It is not within the scope of this text to cover these theoretical approaches. However, we will use the pencil beam and ballooning phenomenon to discuss the behavior of electron beams in a few special situations.

16.8 OBLIQUE INCIDENCE AND DEPTH DOSE

The central-axis depth dose of an electron beam changes with the obliquity of the incident beam with respect to the surface of incidence.[29,30] The standard isodose patterns measured for normal incidence cannot be used for a beam incident on a curved surface without remeasurement or corrections.[31-33] In Figure 16.11a, three pencil beams are shown incident normally on a surface. The three ballooning beams have not yet augmented each other at the shallow depth of point P_1, but they do overlap at the depth of P_2. This should be compared with the oblique incidence illustrated in Figure 16.11b. Here, the pencil beam on the right strikes the surface at a location closer to the source than do the other pencil beams shown, and the interactions spread the electrons to reach point P_1. However, because of the limited range, the pencil beam on the right does not penetrate

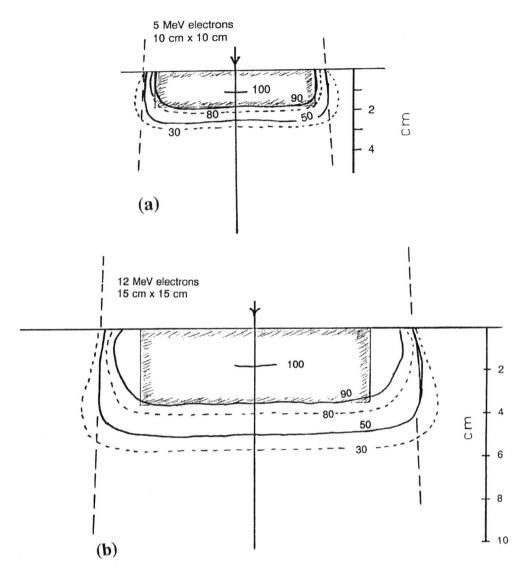

FIGURE 16.9   Narrowing down of the width of the 90% isodose curve with increasing depth for (a) 5-MeV electrons and (b) 12-MeV electrons and two field sizes. The superficial target volumes are shown as shaded rectangles.

to point P_2. Thus, whereas for point P_1 the pencil beam on the right does augment the dose, for point P_2 it does not. In obliquely incident beams, the maximum dose thus moves upward to shallow depths. The depth dose at larger depths becomes less than that for normal incidence. Figure 16.12 compares the central-axis depth dose for an obliquely incident beam with that for a normally incident beam.

The isodose patterns become distorted when the beam is used on a non-flat surface. In Figure 16.13, the surface S is curved. Curve I traces a constant depth from the surface, with the depth chosen to be at 80% depth dose for a normal beam. It will be noticed that the isodose curves have moved closer to the surface where the obliquity is high.

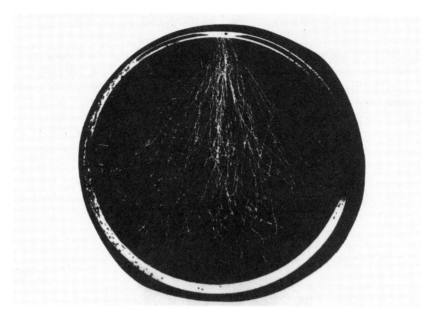

FIGURE 16.10 Cloud chamber image showing the dispersion of an electron pencil beam. (Figure courtesy of Rolf Wideroe.)

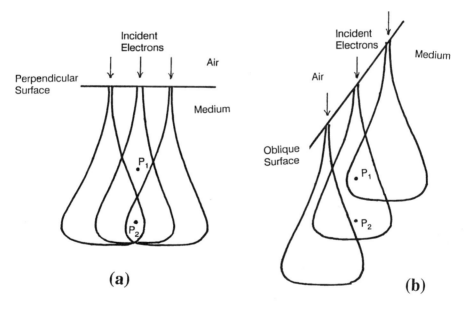

FIGURE 16.11 Superposition of adjacent pencil beams of electrons incident on (a) a perpendicular surface and (b) an oblique surface.

16.9 ELECTRON BEAMS: SOME PRACTICAL CONSIDERATIONS

16.9.1 ELECTRON BEAM OUTPUT FACTORS

The dose output of any electron beam is measured at the depth of the peak dose according to the American Association of Physicists in Medicine (AAPM) Task Group 21 protocol.[34] Because electron beam treatments are usually done with fixed source-to-skin distance (SSD) techniques, the calculation of the monitor units (Mu) can be based on Equation 13.20:

$$\dot{D}_p = CPOR \cdot NPOF\ (A_{dm}) \cdot [PDD(SSD, A_m, d)/100]$$

It is convenient to adjust the sensitivity of the monitoring ionization chamber to obtain a calibrated peak output rate (CPOR) of 1 cGy Mu^{-1} for a chosen standard field size A_{St} (usually 10 cm × 10 cm) and for the standard SSD used. The output factors for any other field size A can be stated as a normalized peak output rate, NPOR(A), as was done for photon beams.

The output factors for electron beams can vary over a wide range as the field changes from a small to a large size. The output of an electron beam can be very sensitive to the position of the photon-collimating diaphragms and the scattered electron fluence from them. We already explained how the field outline at the skin level is defined by the electron penumbra trimmers that extend close to the patient.[35,36] Usually, the geometry of the photon collimator opening and of the electron penumbra trimmers is optimally designed to reduce the variation in the output factors with field size.

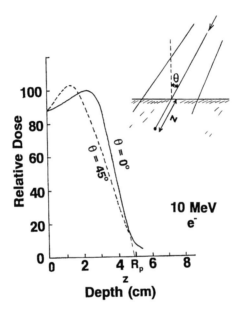

FIGURE 16.12 Comparison of the central-axis depth-dose curves for 10-MeV electrons at normal incidence and incidence at 45° with respect to the entrance surface.

Example 16.1

An electron beam treatment is to be done with 13-MeV electrons, with a field size of 7 cm × 7 cm at SSD = 100 cm. The calibrated peak output rate (CPOR) for a 10 cm × 10 cm field is 1.0 cGy Mu^{-1}, and the normalized peak output factors (NPOF) are as follows:

Field Size (A_0)	NPOF (A_0)
5 cm × 5 cm	0.93
6 cm × 6 cm	0.97
8 cm × 8 cm	0.99
10 cm × 10 cm	1.00
12 cm × 12 cm	1.01
15 cm × 15 cm	1.01

It is desired to deliver a dose of 180 cGy at the level of the 90% depth dose. What should be the Mu and what is the maximum dose per treatment?

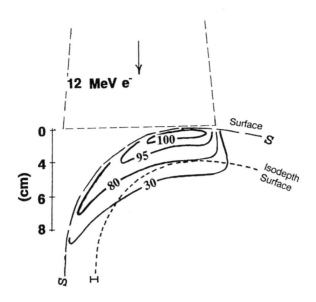

FIGURE 16.13 Isodose distribution for a single electron beam incident on a curved surface.

CPOR $= 1.0$ cGy Mu^{-1}

NPOF for field size 7 cm $\times$ 7 cm $= 0.98$ (from the table above)

PDD $= 90\%$ (as prescribed)

Dose to be delivered $= 180$ cGy

Based on expression (13–20),

Dose rate $=$ CPOR $\times$ NPOF $\times$ PDD/100

$\qquad = 1.0$ cGy Mu$^{-1} \times 0.98 \times (90/100) = 0.882$ cGy Mu^{-1}

Mu to deliver 180 cGy $= 180/0.882 = 204$ Mu

Maximum dose corresponding to PDD $= 100\%$ is 180 cGy $\times (100/90) = 200$ cGy

16.9.2 OUTPUT FACTORS FOR NON-SQUARE FIELDS

For dosimetry of rectangular fields of photon beams, we used the empirical approximation of an equivalent square field. This approach does not work equally well for electron fields. This is because, as we know, the electron beam output is much influenced by the scattered fluence from the beam-defining devices and the air.

It has been determined empirically that the output factor for a rectangular electron field of width W_0 and length L_0 can be derived from the output factors for square fields of sides W_0 and L_0 by the relation[37-39]

$$\text{NPOR}\left(W_0 \times L_0\right) = \left[\text{NPOR}\left(W_0 \times W_0\right) \times \text{NPOR}\left(L_0 \times L_0\right)\right]^{1/2}$$

In irregularly shaped fields produced by placement of shields in the path of the beam, the output rates can be very sensitive to the scattered fluence from the shield itself, depending upon the position of the shield. Any interpretive or approximate method used for deriving the output rate for irregularly shaped fields should be established for routine use only after verification by measurements.[40,41]

16.9.3 FIELD SHAPING AND SELECTIVE SHIELDING

Electron beams are used for treatment of superficial lesions, which the physician can often palpate and outline on the skin. Lead cutouts can be used for shaping of the electron beam portal to the outline drawn. The lead shielding used should be of sufficient thickness to stop the electrons completely.[41-44] A lead shield of inadequate thickness may slow down the energy of the electrons without stopping them. Under such conditions, the scattering events in the high-Z shielding material can actually increase the electron fluence in the region behind the shield and cause up to 30% enhancement of the dose.[43] Figure 16.14a shows an experimental setup that irradiates a photographic film with an electron beam within which different parts have been subjected to different thicknesses of lead shielding. Figure 16.14b shows the image obtained on the film in this setup. It should be noticed that the area under the inadequately thin lead shield on the left part of the image is darker than the unshielded area in the middle of the beam. The area below the thick lead shield on the right side appears light, indicating that it is well shielded. The lead thickness used should be optimal, because over-cautious use of a generous thickness will make the shield unduly heavy and difficult to use.[45]

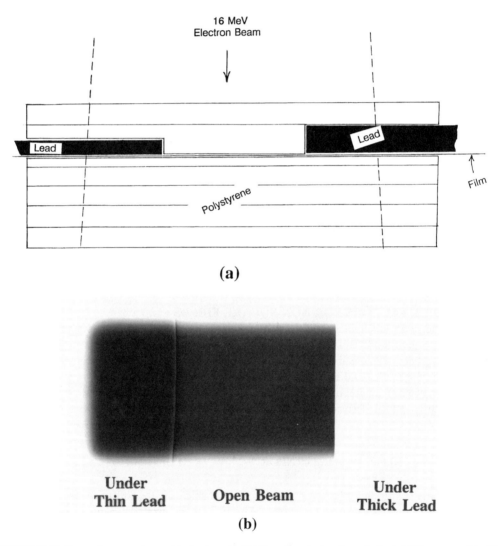

(a)

(b)

Under Thin Lead   **Open Beam**   **Under Thick Lead**

FIGURE 16.14 Dose enhancement caused by inadequate shielding of an electron beam by lead. (a) Placement of the film and the shield in the phantom during irradiation. (b) Film image obtained, showing the variation in the darkening behind inadequate shielding (on the left side), no shielding (in the middle), and adequate shielding (on right side).

There can be an inclination to place a shield behind the target volume in an accessible body cavity, to protect any organ in the exit path of an electron beam. However, this can have an adverse effect of producing dose enhancement in the region above the shield because of the electrons that are back-scattered by the shield.[27,43,46-48] For example, one might want to shield the floor of the mouth while irradiating the tongue by placement of a lead sheet under the tongue. Although the lead layer may be of sufficient thickness to protect the floor of the mouth, the electrons back-scattered from the lead can adversely enhance the dose to the tongue above. Figure 16.15a shows

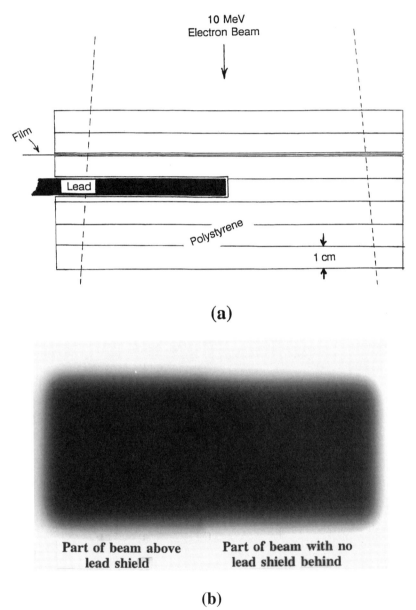

(a)

(b)

FIGURE 16.15 Upstream dose enhancement caused in an electron beam by a high-Z shield placed behind the region treated. (a) Placement of the film and the shield in the phantom during irradiation. (b) Film image obtained, showing the increased darkening on the left side that lay above the shield.

an experimental setup in which a film is irradiated by an electron beam and a part of the beam behind the film is shielded by lead. Figure 16.15b shows the image registered by the film. It could be observed that the area on the left side of the film that lay above the lead shield is darker than the right side. The higher the atomic number Z of the shielding material used, the greater is the back-scattered fluence and the consequent dose enhancement. For 6.4-MeV electrons, it has been reported that lead, copper, and aluminum shields enhanced the dose upstream by about 73%, 33%, and 15%, respectively.[46] Furthermore, the average energy of the back-scattered electrons increases with the atomic number Z of the back-scattering material.[49] For higher values of Z, the dose enhancement becomes observable farther above the shield. Such a dose enhancement by back-scattered electrons from an internal shield is not unique to electron beams. It also applies to shields inserted in beams of kilovoltage X-rays[50] (which may also be used for treatment of superficial lesions [see Section 16.11]) and high-energy photons.[51] One can avoid the undesirable effect of the dose enhancement by covering the internal shield by a layer of a low-Z material of thickness equal to or larger than the range of the back-scattered electrons to absorb them. Without such a preventive measure, the dose enhancement can be significant enough to cause adverse clinical reactions.

16.9.4 EFFECTIVE SSD

At times, it is not possible to set up the patient at the normal SSD, which we will refer to here as SSD_N. This could happen because of interference of a protruding body part (such as the shoulder) with the electron trimmers. An additional air gap g may need to be accepted, giving an extended SSD, SSD_{ext} (= SSD_N + g). The influence of scatter from the collimators and trimmers above the patient in an electron beam makes the focus of electron emission apparently diffuse and uncertain. The output factors measured at the normal SSD cannot be converted to provide the output factors for the SSD_{ext} by a simple inverse-square factor based on distance. However, inverse-square corrections can be applied by determination of an effective SSD, which we will refer to here as SSD_{eff}, because the fall-off of the fluence with distance in an electron beam occurs as if there were an effective point of electron emission.[52,53] If $(OR)_N$ (in cGy Mu^{-1}) is the peak output rate at the depth d_m, with SSD = SSD_N, the peak output rate, $(OR)_{ext}$, at the depth d_m, with SSD = SSD_{ext}, can be derived by a relation of the form

$$(OR)_{ext} = (OR)_N \left[\frac{(SSD_{eff} + d_m)}{(SSD_{eff} + g + d_m)} \right]^2$$

The value of SSD_{eff} should be determined experimentally by actual measurement of the output rates for different values of the gap g. A plot of the square root of the ratio $(OR)_N/(OR)_{ext}$ vs. g has a slope equal to $1/(SSD_{eff} + d_m)$, as shown in Figure 16.16. The method for deriving the output at the extended SSD should be used with caution and should be limited to small values of g, up to about 10 cm. The SSD_{eff} is a function of electron energy, field size, and the actual scatter geometry, which can vary from machine to machine. For small field sizes, the SSD_{eff} is much shorter than the SSD indicated during setup. In one case, as the field size changed from 6 cm × 6 cm to 25 cm × 25 cm, the SSD_{eff} changed from 70 cm to 95 cm, whereas the actual setup indicated an SSD of 100 cm.

Example 16.2

A 10-MeV electron beam has an output rate of 0.98 cGy Mu^{-1} at the depth of the peak dose when used at the normal setup with SSD_N = 100 cm. For one patient, it becomes necessary to use an extended SSD_{ext} of 105 cm. The beam is known to have an SSD_{eff} of 80 cm. Compare the two output rates obtained by use of SSD_{eff} and SSD_N for estimating the inverse-square divergence. Use d_m = 2.5 cm.

In this case, g = 5 cm; d_m = 2.5 cm; SSD_{eff} = 80 cm; and output at SSD_N = 0.98 cGy Mu^{-1}.

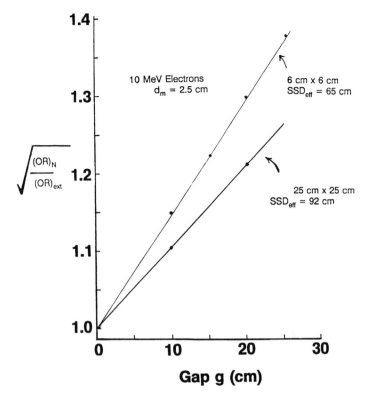

FIGURE 16.16 Plot of the square root of the ratio of electron beam output rates with distance **g** for derivation of SSD_{eff}. The gap g is the distance between the SSD used for the measurements and SSD_N.

(i)   Inverse-square correction for $SSD_{eff} = 80$ cm:

$$\left[\frac{\left(SSD_{eff} + d_m\right)}{\left(SSD_{eff} + g + d_m\right)}\right]^2 = \left[\frac{80 + 2.5}{80 + 5 + 2.5}\right]^2 = 0.889$$

Estimated output rate for SSD of 105 cm = 0.98 cGy Mu^{-1} × 0.889 = 0.871 cGy Mu^{-1}.

(ii)   Inverse-square correction for the normal $SSD_N = 100$ cm:

$$\left[\frac{\left(SSD_N + d_m\right)}{\left(SSD_N + g + d_m\right)}\right]^2 = \left[\frac{100 + 2.5}{100 + 5 + 2.5}\right]^2 = 0.909$$

Estimated output rate for SSD of 105 cm = 0.98 cGy Mu^{-1} × 0.909 = 0.891 cGy Mu^{-1}.

Note that, even for a small value of **g** of 5 cm, the two calculated outputs differ by about 2% in the above example.

16.9.5 AGREEMENT OF LIGHT FIELD AND RADIATION FIELD

The projection of the collimating aperture by the localization light beam generally indicates a beam cross section that appears as if the beam emerged from a point. However, we just discussed that the electron fluence falls off with distance as if the source were at an effective SSD. These two facts together mean that the assumption that the light beam outline can represent the radiation beam outline cannot be taken for granted as readily for electrons as for photons. Figures 16.17a, b, and c show the photographic images of the cross section of an electron beam at the standard

SSD used and at two other distances applicable for two values of the air gap g. The extension of the light field edges is indicated by straight lines (marked X and Y) outside the beam. It can be seen that the beam edges become diffuse with increasing g. On the other hand, the edges for photon beams, as illustrated in Figure 16.17d, e, and f, follow the light beam indication closely. For electron beams, if the patient is set up at an extended distance, the light beam outline seen on the patient's surface cannot be taken to represent the outline of the beam. Furthermore, if any lead shield or block is placed far above the patient, the shadow of the light field cannot truly indicate a shielded region. The blocking or field shaping should be done close to the patient's body surface to be effective.

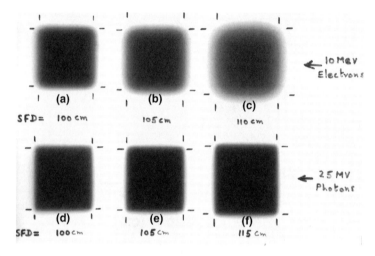

FIGURE 16.17 Agreement of light field and radiation field, as obtained on a photographic film at the normal treatment distance, and with the distance 5 cm and 10 cm larger than normal. (a), (b), and (c) are for a 10-MeV electron beam; (d), (e), and (f) are for a 25-MV photon beam. The corners of the light field are indicated by the lines made with a ballpoint pen on the emulsion.

16.10 INFLUENCE OF INHOMOGENEITIES

The dose at any point in an electron beam is not only dependent upon the path traversed by the ray connecting that point to an apparent or virtual source position. Structures (or inhomogeneities) in the regions lateral to the ray and above the point of dose calculation can also affect the fluence reaching the point. The influence of any structure can depend in a complicated way on its shape and size, the electron density, and the scattering power as governed by the atomic number. This phenomenon was known and studied already during the early years of the practice of electron therapy.[54-58] More recently, this subject has been addressed with several theoretical models.[15,19,21,24,59,60]

Here, we endeavor to explain the phenomenon brought about by the inhomogeneities by using the conditions shown in Figure 16.18. Figure 16.18a shows a uniform water-equivalent medium within which a volume is replaced by air in Figure 16.18b and by bone in Figure 16.18c. Four points, P_1, P_2, P_3, and P_4, have been chosen at the same depth, d, from the surface. Figure 16.18a shows how the medium overlying P_2 scatters electrons onto P_3 and vice versa. The scattered amount from above P_2 to P_3 and vice versa is the same, because the media above P_2 and P_3 are identical. The fluence (and hence the dose) at P_2 and P_3 is the same also.

In Figure 16.18b, the amount of scatter in the medium above P_2 is the same as before, but the air above P_3 does not deflect as many electrons that reach P_2. The reduced number of interactions in air also lets more electrons reach P_3. As a consequence, the dose at P_3 will be increased at the expense of the dose at P_2. The change in the scattering behavior with the change in medium does not influence the dose at P_1, because it is located too far laterally from the edge of the inhomogeneity. The dose at P_1 will thus be the same as that in Figure 16.18a. Point P_4 is likewise located too far

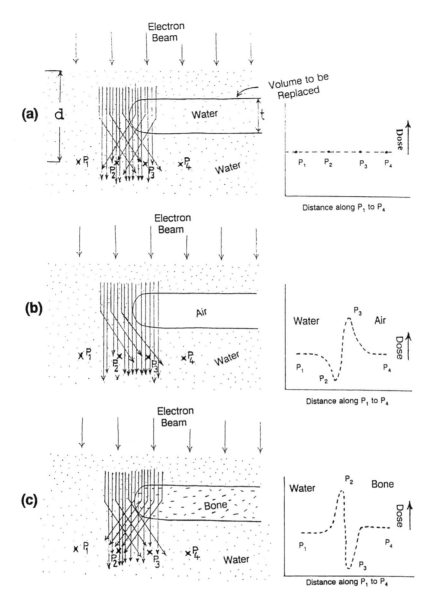

FIGURE 16.18 Dispersion of electrons by the edge of an inhomogeneity. (a) A uniform water-equivalent medium with a volume as marked. This volume is replaced by air in (b) and by bone in (c). The expected dose profiles through points P_1, P_2, P_3, and P_4 are shown on the right.

laterally from the edge of the inhomogeneity to be influenced by the edge scatter. However (assuming that the density of air is almost zero), the dose at P_4, which is located directly underneath the air cavity, will correspond to an effective depth of $(d - t)$. The dose at P_3 is higher than that at P_4 because P_3 receives more scatter from the high-density medium above P_2. The cross-beam dose profile expected to be obtained below the transition interface is shown on the right side of Figure 16.18b.

In Figure 16.18c, the air is replaced by bone. In bone, due to its high density, the scattering events are more numerous than those in water. The dose at P_2 increases because of the increased amount of scatter from bone, and the dose at P_3 consequently is reduced. The dose profile expected to be obtained below the transition interface is shown on the right side of Figure 16.18c. Thus, the inhomogeneities in electron beams can cause hot spots and cold spots downstream from any transition edge. The dose pattern is difficult to predict and quantify (although this is possible theoretically).[19] An example of the effect of a high-density (lead) inhomogeneity is shown in Figure 16.14. The dense and light regions below the edge of the lead in the film are attributable to the phenomenon described above.

If the point of calculation is considerably displaced laterally (i.e., at least by an electron range) from any transition edge, one can evaluate the dose by estimating a coefficient of equivalent thickness (CET). This is referred to as the "infinite-limit" approximation and can be applied to point P_4 in our example. The CET is defined as the ratio of the linear thickness of water to the linear thickness of an inhomogeneity, with the two thicknesses chosen to produce the same degrees of electron transmission and absorption. This means that the CET for any material is given approximately by the ratio of the linear stopping power of the material to that of water. In Figure 16.18c, P_4 is at an effective water-equivalent depth, d_{eff}, given by

$$d_{eff} = \left[d + t \left(CET_{bone} - 1 \right) \right]$$

where CET_{bone} is the CET for bone. The percent depth dose (PDD) read for the depth d_{eff} from the standard depth dose tables cannot be used as such for point P_4 without an additional inverse-square distance correction. This is because the standard PDD value applies to a point at a distance ($SSD_N + d_{eff}$) from the source, but the actual distance of point P_4 is ($SSD_N + d$). Thus,

$$PDD \text{ at } P_4 = \left(PDD \text{ read for } d_{eff} \right) \times \left[\frac{SSD_N + d_{eff}}{SSD_N + d} \right]^2$$

In general, the value of the CET can vary with depth and beam energy. The above expression does not address the details of the perturbations caused by the presence of an inhomogeneity. Calculation models based on pencil beam dispersion by multiple coulomb scattering are better suited to solution of the problem.[15,19,21,24,26,59,60] By modern computed tomography (CT), the theoretical models can directly utilize the detailed patient anatomy provided by the pixel-to-pixel variation of the CT numbers.[15,26]

16.11 COMPARISON OF KILOVOLTAGE X-RAY AND ELECTRON BEAMS

It is interesting to compare the relative merits of electron beams and kilovoltage X-ray beams for treatment of superficial lesions. Figure 16.19 compares the doses delivered by electron beams of three different energies with that for a 250-kV X-ray beam (2.5 mm Cu HVT). For a selected maximum target depth of 3 cm, it is seen that the 10-MeV electron beam and the X-ray beam provide dose distributions that are nonuniform to the same degree within the target volume. However, the X-ray beam delivers a much higher exit dose beyond the target depth. In addition, we recall (from our discussions in Chapters 11 and 14), that a 1.5 to 4 times higher dose can result in bone compared to soft tissue with low-energy X-rays. The mass stopping power (and hence the energy absorbed per unit mass) is not too different between bone and soft tissue for electrons. For 10-MeV electrons, the mass stopping power of soft tissue and bone is 1.974 and 1.835 MeV cm^2 g^{-1}, respectively. This implies that an 8% higher dose will be delivered to soft tissue than to bone if both are irradiated with the same electron fluence.

Some advantages of X-ray beams over electron beams in certain situations have also been noted.[61,62] These advantages include a higher skin dose, gradual fall-off of the dose on the exit side to cover uncertain tumor extensions, the possibility of using very small field sizes without compromising the coverage, the adequacy of thinner lead cutouts (of only a few millimeters) for field shaping, thinner inserted lead shields for protection of tissues on the exit side of the beam, a smaller thickness (only a few millimeters) of plastic needed on any inserted lead shielding to absorb the

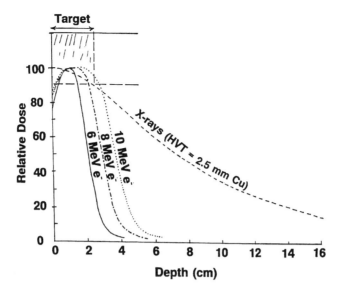

FIGURE 16.19 Depth dose curves for electron beams of 6, 8, and 10 MeV energies and a 2.5-mm HVT kilovoltage X-ray beam for treatment of a 3-cm thick superficial target volume.

back-scattered electrons for prevention of dose enhancement to tissues overlying the shield, and a lower overall cost of the radiation generator.

16.12 TOTAL-SKIN ELECTRON TREATMENT

In certain clinical situations, a radiation dose may need to be delivered to the superficial cutaneous tissues of the entire body. The need to cover the entire body will require a very large beam cross section, with good uniformity of electron energy and fluence within it. Such large field sizes are possible only at very large treatment distances, making use of the entire treatment room.

In a different approach, a beam collimated to produce a narrow strip of radiation beam has been used for scanning across the patient.[63] The techniques and dosimetry of carrying out total-skin electron irradiation can be very involved. The reader should study the comprehensive reviews listed in References 64 and 65.

Figure 16.20a shows a geometry in which oblique beam orientations are employed to provide large coverage. Two different oblique orientations are shown, and these can be used alternately, making the total fluence uniform. The uniformity of electron fluence within the field is improved further by placement of a plastic sheet, which acts as a scatterer of electrons between the source and the patient, so as to diffuse the beam and improve the uniformity. However, it also degrades the beam energy.

The depth dose characteristics of the electron beam as documented for the usual treatment distance cannot be applied to the total-skin irradiation setup. The presence of the lucite scatterer, together with the beam obliquity with respect to the patient's surface, can annul the dose build-up at the skin. In fact, the selection of the beam energy, and of the thickness and position of the scatterer, should be done with the objective of producing acceptable dose uniformity and depth dose. It is necessary to diffuse the self-shielding and shadowing effects of one part of the body on another to avoid cold spots. Some have used a pedestal and rotation of the patient during the treatment. One technique,[66] developed at Stanford, uses six different orientations of the patient, as illustrated in Figure 16.20b, with three beams used each day. The patient's extremities should be extended and exposed at different orientations as well. It might be necessary to boost the dose to selected body parts, such as the armpits and feet, in a follow-up treatment. Selective shielding of the eyes or other sensitive areas can be employed.

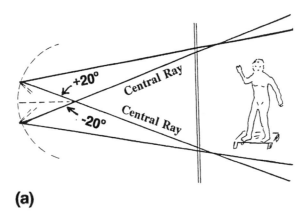

(a)

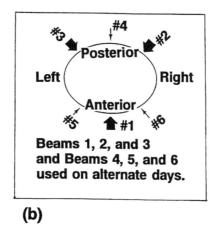

(b)

FIGURE 16.20 Total-skin electron beam irradiation. (a) Beams at ±20° inclinations with the patient at a very large distance and an acrylic scatterer in the beam. (b) Six different patient orientations are used for diffusion of nonuniformity.

16.13 INTRAOPERATIVE ELECTRON THERAPY

In intraoperative radiotherapy (IORT), the radiation beam is directed through a surgical opening for treatment of an internal target site.[67-73] The normally overlying body tissues are thus spared from exposure to radiation. A large single dose of radiation is usually delivered by an electron beam. Here we attempt to give only a very brief overview.

IORT requires a special collimating system (Figure 16.21), which usually consists of (i) a large cylindrical collimator made of stainless steel that is attached to the front face of the machine, and (ii) interchangeable applicators or "cones" of cylindrical or elliptical cross section, made of metal or transparent plastic. (Some IORT systems do not use rigid fastening to the machine.) The cylindrical steel collimator shown in Figure 16.21 can incorporate a viewing mechanism with a mirror for obervation of the tumor site during setup. The applicators have a wall thickness of 3 to 5 mm and are 20 to 40 cm long. Because most of the electrons travel in straight lines, the leakage through the walls is negligible. The diameters of the applicators range from 3.0 cm to 12 cm. On the beam exit end, the applicator can have either a flat or a beveled end. The output rate and the depth dose distributions of all IORT applicators should be measured individually and should be available prior to their use.

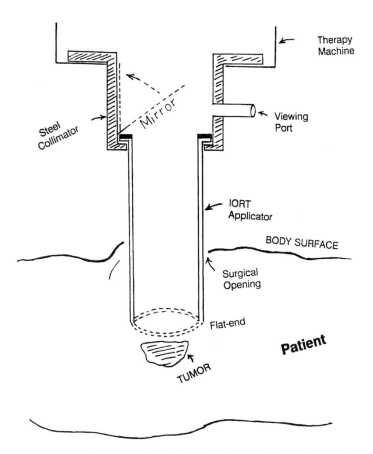

FIGURE 16.21 Schematic diagram of an electron beam irradiating a deep-seated tumor intraoperatively. An applicator is inserted through a surgical incision.

16.14 ELECTRON ARC THERAPY

Electron arc therapy can be used for treatment of a large superficial layer of a target volume on a curved body surface. However, the planning for arc treatment with electrons is more complex than that with photons.[74-81] We will discuss it only briefly, mainly to indicate its complexity. Users wishing to practice arc therapy should do a more detailed study based on the references cited.

Patients are not perfect cylinders. The output rate of an arc changes with the radius of curvature of the surface irradiated. If the surface curvature changes gradually along the longitudinal axis of the patient, there will be a corresponding change in the dose delivered by the arc. By use of custom-designed secondary collimators that produce a field of trapezoidal shape, the uniformity of the dose can be improved.

Figure 16.22a shows two transverse sections, TS_1 and TS_2, which may be located in two different planes of a patient's body. The target volumes in these two sections with different radii are identified as T_1 and T_2. The points I_1 and I_2 in the two sections are such that circles drawn with these points as the origins nearly match the body outlines at the two levels. The radii of curvature are R_1 and R_2 for the two sections. The beam can rotate around only one axis. This requires manipulation of the patient support system (i.e., couch rotation and a patient tilt) to bring points I_1 and I_2 into line and in alignment with the isocentric axis of rotation I of the treatment apparatus. The expected result is shown in Figure 16.22b, where the two sections have been overlaid so that I_1 coincides with I_2 at I. The arc of the beam should span a larger area than needed to cover the target surface. The edges of the arc can be custom-trimmed by placement of lead shields on the skin. The field width chosen should be sufficiently small to have minimum obliquity and surface curvature within itself in all directions, but large enough to give a good output rate. A field width of about 5 cm may achieve this in many actual situations. The peak output rate for the arc is sensitive to the field width. For a chosen field width, with an increase in the angle of arc, an equilibrium output rate is reached in the central region covered by the arc. The output rate for the arc is determined by placement of the single-electron-beam isodose curve along several adjacent radii and integrating of the doses. This can be done manually or by computer. Uniformity of dose delivery is achieved by designing the shape of the trapezoidal secondary collimator to suit the body shape, as explained next.

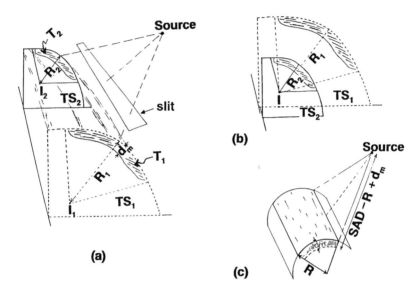

FIGURE 16.22 Planning of electron arc therapy. (a) Illustration of changing body size along the length of the patient. Points I_1 and I_2 have been identified as centers of circles of radii R_1 and R_2 that nearly approximate the surfaces in body sections TS_1 and TS_2. The field is shaped by a slit. (b) The body is aligned by couch rotation and patient tilt so that centers I_1 and I_2 coincide with the axis of rotation of the beam, I. (c) A cylindrical surface treated with an arc.

The electron fluence is spread out in two directions: in the plane of rotation and perpendicular to it (Figure 16.22a and b). Hence, the dose delivered by the arc is influenced by the radius of curvature R of the treated body section in two ways. First, in the plane of rotation, because the arc length is proportional to R, the fluence dilution is greater for a larger radius. The peak dose is therefore proportional to $1/(R - d_m)$. Thus, a large R means a low dose rate. Next, when we look at a cylindrical surface in the direction perpendicular to the plane of rotation, a large radius presents the surface closer to the electron source than does a small radius (Figure 16.22c). In this perpendicular direction, the spread of the beam is proportional to the distance (SAD − R + d_m), and the fluence is inversely proportional to that distance. Combining both, we obtain

$$\text{Dose} \propto \frac{1.0}{\left(R - d_m\right) \times \left(\text{SAD} - R + d_m\right)}$$

If the peak doses are D_1 and D_2 in sections TS_1 and TS_2, from the above reasoning, we obtain the ratio

$$\frac{D_1}{D_2} = \frac{\left(R_2 - d_m\right) \times \left(\text{SAD} - R_2 + d_m\right)}{\left(R_1 - d_m\right) \times \left(\text{SAD} - R_1 + d_m\right)}$$

Because the output increases with the field width, the difference between D_1 and D_2 can be improved if one uses different field widths for the two sections. In fact, a slit that produces a field of trapezoidal cross section, as shown in Figure 16.22a, can be designed to narrow the field width progressively from large to small body sections.

The depth dose characteristics of an arc are different from those of a fixed beam of the same electron energy. The cross-firing in the arcs reduces the skin dose and increases the depth of the peak dose.

In an alternate approach to arc therapy, the arc is replaced by several adjacent stationary beams.[82-85] This is also referred to as "pseudo-arc technique." In the implementation of this technique, care should be exercised to avoid cold or hot spots at the junction between adjacent beams.

16.15 ADJACENT ELECTRON FIELDS

It is desirable to keep in mind the behavior of the isodose curves along the edges of electron beams when several such beams are juxtaposed. In electron beams, the isodose curves of high denominations (above 70%) curve from the beam edge inward to become narrower with increasing depth. However, the lower-denomination isodose curves (below 30%) expand in width and balloon outward with increasing depth. The fact that electron beam isodose curves do not follow the geometric edge of the beam causes special problems when adjacent electron fields are to be matched with skin gaps or appropriate relative beam orientations.[86-88] Generally, it is desirable to encompass the entire surface region to be treated by a single electron beam of large cross section. However, situations can occur where it may be advantageous to split the target volume and treat it with two different beams.

Figure 16.23a illustrates two adjacent sites treated with 7-MeV and 16-MeV electron beams. Here, the split is used to tailor the energy of the two beams to suit the difference in depth of the target volume. The beams are shown positioned with the light fields of the two beams (which, by definition, are also the 50% dose with respect to the central-axis dose) abutting on the body surface. The combined isodose distribution for this situation is one of "no skin gap," as shown in Figure 16.23b. Figures 16.23c and d give the dose distributions when 0.5-cm and 1.0-cm skin gaps are used.

A similar problem of beam placement can occur whenever an electron beam is juxtaposed to a site treated by photon beams. Because photon beams are often used as parallel opposed beams, there can be an exiting and an entering photon beam at the surface of match. Situations such as these may call for a careful trade-off between hot and cold spots. Some investigators have reported the use of "penumbra producers" to perturb the penumbra and improve the match.[89-92]

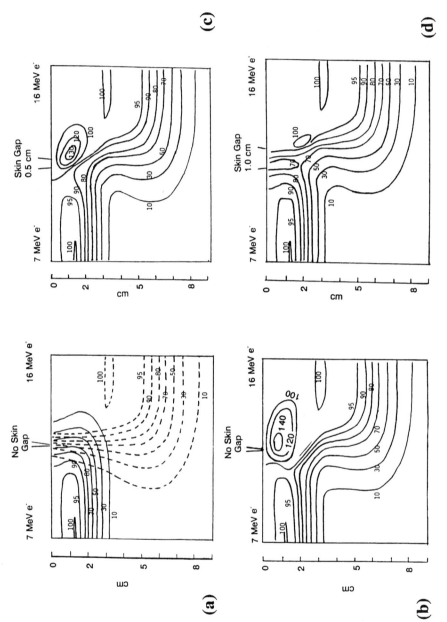

FIGURE 16.23 Illustration of treatment of adjacent sites with electron fields of different energies. (a) Isodose curves of individual beams shown juxtaposed, with no skin gap between the geometric edges. (b), (c), and (d) show combined isodose curves for no skin gap, 5-mm skin gap, and 1.0-cm skin gap, respectively.

REFERENCES

1. Moliere, G., Theorie der Streuung schneller geladener Teilchen II, Mehrfach- und Vielfachstreuung, Z. Naturforsch., Vol 3a, p78-97, 1948.
2. Bethe, H.A., Rose, M.E., and Smith, L.P., The multiple scattering of electrons, Proc. Am. Philos. Soc., Vol 78, p573-585, 1938.
3. Heitler, W., The Quantum Theory of Radiation, Third Edition, p414, Oxford University Press, London, 1954.
4. Scott, W.T., The theory of small-angle multiple scattering of fast charged particles, Rev. Mod. Phys., Vol 35, p2-313, 1963.
5. Lanzl, L.H., Fundamental interactions of electrons with water, p21-24, in Proceedings of the Symposium on Electron Dosimetry and Arc Therapy, Paliwal, B. (Ed.), American Institute of Physics, New York, 1982.
6. Lanzl, L.H., Electron pencil beam scanning and its application in radiation therapy, p55-66, in Frontiers of Radiation Therapy, Oncology, Vol 2, Karger, Basel, 1968.
7. Mandour, M.A., and Harder, D., Systematic optimization of the double scatterer system for electron beam field flattening, Strahlentherapie, Vol 154, p328-322, 1978.
8. Lax, I., and Brahme, A., On the collimation of high energy electron beams, Acta Radiol. Oncol., Vol 19, p199-207, 1980.
9. Markus, B., Energie-Bestimmung schneller Elektronen auf Tiefendosiskurven, Strahlentherapie, Vol 116, p280-286, 1961.
10. Perry, D.J., and Holt, J.G., A model for calculating the effects of small inhomogeneities on electron beam dose distributions, Med. Phys., Vol 7, p207-215, 1980.
11. Hogstrom, K.R., and Mills, M.D., Electron beam dose calculations, Phys. Med. Biol., Vol 26, p445-459, 1981.
12. Werner, B.L., Khan, F.M., and Diebel, F.C., Model for calculating electron beam scattering in treatment planning, Med. Phys., Vol 9, p180-187, 1982.
13. Jette, D., Pagnamenta, A., Lanzl, L.H., and Rozenfeld, M., The application of multiple scattering theory to therapeutic electron dosimetry, Med. Phys., Vol 10, p141-146, 1983.
14. Storchi, P.R.M., and Huizenga, H., On a numerical approach of the pencil beam model, Phys. Med. Biol., Vol 30, p467-473, 1985.
15. Kirsner, S.M., Hogstrom, K.R., Kurup, R.G., and Moyers, M.F., Dosimetric evaluation in heterogeneous tissue of anterior electron beam irradiation for treatment of retinoblastoma, Med. Phys., Vol 14, p772-779, 1987.
16. Lax, I., Brahme, A., and Andreo, P., Electron beam dose planning using Gaussian beams, Acta Radiol. Suppl., 364, Vol 36, p49-59, 1983.
17. McParland, B.J., Cunningham, J.R., and Woo, M.K., The optimization of pencil beam widths for use in an electron pencil beam algorithm, Med. Phys., Vol 14, p489-497, 1988.
18. Jette, D., Electron dose calculation using multiple-scattering theory. A Gaussian multiple-scattering theory, Med. Phys., Vol 15, p123-137, 1988.
19. Jette, D., Lanzl, L.H., Pagnamenta, A., Rozenfeld, M., Bernard, D., Kao, M., and Sabbas, A.M., Electron dose calculation using multiple scattering theory: Thin planar inhomogeneities, Med. Phys., Vol 16, p712-725, 1989.
20. Huizenga, H., and Storchi, P.R.M., Numerical calculations of energy deposition of broad high energy electron beams, Phys. Med. Biol., Vol 34, p1371-1396, 1989; Corrigendum, Phys. Med. Biol., Vol 35, 1445, 1990.
21. Jette, D., Electron dose calculation using multiple-scattering theory: Localized inhomogeneities — a new theory, Med. Phys., Vol 18, p123-132, 1991.
22. McLellan, J., Sandison, G.A., Papiez, L., and Huda, W., A restricted angular scattering model for electron penetration in dense media, Med. Phys., Vol 18, p1-6, 1991.
23. Shiu, A.S., and Hogstrom, K.R., Pencil beam redefinition algorithm for electron dose distributions, Med. Phys., Vol 18, p7-18, 1991.
24. Jette, D., and Walker, S., Electron beam dose calculation using multiple scattering theory: Evaluation of a new model for inhomogeneities, Med. Phys., Vol 19, p1241-1254, 1992.
25. Petti, P.L., Differential pencil beam dose calculation for charged particles, Med. Phys., Vol 19, p137-149, 1992.
26. Al-Beteri, A.A., and Raeside, D.E., Optimal electron beam treatment planning for retinoblastoma using a new three-dimensional Monte Carlo based treatment planning system, Med. Phys., Vol 19, p125-135, 1992.
27. Morawska-Kaczynska, M., and Huizenga, H., Numerical calculations of energy deposition by broad high-energy electron beams, Phys. Med. Biol., Vol 37, p2103-2106, 1992.
28. Shiu, A.S. et al., Verification data for electron beam dose algorithms, Med. Phys., Vol 19, p623-636, 1992.
29. McKenzie, A.L., Air-gap correction in electron treatment planning, Phys. Med. Biol., Vol 24, p628-635, 1979.
30. Ekstrand, K.E., and Dixon, R.L., Obliquely incident electron beams, Med. Phys., Vol 9, p276-278, 1982.
31. Biggs, P.J., The effect of beam angulation on central axis depth dose for 4–29 MeV electrons, Phys. Med. Biol., Vol 29, p1089-1096, 1984.
32. Khan, F.M., Deibel, F.C., and Soleimani-Meigooni, A., Obliquity correction for electron beams, Med. Phys., Vol 12, p749-753, 1985.
33. Ulin, K., and Sternick, E.S., An isodose shift technique for obliquely incident electron beams, Med. Phys., Vol. 16, p905-910, 1989.

34. Task Group 21, Radiation Therapy Committee, American Association of Physicists in Medicine, A protocol for the determination of absorbed dose from high-energy photon and electron beams, Med. Phys., Vol 10, p741-771, 1983.

35. Biggs, P.J., Boyer, A.L., and Doppke, K.P., Electron dosimetry of irregular fields on the Clinac-18, Int. J. Radiat. Oncol. Biol. Phys., Vol 5, p433-440, 1979.

36. Purdy, J.M., Choi, M.C., and Feldman, A., Lipowitz metal shielding thickness for dose reduction of 6–20 MeV electrons, Med. Phys., Vol 7, p251-253, 1980.

37. Mills, M.D., Hogstrom, K.R., and Almond, P.R., Prediction of electron beam output factors, Med. Phys., Vol 9, p60-68, 1982.

38. McParland, B.J., A parametrization of the electron beam output factors for a 25 MeV linear accelerator, Med. Phys., Vol 14, p666-669, 1987.

39. McParland, B.J., A method of calculating output factors for arbitrarily shaped electron fields, Med. Phys., Vol 16, p88-93, 1989.

40. McParland, B.J., An analysis of equivalent fields for electron beam central axis dose calculation, Med. Phys., Vol 19, p901-906, 1992.

41. Choi, M.C., Purdy, J.A., Gerbi, B.J., Abrath, F.G., and Glasgow, G.P., Variation in output factors caused by secondary blocking for 7–16 MeV electron beams, Med. Phys., Vol 6, p137-139, 1979.

42. Giarattano, J.C., Duerkes, R.J., and Almond, P.R., Lead shielding thickness for dose reduction of 7-20 MeV electrons, Med. Phys., Vol 2, p336-337, 1975.

43. Khan, F.M., Moore, V.C., and Levitt, S.H., Field shaping in electron therapy, Br. J. Radiol., Vol 49, p883-886, 1976.

44. Khan, F.M., Werner, B.L., and Deibel, F.C., Lead shielding for electrons, Med. Phys., Vol 8, p712-713, 1981.

45. Asbell, S.O., Sill, J., Lightfoot, D.A., and Brady, N.L., Individualized eye shield for use in electron beam therapy as well as low energy photon irradiation, Int. J. Radiat. Oncol. Biol. Phys., Vol 6, p519-521, 1980.

46. Saunders, J.E., and Peters, V.G., Backscattering from metals in superficial therapy with high energy electrons, Br. J. Radiol., Vol 47, p467-470, 1974.

47. Gagnon, W.F., and Cundiff, J.H., Dose enhancement from back-scattered radiation at tissue metal interfaces irradiated with high energy electrons, Br. J. Radiol., Vol 53, p466-470, 1980.

48. Klavenhagen, S.C., Lambert, G.D., and Arbari, A., Backscattering in electron therapy for energies between 3 and 35 MeV, Phys. Med. Biol., Vol 27, p363-373, 1982.

49. Frank, H., Zur Vielfachstreuung und Rückdiffusion schneller Elektronen nach Durchgang durch dicke Schichten, Z. Naturforsch., Vol 14a, p247-261, 1959.

50. Bjarngard, B.E., McCall, R.C., and Berstein, I.A., Lithium fluoride teflon thermoluminescent dosimeters, p308-316, in Proceedings of First International Conference on Luminescence Dosimetry, Stanford, Attix, F.H. (Ed.), Conference no. 650637, U.S. Atomic Energy Commission, Washington, D.C., 1967.

51. Dutreix, J., and Bernard, M., Dosimetry at interface for high-energy x and γ rays, Br. J. Radiol., Vol 39, p205-210, 1966.

52. Khan, F.M., Sewchand, W., and Levitt, S.H., Effect of air space on depth dose in electron beam therapy, Radiology, Vol 126, p249-252, 1978.

53. Jamshedi, A., Kuchnir, F.J., and Reft, C.S., Determination of the source position for the electron beams from a high energy linear accelerator, Med. Phys., Vol 13, p942-948, 1986.

54. Laughlin, J.S., High-energy electron treatment planning for inhomogeneities, Br. J. Radiol., Vol 38, p143-147, 1965.

55. Boone, M.L.M., Jardine, J.H., Wright, A.E., and Tapley, N., High-energy electron dose perturbations in the regions of tissue heterogeneity. I. In vivo dosimetry, Radiology, Vol 88, p1136-1145, 1967.

56. Almond, P.R., Wright, A.E., and Boone, M.L.M., High-energy electron dose perturbations in regions of tissue heterogeneity. II. Physical models of tissue heterogeneities, Radiology, Vol 88, p1146-1153, 1967.

57. Pohlit, W., Calculated and measured dose distributions in inhomogeneous materials and in patients, Ann. N.Y. Acad. Sci., Vol 161, p189-197, 1969.

58. Brenner, M., Karjalainen, P., Rytila, A., and Jungar, H., The effects of inhomogeneities on dose distribution of high-energy electrons, Ann. N.Y. Acad. Sci., Vol 161, p189-197, 1969.

59. Shrott, K.R., Ross, C.K., Bielajew, A.F., and Rogers, D.W.O., Electron beam dose distributions near standard inhomogeneities, Phys. Med. Biol., Vol 31, p235-249, 1986.

60. Hogstrom, K.R., Dosimetry of electron heterogeneities, p532-561, in Radiation Oncology Physics — 1986, Medical Physics Monograph 15, Keriakes, J.G., Elson, H.R., and Born, C.G., (Eds.), American Institute of Physics, New York, 1987.

61. Amdur, R.J., Kalbaugh, K.J., Ewald, L.M., Parsons, J.T., Mendenhall, W.M., Bova, F.J., and Million, R.R., Radiation therapy of skin cancer near the eye: Kilovoltage X-rays versus electrons, Int. J. Radiat. Oncol. Biol. Phys., Vol 23, p769-779, 1992.

62. Lovett, R.D., Perez, C.A., Shapiro, S.J., and Garcia, D.M., External irradiation of epithelial skin cancers, Int. J. Radiat. Oncol. Biol. Phys., Vol 19, p235-242, 1990.

63. Williams, P.C., Hunter, R.D., and Jackson, S.M., Whole body electron therapy in mycosis fungoides — a successful translational technique achieved by modification of an established linear accelerator, Br. J. Radiol., Vol 52, p302-307, 1979.

64. Task Group 30, AAPM Monograph 23, Total Skin Electron Therapy and Dosimetry, American Association of Physicists in Medicine, Radiation Therapy Committee, Report of Task Group 30, American Institute of Physics, New York, 1988.

65. Almond, P.R., Total skin electron irradiation and dosimetry, p296-332, in Radiation Oncology Physics — 1986, Medical Physics Monograph 15, Keriakes, J.G., Elson, H.R., and Born, C.G., (Eds.), American Institute of Physics, New York, 1987.

66. Page, V., Garner, A., and Karzmark, C.J., Patient dosimetry in electron treatment of large superficial lesions, Radiology, Vol 94, p635-641, 1970.

67. Goldson, A.L., Preliminary clinical experience with intraoperative radiotherapy, J. Natl. Med. Assoc., Vol 70, p493-495, 1978.

68. Biggs, P.J., Epp, E.R., Ling, C.L., Novack, D.H., and Michaels, H.B., Dosimetry, field shaping and other considerations for intraoperative electron therapy, Int. J. Radiat. Oncol. Biol. Phys., Vol 7, p875-884, 1981.

69. McCullough, E.C., and Anderson, J.A., The dosimetric properties of an applicator system for intra-operative electron-beam therapy utilizing a Clinac-18 accelerator, Med. Phys., Vol 9, p261-268, 1982.

70. McCullogh, E.C., and Biggs, P.J., Intraoperative electron therapy, p333-347, in Radiation Oncology Physics — 1986, Medical Physics Monograph 15, Keriakes, J.G., Elson, H.R., and Born, C.G., (Eds.), American Institute of Physics, New York, 1987.

71. Hogstrom, K.R., Boyer, A.L., Shiu, A.S., Ocharn, G., Kirsher, S.M., Krispel, F., and Rich, T., Design of metallic electron beam cones for an intraoperative therapy linear accelerator, Int. J. Radiat. Oncol. Biol. Phys., Vol 18, p1227-1332, 1990.

72. Nelson, C.E., Cook, R., and Rafkel, S., The dosimetric properties of an intraoperative radiation therapy applicator system, Med. Phys., Vol 16, p794-799, 1989.

73. Dobblebower, R.R. and Abe, M. (Eds.), Intraoperative Radiation Therapy, CRC Press, Boca Raton, Florida, 1989.

74. Leavitt, D.D., Peacock, L.M., Gibbs, F.A., and Stewart, J.R., Electron arc therapy: Physical measurements and treatment planning techniques, Int. J. Radiat. Oncol. Biol. Phys., Vol 11, p985-999, 1985.

75. Hogstrom, K.R., and Leavitt, D., Dosimetry of arc electron therapy, p265-295, in Radiation Oncology Physics — 1986, Medical Physics Monograph 15, Keriakes, J.G., Elson, H.R., and Born, C.G., (Eds.), American Institute of Physics, New York, 1987.

76. Khan, F.M., Calibration and treatment planning of electron beam arc therapy, p249-266, in Electron Dosimetry and Arc Therapy, Proceedings of Symposium, Paliwal, B. (Ed.), American Institute of Physics, New York, 1982.

77. Levitt, D.D., Stewart, J.R., Moeller, J.H., and Early, L., Optimization of electron arc therapy by multi-vane collimator control, Int. J. Radiat. Oncol. Biol. Phys., Vol 16, p489-496, 1989.

78. Lam, K.S., Lam, W.C., O'Neill, M.J., and Zinreich, E., Electron arc therapy: Beam data requirements and treatment planning, Clin. Radiol., Vol 38, p379-383, 1987.

79. Pla, M., Podgorsak, E.B., Pla, C., and Freeman, C.R., Determination of secondary collimator shape in electron arc therapy, Phys. Med. Biol., Vol 38, p999-1006, 1993.

80. Pla, M., Pla, C., and Podgorsak, E.B., The influence of beam parameters on percentage depth dose in electron arc therapy, Med. Phys., Vol 15, p49-55, 1988.

81. Pla, M., Podgorsak, E.B., Freeman, C.R., Souhami, L., and Guerra, J., Physical aspects of the angle β concept in electron arc therapy, Int. J. Radiat. Oncol. Biol. Phys., Vol 20, p1331-1339, 1991.

82. Boyer, A.L., Fullerton, G.D., and Mira, J.G., An electron beam pseudoarc technique for irradiation of large areas of chest wall and other curved surfaces, Int. J. Radiat. Oncol. Biol. Phys., Vol 8, p1969-1974, 1982.

83. McKenzie, M.R., Freeman, C.R., Pla, M., Guerra, J., Souhami, L., Pla, C., and Podgorsak, E.B., Clinical experience with pseudoarc therapy, Br. J. Radiol., Vol 66, p234-240, 1993.

84. Boyer, A.L., Fullerton, G.D., Mira, J.G., and Mok, E.C., An electron beam pseudo arc technique, p267-293, in Electron Dosimetry and Arc Therapy, Proceedings of Symposium, Paliwal, B. (Ed.), American Institute of Physics, New York, 1982.

85. Pla, M., Podgorsak, E.B., and Pla, C., Electron dose rate and photon contamination in electron arc therapy, Med. Phys., Vol 16, p692-697, 1989.

86. Bagne, F., Adjacent fields of high-energy X-rays and electrons, Phys. Med. Biol., Vol 23, p1186-1191, 1978.

87. Bhaduri, D., Choi, M.C., Weaver, J., and Agarwal, S.K., Matching of electron fields on flat surfaces, J. Am. Assoc. Med. Dosim., Vol 9, p12-16, 1984.

88. Frass, B.A., Tepper, J.E., Glatstein, E., and van de Geijn, J.A., Clinical use of a matchline wedge for adjacent megavoltage radiation field line matching, Int. J. Radiat. Oncol. Biol. Phys., Vol 9, p209-216, 1983.

89. Kalend, A., Zwicker, R.D., Wu, A., and Sternick, E.S., A beam edge modifier for abutting electron fields, Med. Phys., Vol 12, p793-798, 1985.

90. Kurup, R.G., Wang, S., and Glasgow, G.P., Field matching of electron beams using plastic wedge penumbra generators, Phys. Med. Biol., Vol 37, p145-153, 1992.

91. Kurup, R.G., Glasgow, G.P., and Leybovich, L.B., Design of electron beam wedges for increasing penumbra abutting fields, Phys. Med. Biol., Vol 38, p667-674, 1993.

92. Papiez, E., Dunscombe, P.B., and Malakar, K., Matching photon and electron fields in the treatment of head and neck tumors, Med. Phys., Vol 19, p335-341, 1992.

ADDITIONAL READING

1. Task Group 25, Radiation Therapy Committee, American Association of Physicists in Medicine, Clinical Electron Beam Dosimetry, Med. Phys., Vol 18, p73-109, 1991.
2. ICRU Report 35, Radiation Dosimetry: Electron Beams with Energies Between 1 and 50 MeV, International Commission on Radiological Units and Measurements, Bethesda, Maryland, 1984.
3. Klavenhagen, S.C., Physics of Electron Beam Therapy, HPA Medical Physics Handbook 13, Adam Hilger, Bristol, 1985.
4. Keriakes, J.G., Elson, H.R., and Born, C.G. (Eds.), Radiation Oncology Physics — 1986, Medical Physics Monograph 15, American Institute of Physics, New York, 1987.
5. Paliwal, B. (Ed.), Electron Dosimetry and Arc Therapy, Proceedings of Symposium, American Institute of Physics, New York, 1982.
6. Almond, P.R., Radiation physics of electron beams, in Clinical Applications of Electron Beams, Tapley, N. (Ed.), John Wiley & Sons, New York, 1976.
7. Acta Radiologica, Supplement 364, 1983, Computed Electron Beam Dose Planning, Proceedings of a Conference at the Dept. of Radiation Physics, Karolinska Institute, Stockholm, Sweden, 1982.
8. Vaeth, J.M., and Meyer, J.L. (Eds.), The Role of High Energy Electrons in the Treatment of Cancer, Karger, Basel, 1991.
9. Jayaraman, S., Pathways and pitfalls in treatment planning with external beams: the role of the clinical physicist, Radiographics, Vol 8, p.1147-1170, 1988.

Chapter 17

PHYSICS OF THE USE OF SMALL SEALED SOURCES IN BRACHYTHERAPY

17.1 BRACHYTHERAPY

Brachytherapy is a method of radiation treatment in which discrete radiation sources are placed in close proximity to or within the tissues to be treated. The prefix "brachy" means "short-range" in Greek. The word "endocurie therapy" also has been in use ("endo" = within). Most of these treatments are performed with photons; in a few situations, beta particles and neutrons are used. The brachytherapy sources may be in the form of radioactive seeds or linear capsules. These sources generally contain a small amount of radioactive material within a metallic capsule having a wall of 0.1 to 1 mm thickness. The container keeps the radioactive material from entering the patient's tissues or body fluids during its use. It also prevents contamination of the surroundings with radioactivity during source storage and handling.

In early brachytherapy practice,[1] naturally occurring radium encapsulated in platinum was used as the source of radiation. Martin and Martin,[2] in 1959, documented pictorially the regression of several tumors treated with gamma rays emanating from radium needles. Radium, however, has the major disadvantage that its decay product, radon, is a gas. Thus, any breach in a radium container can result in leakage of radon gas into the atmosphere. The diffusing radon can spread, decay further into its own radioactive daughter products, and contribute to widespread radioactive contamination.[3] All radium sources need to be tested frequently for radon leaks.

Since artificially produced radionuclide sources became available, they have been favored as substitutes for radium.[4-6] In general, all brachytherapy sources should be tested to ensure the integrity of their encapsulation and thus to avoid the spread of radioactivity.[7,8] In some localities, regulations stipulate the frequency with which sealed sources should be tested for leakage.

Some beta sources are also used in brachytherapy for treatment of superficial lesions.[9-12] However, most common brachytherapy applications make use of the dose delivered by the penetrating photons emitted from radioactive sources. Another purpose served by the capsule, apart from helping to contain the radioactive material, is that it is thick enough to absorb any short-range beta particles emitted by the source. The useful radiation fluence is made up mostly of gamma rays, and also of characteristic X-rays emitted incidental to the atomic and nuclear transitions. In addition, there is a contribution by characteristic X-rays and bremsstrahlung produced in the source capsule. However, these usually form a negligible component. Table 17.1 lists the characteristics of several radionuclides for use in brachytherapy. In this chapter, we discuss the dosimetry of the gamma ray sealed sources used in brachytherapy and the problem of planning the dose distribution in brachytherapy for controlled delivery of the radiation dose.

17.2 CATEGORIES OF APPLICATIONS

Brachytherapy can be classified broadly into three categories: surface, interstitial, and intracavitary applications.

In *surface* applications, a block of wax, dental compound, or any near–tissue-equivalent plastic material is molded to form a layer of uniform thickness. The molded layer is placed on a body surface that bears a superficial lesion to be irradiated, as shown in Figure 17.1. An outline is drawn with a margin around the lesion, identifying the "target area" for the treatment. The sources are distributed on the top surface of the mold over a "source area." The thickness of the mold, **h**, is referred to as the treatment distance. For practical treatments, on many occasions, **h** is chosen to be 0.5 cm; at other times, it may be an integral multiple of 0.5 cm. The value of **h** influences the

TABLE 17.1
Physical Properties of Radionuclide Sources Used in Brachytherapy

Element	Source isotope	Beta(s) $(E_\beta)_{max}$ (keV)	Energy Range of Photons (keV)	Mean Photon Energy (keV)	Half-Life T_h	HVT in Lead (mm)	TVT in Lead (mm)	Exposure Rate Constant (Γ_x) ($\mu C\ kg^{-1}\ cm^2\ MBq^{-1}\ h^{-1}$) [$R\ cm^2\ mCi^{-1}\ h^{-1}$]	Air-kerma Rate Constant (Γ_{ak}) ($\mu Gy\ cm^2\ MBq^{-1}\ h^{-1}$)	Dose Rate Constant (Λ) ($cGy\ h^{-1}$)/($(cGy\ cm^2\ h^{-1})$)[a]
Photon Sources										
Radium	226Ra	17–3260	47–2440	830	≈1600 years	14	42	58.2 [8.35][b]	1971	1.10
Radon	222Rn	17–3260	47–2440	830	3.8 d	14	42	58.2 [8.35]	1971	1.10
Gold	198Au	29–1370	412–1088	416	2.7 d	3	11	16.3 [2.34]	552	1.13
Cobalt	60Co	313	1170,1330	1250	5.26 years	11	46	90.5 [12.98]	3064	1.11
Cesium	137Cs	514,1170	662	662	30 years	6	22	22.9 [3.28]	774	1.11
Tantalum	182Ta	180–514	43–1453	670	115 d	12	39	54.0 [7.75]	1829	1.13
Iridium	192Ir	240–670	136–1062	380	74 d	3	12	32.7 [4.69]	1107	1.12
Iodine	125I	None	27–35	29	59.6 d	0.025	0.1	10.11 [1.45]	342	0.90
Palladium	103Pd	None	20–23	21	17 d	0.008	0.03	10.32 [1.48]	349	0.74
Americium	241Am	None	60	60	432 years	0.125	0.4	0.850 [0.122]	28.8	—
Samarium	145Sm	None	38–61	41	340 d	0.06	0.2	6.17 [0.885]	209	—
Ytterbium	169Yb	None	49–308	93	32 d	0.2	0.7	12.55 [1.8]	425	1.19
Beta Sources										
Strontium	90Sr & 90Y	540 & 2270	None	None	28.9 years & 64 h					
Phosphorous	32P	1710	None	None	14.3 d					
Ruthenium	106Ru & 107Rh	39 & 3540	None & 500 (in 21% of decay and other photons of energies up to 1550 in very low intensities)	None	368 d & 40 sec					

Note: Data subject to continuous revisions and update. The above values are assembled by the authors based on various references 6, 27 to 31 (including Jani, S.K., Handbook of Dosimetry Data for Radiotherapy, CRC Press, Boca Raton, Florida, 1993, and their own calculations and estimates).

[a] Estimated for an ideal point source with isotropic emission. Actual sources may have a range of values.

[b] Applicable for radium sources filtered by 0.5 mm Pt. Assumes 0.988 mCi/mg Ra.

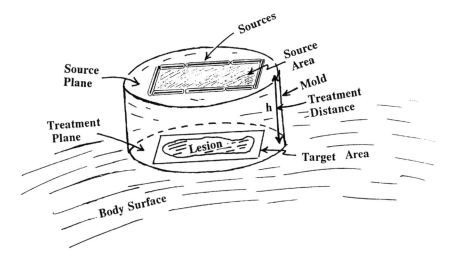

FIGURE 17.1   A surface application with discrete sources arranged on top of a mold.

dose fall-off with depth within the lesion. The smaller the value of **h**, the steeper the dose fall-off with depth from the skin. Surface application is not suitable for lesions deeper than a few millimeters.

For thick lesions, an *interstitial* application, in which the sources are implanted or embedded directly in the lesion, is favored. Such an application is called an implant. The simplest of these is a single-plane implant, in which sources are spread over an area in one plane within the slab of tissue to be treated. It is obvious that the dose rate will be high in the implant plane (i.e., the source plane) and fall off at distances away from it. It has traditionally been assumed that sources implanted in a plane can adequately irradiate tissues located up to 0.5 cm away from it, as illustrated in Figure 17.2a. Thus, the target volume for a single-plane implant is regarded to be a slab of tissue of 1 cm thickness extending up to 0.5 cm on either side of the implant plane.

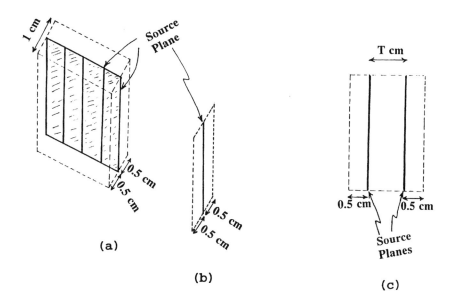

FIGURE 17.2   Size of the target volumes for planar implants. (a) A single-plane implant in a three-dimensional view. (b) End-on view of a single-plane implant. (c) End-on view of a two-plane implant with an interplanar spacing T.

For treatment of lesions thicker than 1 cm, a two-plane implant of sources in two parallel planes can be considered. With the assumption that any plane implant can treat up to a distance of 0.5 cm, implants in two planes separated by T cm can irradiate a target volume of thickness (T + 1) cm, as illustrated in Figure 17.2c. If the two source planes are 1.0 cm apart, the target thickess will be 2 cm. With a separation of 1.0 to 2.0 cm between the two source planes, a two-plane implant can treat a slab of 2.0 to 3.0 cm thickness.

Use of two-plane separations of more than 1.5 cm can create low-dose regions midway between the source planes. For larger thicknesses, the use of more than two planes of sources may be appropriate. The implant is then called a volume implant. The implanted volume can be of any chosen shape — rectangular, cylindrical, spherical, or ellipsoidal — so as to cover the lesion and the target volume.

If sources are implanted for a specified duration of irradiation and then removed, the implant is a temporary implant. The term "removable implant" is also sometimes used. In some instances, short-lived radionuclide sources may be implanted and left permanently in the body to decay. Such an implant is called a permanent implant.

In *intracavitary* insertions, the sources are positioned in accessible body cavities to irradiate lesions located there. Tumors that grow around the uterine and vaginal cavities have been success-fully irradiated by intracavitary insertions of radioactive sources. Lesions in esophageal and bron-chial passages have also been treated by insertion of tubes and placement of sources. These techniques are sometimes referred to as "intraluminal" therapy.

In the early practice of brachytherapy, radium needles were pushed directly into tissues as implants. For intracavitary insertions, catheters and applicators loaded with radioactive sources were inserted into the patient. Thus, the applicators were "preloaded" with the sources prior to insertion into the patient. Because the procedure involved handling of applicators that already contained the radioactive sources, the personnel was exposed to radiation even during the time of insertion and positioning of the sources in the cavities. In contrast, in modern practice, afterloading techniques have become common.[13-20] In these techniques, empty guides or catheters, without radioactive sources, are first inserted and positioned in the patient. Thus, in the early part of the procedure of handling the catheters, radiation exposure to personnel is avoided. After making sure that the catheters are properly positioned, one can promptly load the radioactive sources into them. The simplest approach is manual insertion of the sources, which are held with a handle.

Sophisticated remote-handling apparatus has also become available for source insertion and retrieval. These devices steer the sources into the catheters and retrieve them after a preassigned period of irradiation.

17.3 SOURCE STRENGTH OF BRACHYTHERAPY SOURCES

17.3.1 NEED FOR SPECIFICATION OF SOURCE STRENGTH

An institution may possess several sources that are identical in physical size, construction, and the radionuclide contained, but each of the individual sources may give different fluence yields, i.e., the sources may be of different strengths. This is analogous to having electric bulbs of different wattages providing distinct luminescence yields. Each brachytherapy source has a specified source strength that is used for the calculation of dose rate. The source strength is generally specified in a certificate issued by the source supplier. It is possible to state the source strength in terms of one of several interrelated physical quantities. These quantities are radium-equivalent mass, absolute activity, apparent activity, and air-kerma yield rate. The numerical relationships of the source strengths as specified by these quantities for brachytherapy sources in common use are given in Reference 21. It is currently recommended that the physical quantity to be preferred for specifying the source strength is the air-kerma yield rate.[22] The unit in which the source strength is specified should be traceable to the standards maintained by the national and international standardization laboratories.

17.3.2 SPECIFICATION BY RADIUM-EQUIVALENT MASS

In the early practice of brachytherapy, radium* was the predominant source in use. The radium sources were assayed in terms of the actual mass of radium contained (in milligrams). The standard radium sources were contained in 0.5 mm thick platinum (with 10% iridium) capsules. The radium source strength was specified in milligrams and was intended to be used together with a radium exposure rate constant $\Gamma_x = 8.25$ R cm^2 mg^{-1} h^{-1} (i.e., equivalent to $\Gamma_{ak} = 8.25 \times 0.873 = 7.20$ cGy cm^2 mg^{-1} h^{-1}; see Section 11.8), which applied specifically to radium sources in containers having a 0.5-mm platinum wall thickness.

Using the mass for specification of source strength was possible with radium, because all of the radium nuclides without exception are radioactive. However, in artificially produced radioactive materials, only a certain percentage of the target nuclides are activated and become radioactive (see Section 5.4). Thus, the mass is not a direct measure of the radioactivity contained. However, if the exposure rate (or air-kerma rate) from such a non-radium source is compared with that from a radium source of known mass, its strength (i.e., radioactivity) in terms of radium-equivalent mass can be assessed.

A reentrant ionization chamber, shown schematically in Figure 17.3, is a device that is useful for rapid verification of the source strength in hospital settings. The chamber has a well-type receptacle for the source. The ion-collection volume of the chamber surrounds the source in almost all directions, except in the direction toward the opening of the well.

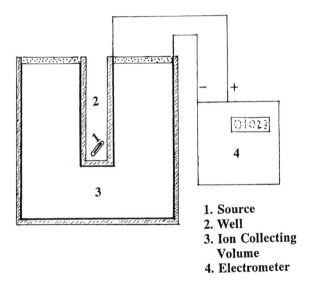

1. Source
2. Well
3. Ion Collecting Volume
4. Electrometer

FIGURE 17.3 A reentrant ionization chamber useful for source strength intercomparisons.

Let us say that a standard radium source of strength S_{stmg} mg is placed in the receptacle and a reading of the ionization current, R_{st}, is obtained. Next, the source is replaced by the non-radium source to be assayed in the same geometry, and a reading, R, is obtained. The milligram radium equivalent (mgRaeq), S_{mg} (0.5 mm PtIr), of the assayed source is

$$S_{mg} = \frac{R}{R_{st}} S_{stmg} \quad \text{mgRaeq (in a 0.5-mm PtIr capsule)} \qquad (17\text{--}1)$$

---

* Radium in medicine typically means ^{226}Ra.

The value S_{mg} stated in mgRaeq units (in a 0.5-mm PtIr capsule) can be used together with the radium exposure rate constant $(\Gamma_x)_{Ra} = 8.25$ R cm^2 mg^{-1} h^{-1} to yield the exposure rate, $\dot{X}_{air}$, at a distance r from the source in air, as follows:*

$$\dot{X}_{air} = \frac{(\Gamma_x)_{Ra} \cdot S_{mg}}{r^2} \qquad (17\text{--}2)$$

A similar equation can be used with the air-kerma rate constant for radium, $(\Gamma_{ak})_{Ra} = 7.70$ cGy cm^2 mg^{-1} h^{-1}, to give the kerma rate in air, $\dot{k}_{air}$, at a distance r from the source by the relation

$$\dot{k}_{air} = \frac{(\Gamma_{ak})_{Ra} \cdot S_{mg}}{r^2} \qquad (17\text{--}3)$$

The use of a reentrant chamber as described above, however, has some limitations.[23,24]

17.3.3 SPECIFICATION BY ACTIVITY

The most fundamental physical quantity that specifies the strength of a source is its absolute disintegration rate (i.e., activity), S_{act}. For example, S_{act} may be stated to be 100 MBq. If it is a point source having a capsule that filters the radiation by a factor A_{enc}, then the air-kerma rate, $\dot{k}_{air}$, at a distance r from the source is given by

$$\dot{k}_{air} = \frac{\Gamma_{ak} S_{act} A_{enc}}{r^2} \qquad (17\text{--}4)$$

where Γ_{ak} is the air-kerma rate constant for the radionuclide composing the source (see Section 11.8). Although the activity S_{act} is fundamental in its nature, specification in terms of it can cause discrepancies in dosimetry and hence is not recommended. This is because, in practice, the activity is often derived indirectly, based on an exposure or air-kerma rate measurement. The vendor may report the value of S_{ak} to the user in a certificate, but may actually have measured $\dot{k}_{air}$ and derived the value of S_{act} through Equation (17--4) by assuming certain values for Γ_{ak} and A_{enc}. The user, in turn, cannot use the reported value of S_{act} for practical dosimetry without assigning values for Γ_{ak} and A_{enc}. The method or the references by which he selects these values may disagree with those which the source vendor adopted, thus leaving room for a discrepancy between $\dot{k}_{air}$ as derived by the vendor and that derived by a user. A part of this problem is solved if the vendor derives and reports to the user an apparent activity, S_{app}, given by

$$S_{app} = (S_{act} \cdot A_{enc}) = \frac{r^2 \dot{k}_{air}}{\Gamma_{ak}} \qquad (17\text{--}5)$$

Using S_{app} (instead of S_{act}) allows the user to depend on the published references for Γ_{ak} only. However, Γ_{ak} values have been calculated and reported differently for many radionuclides by various investigators. Thus, the possibility for an inconsistency in the selection of Γ_{ak} and the derivation of $\dot{k}_{air}$ remains.

17.3.4 SPECIFICATION BY AIR-KERMA RATE YIELD

The source strength can be specified in terms of the kerma rate, $\dot{k}_{air}$, in air at a particular distance **r** from the source, with the source in free space.[22] The air-kerma rate yielded by the source value can be expressed as normalized at a unit distance of 1 cm or 1 m from the source. That is, the air-kerma strength, S_{ak}, of a source is defined to be such that

---

* A dot placed over any quantity such as $\dot{X}$ or $\dot{k}$ indicates the time rate of change of that quantity.

$$\dot{k}_{air} = \frac{S_{ak}}{r^2} \qquad (17\text{--}6)$$

or
$$S_{ak} = \dot{k}_{air}\, r^2 \qquad (17\text{--}7)$$

In writing the above equations, we have assumed that the source is a point isotropic source giving the same k_{air} at a distance **r** in all directions. Linear sources have nonisotropic emissions. For these, a source strength S_{ak} can be based on the convention that the value of $\dot{k}_{air}$ is measured at a point along the mid-perpendicular line of the source at a distance very much larger than the active length of the source. It is apparent from (17–4) and (17–7) that

$$S_{ak} = \Gamma_{ak}\, S_{act}\, A_{enc} \qquad (17\text{--}8)$$

17.3.5 SPECIFICATION BY WATER-KERMA RATE YIELD

The source strength can be specified also in terms of the kerma rate, $\dot{k}_{water}$, yielded in water at a stated distance r from the source, with the source in free space. Again, the value can be presented as normalized at a unit distance of 1 cm or 1 m from the source. That is, the water-kerma strength, S_{wk}, of a source is given by

$$S_{wk} = \dot{k}_{water}\, r^2 \qquad (17\text{--}9)$$

S_{wk} and S_{ak} are related by

$$\frac{S_{wk}}{S_{ak}} = \frac{[\mu_{tr}/\rho]_{water}}{[\mu_{tr}/\rho]_{air}} \qquad (17\text{--}10)$$

17.4 SOURCE STRENGTH AND TIME PRODUCT

17.4.1 SIGNIFICANCE

The dose delivered in any particular brachytherapy application increases in direct proportion to both the source strength employed and the duration of irradiation. The dose delivered to the patient can be controlled by either or both of these. For delivery of a given dose, sources of low strength can be used over a long treatment time, or sources of high strength can be employed for a correspondingly shorter time. Thus, the product of source strength and time of irradiation can serve as a single index of treatment. Brachytherapy dosage tables have been published giving the value of this index for the delivery of a stated dose for different source arrays, with the stated dose conforming to a particular definition or system. The systems or approaches are explained in Section 17.9.

17.4.2 MILLIGRAM HOURS OF TREATMENT

The dosage tables published for radium sources in the past used milligram hours (mgh) as the treatment index. In general, if a source of strength S_{mg} is used for T hours, the mgh is $S_{mg} \times T$. If an array of **m** sources with source strengths $(S_{mg})_1$, $(S_{mg})_2$, ..., $(S_{mg})_m$ is used over an irradiation period T, the total mgh is the following sum:

$$\left[\left(S_{mg} \right)_1 + \left(S_{mg} \right)_2 + \ldots + \left(S_{mg} \right)_m \right] \times T \ \text{mgh}$$

17.4.3 AIR-KERMA YIELD OF TREATMENT

If the source strength is evaluated in air-kerma rate yield in cGy cm^2 h^{-1}, the product of source strength and time becomes cGy cm^2. We will call this the air-kerma yield of treatment. It is an overall index of both the source strength employed and the time of irradiation. In general, if a source of strength S_{ak} (cGy cm^2 h^{-1}) is used for T hours of irradiation, the corresponding air-kerma yield of treatment is

$$\left(S_{ak} \text{ cGy cm}^2 \text{ h}^{-1} \times Th\right) = \left(S_{ak} \times T\right) \text{ cGy cm}^2$$

If it is an array of **m** sources with source strengths $(S_{ak})_1$, $(S_{ak})_2$, ..., $(S_{ak})_m$, used over an irradiation period T, the corresponding air-kerma yield is the following sum:

$$\left[\left(S_{ak}\right)_1 + \left(S_{ak}\right)_2 + ... + \left(S_{ak}\right)_m\right] \times T \text{ cGy cm}^2$$

Example 17.1

Early tables of radium dosage presented the data as milligram hours required to deliver an exposure of 1000 R. A radium exposure rate constant of $\Gamma_x = 8.40$ R cm^2 mg^{-1} h^{-1} was used. All calculations were done in air, ignoring tissue attenuation, scatter, and filtration in the capsule. It has been determined that the milligram hours will increase, on the average, by a factor of 1.015 if these effects are allowed for.[25] Derive the factor by which the milligram hours for 1000 R can be converted to air-kerma yield (cGy cm^2) for delivery of a dose of 1 cGy to water. (Given: 1 R = 2.58 $\times$ 10^{-4} C kg^{-1}, W = 33.85 J C^{-1}, $(f_{xd})_{water} = 0.965$ cGy R^{-1} for radium gamma rays.)

The exposure yield calculated for 1 mgh of radium irradiation was

$$\Gamma_x \times 1 \text{ mgh} = 8.40 \text{ R cm}^2 \text{ mg}^{-1} \text{ h}^{-1} \times 1 \text{ mgh} = 8.40 \text{ R cm}^2$$

The corresponding air-kerma yield is

$$8.40 \text{ R cm}^2 \times 2.58 \times 10^{-4} \text{ C kg}^{-1} \text{ R}^{-1} \times 33.85 \text{ J C}^{-1}$$
$$= 8.4 \times 8.733 \times 10^{-3} \text{ J kg}^{-1} \text{ cm}^2$$
$$= 7.336 \text{ cGy cm}^2$$

In addition, an exposure of 1000 R is equivalent to a dose of

$$1000 \text{ R} \times \left(f_{xd}\right)_{water} = 1000 \text{ R} \times 0.965 \text{ cGy R}^{-1} = 965 \text{ cGy}$$

Furthermore, to allow for attenuation and scatter in tissue and filtration in the capsule, the milligram hours should be increased by 1.015. Hence, M mgh for delivery of 1000 R in the early data becomes:

$$M \text{ mgh} \times 1.015 \times \left(7.336 \text{ cGy cm}^2/\text{mgh}\right) \times \left(1/965 \text{ cGy}\right)$$
$$= \left[7.716 \times 10^{-3} \text{ M}\right] \text{ cGy cm}^2 \text{ air-kerma yield for delivery of 1 cGy in water}$$

In more recent times, dosage tables giving milligram hours for 1000 cGy have been published for Γ_x of 8.25 R cm^2 mg^{-1} h^{-1}, $(f_{xd})_{tissue}$ of 0.957 cGy R^{-1}. These also allowed for tissue attenuation and filtration. For such cases, M mgh for 1000 cGy will convert to

$$\left(M \text{ mgh}/1000 \text{ cGy}\right) \times 8.25 \text{ R cm}^2 \text{ mg}^{-1} \text{ h}^{-1} \times 2.58 \times 10^{-4} \text{ C kg}^{-1} \text{ R}^{-1}$$

$$\times 33.85 \text{ J C}^{-1} \times \left[0.957 \text{ cGy R}^{-1}/0.965 \text{ cGy R}^{-1}\right]$$

$$= \left[7.145 \times 10^{-3} \text{ M}\right] \text{ cGy cm}^2 \text{ for delivery of 1 cGy in water}$$

17.5 DOSIMETRY OF A POINT SOURCE IN WATER

17.5.1 THEORETICAL APPROACH

A theoretical formula can be developed for the dosimetry of an ideal point source which (i) has a radioactive volume of near-zero dimensions and (ii) emits radiation isotropically. Such an ideal source S that has a source strength S_{ak} and has an encapsulation is shown located in air in Figure 17.4a and in water in Figure 17.4b. In the latter case, the attenuation and scatter in water make the situation comparable to that in a patient. Point P is at distance r from the source. The dose rate, $\left(\dot{D}_P\right)_{in\,air}$ to a mass of water large enough to provide charged-particle equilibrium (see Section 11.7.2) surrounded by air at P is

$$\left(\dot{D}_P\right)_{in\,air} = \dot{k}_{air}\left(f_{akmd}\right)_{water} = \frac{S_{ak}}{r^2} \cdot \left(f_{akmd}\right)_{water} \tag{17--11}$$

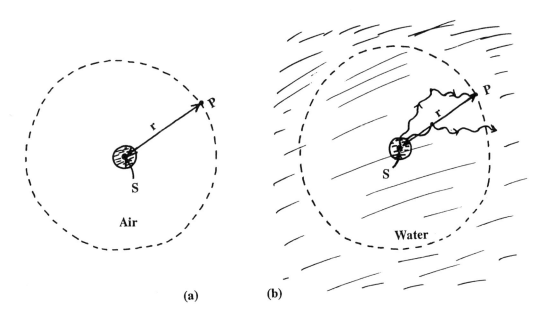

FIGURE 17.4 An encapsulated point source (a) in air under minimum attenuation and scatter conditions, (b) in water with attenuation loss and scatter gain.

where $(f_{akmd})_{water}$ is the air-kerma to medium-dose conversion factor, the medium being water. Values of $(f_{akmd})_{water}$ at different photon energies are given in Table 17.2.

To derive the dose rate in water, $\left(\dot{D}_P\right)_{in\,water}$ at point P at distance r from the source, we modify the calculated $\left(\dot{D}_P\right)_{in\,air}$ to allow for attenuation and scatter in water. We will refer to this factor as the water perturbation correction (WPC). The WPC is a function of the distance r from the source and is defined by the ratio

$$\text{WPC}(r) = \frac{\text{dose (to water) at distance r in water}}{\text{dose (to water) at distance r in air}} = \frac{\left(\dot{D}_P\right)_{in\,water}}{\left(\dot{D}_P\right)_{in\,air}}$$

TABLE 17.2
Air-Kerma To Water Dose Conversion Factors

Photon Energy (keV)	Factor $(f_{akmd})_{water}$[a]
30	1.007
50	1.030
100	1.094
600	1.111
800	1.111
1000	1.104
1500	1.102

[a] Given by the ratio $\dfrac{\left[\bar{\mu}_{ab}/\rho\right]_{water}}{\left[\bar{\mu}_{tr}/\rho\right]_{air}}$.

Thus, the dose rate, $\left(\dot{D}_P\right)_{in\,water}$, at P when the source is immersed in water is

$$\left(\dot{D}_P\right)_{in\,water} = \dot{k}_{air} \cdot \left(f_{akmd}\right)_{water} \cdot WPC(r) = \frac{S_{ak}}{r^2} \cdot \left(f_{akmd}\right)_{water} \cdot WPC(r) \qquad (17\text{--}12)$$

The values of WPC(r) have been studied by different investigators with both theoretical and experimental methods. The values given in Table 17.3 are indicative of the trend and relative magnitudes of the perturbation corrections (as compiled by the authors of this book based on published results)[26] for various isotopes in common use. Among the sources listed in Table 17.3, all except ^{103}Pd emit photons of high energy (several hundred kiloelectron volts). We can explain why the WPC for these high-energy emitters remains so close to unity, particularly at distances within 3 cm of the source. Water is a denser medium than air. Hence, there is a reduction in the primary photon fluence reaching point P in water compared to air due to attenuation along the ray SP in Figure 17.4. However, in the denser medium of water, more scattering events also occur all around compared to air. Thus, the scattered photon fluence reaching point P is greater in water than in air. Overall, in water at distances close to the source, the reduction in the primary fluence through attenuation is nearly balanced by the increased scatter fluence. At large distances from the source, the WPC values are significantly below unity. For ^{125}I and ^{103}Pd, which emit photons of particularly low energies (in the 20- to 30-keV range), the Compton scatter events are fewer, and consequently the WPC values are very low even at short distances. Overall, at close distances of interest in brachytherapy, the geometric inverse-square fall-off of intensity becomes a more significant factor than the WPC. This is because the bulk of the dose delivered to any point is likely to be contributed by the sources located near that point.

A point-source approximation may be valid for the dosimetry of many radioactive-seed implants. The isodose surfaces from an ideal point source are concentric spheres which almost follow the inverse-square law at distances close to the source. The water perturbation corrections cause a deviation from strict adherence to the inverse-square law. Such deviations become significant at distances of several centimeters from the source.

If $\dot{D}\left(r_0\right)$ and $\dot{D}(r)$ are the dose rates at a reference distance r_0 close to the source and at a distance r, respectively, a radial function g(r) is defined by the ratio

$$g(r) = \frac{\dot{D}(r)r^2}{\dot{D}(r_0)r_0^2} \qquad (17\text{--}13)$$

TABLE 17.3
Water Perturbation Corrections (WPC) for Different Radionuclides Used in Brachytherapy

Source Nuclide	Distance from Source (cm)									
	0.5	1.0	2.0	3.0	4.0	5.0	6.0	8.0	10.0	
^{226}Ra	0.999	0.994	0.985	0.972	0.957	0.945	0.915	0.894	0.860	*
^{137}Cs	1.004	1.000	0.989	0.978	0.966	0.952	0.936	0.913	0.856	*
^{192}Ir	0.994	1.017	1.018	1.017	1.013	1.006	0.997	0.968	0.925	**
^{60}Co	0.991	0.986	0.974	0.958	0.940	0.919	0.897	0.852	0.813	*
^{198}Au	1.027	1.023	1.017	1.012	1.006	0.997	0.987	0.954	0.901	*
^{103}Pd	0.974	0.725	0.391	0.209	0.113	0.065	0.038	—	—	**

* Average of several published values based on Meisberger et al.[26]
** From Meigooni, A.S. et al.[31]

The value of g(r) is a measure of the lack of conformity to the inverse-square fall-off caused by absorption and scatter in the medium. Thus, g(r) is a measure of the penetration of radiation in tissue (or water). The functions g(r) and WPC(r) are related by

$$g(r) = \left[\mathrm{WPC}(r) \big/ \mathrm{WPC}(r_0) \right]$$

The reference distance r_0 is usually 1.0 cm. Values of g(r) for several source nuclides are given in Table 17.4.

TABLE 17.4
Values of g(r) for Different Radioisotope Sources

Source Nuclide	Distance from source r (cm)							
	1.0	2.0	3.0	4.0	5.0	6.0	8.0	10.0
^{137}Cs	1.00	0.99	0.98	0.97	0.96	0.95	0.91	0.88
^{192}Ir	1.00	1.03	1.00	0.97	0.97	0.97	0.94	0.87
^{198}Au	1.00	1.01	1.01	1.01	1.01	1.01	0.98	0.95
^{125}I*	1.00	0.85	0.655	0.50	0.36	0.275	0.18	—
^{103}Pd	1.00	0.54	0.29	0.16	0.09	0.05	—	—
^{145}Sm	1.00	1.02	0.97	0.92	0.87	0.78	0.61	0.44
^{169}Yb	1.00	1.10	1.18	1.21	1.23	1.23	1.17	1.10

* Values presented here are average for two different source models.

Reproduced from Jani, S.K., p161, Handbook of Dosimetry Data for Radiotherapy, CRC Press, Boca Raton, Florida, 1993.

17.5.2 AAPM AND ICWG EMPIRICAL APPROACH FOR DOSIMETRY OF RADIOACTIVE SEEDS

Radioactive seeds used in practice may have a finite length of 2 to 3 mm. In addition, the radioactive seeds available commercially are not quite isotropic in their physical construction or radiation emission.[27-31] These facts were recognized by an Interstitial Collaborative Working Group (ICWG) that was sponsored by the U.S. National Cancer Institute and a task group appointed by the American Association of Physicists in Medicine (AAPM).[6,27,28] They outlined an empirical dose calculation approach, which we describe next.

In general, one may want to calculate the dose rate $\dot{D}(r, \phi)$ at a point P which is on a radial line at an angle ϕ with respect to the perpendicular to the source and at a distance r from its center, as shown in Figure 17.5. A reference point R is located at $r_0 = 1$ cm and $\phi = 0$, and the dose rate at R per unit air-kerma strength is Λ. Λ, called the dose rate constant, is a characteristic value for a source of a particular design or construction. Its value is to be determined by an experimental measurement on a reference source that has a known source strength, $(S_{ak})_{ref}$, and is of identical construction and design. That is,

$$\Lambda = \left[\dot{D}\left(r_0 = 1\,\text{cm},\ \phi = 0\right) \middle/ \left(S_{ak}\right)_{ref} \right] \tag{17-14}$$

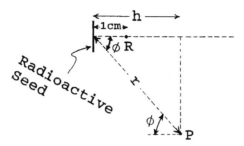

FIGURE 17.5   Radial distance r and polar angle ϕ defining the location of point P with respect to the center and axis of a source. R is a reference point on the mid-perpendicular line of the source.

For another source that has an air-kerma strength S_{ak}, the dose rate at R is

$$\dot{D}\left(r_0 = 1\,\text{cm},\ \phi = 0\right) = \Lambda\,S_{ak} \tag{17-15}$$

The dose rate, $\dot{D}(r, \phi)$, at any other point such as P at location (r,ϕ) can be calculated by the relation

$$\dot{D}(r,\ \phi) = \Lambda \times S_{ak} \times \frac{G(r,\ \phi)}{G\left(r_0 = 1\,\text{cm},\ \phi = 0\right)} \times g(r) \times F(r,\ \phi) \tag{17-16}$$

where $G(r,\phi)$ is the geometric term $(= 1/r^2)$ that accounts for inverse-square fall-off (as would apply for an ideal point source); $g(r)$ is the radial function that allows for photon absorption and scatter in water along the direction $\phi = 0$; and $F(r,\phi)$ is a dimensionless factor that is included as a correction for anisotropy and is normalized to be 1.0 at the angle $\phi = 0$.

For an ideal point-isotropic source, for a point at 1 cm distance from the source, and for all values of ϕ, we can substitute in (17–16):

$$r = 1\,\text{cm};\ g(r) = 1;$$

$$\frac{G(r,\ \phi)}{G\left(r_0 = 1\,\text{cm},\ \phi = 0\right)} = 1;\ \text{and}\ F(r,\ \phi) = 1$$

Hence, the dose rate at this point is

$$\dot{D}(r = 1\,\text{cm},\ \phi) = \Lambda \times S_{ak}$$

From (17–11), we obtain

$$\dot{D}(r = 1\,\text{cm},\ \phi = 0) = S_{ak} \times \left(f_{akmd}\right)_{water} \times \text{WPC}(r = 1.0\,\text{cm})$$

A comparison of the above two expressions gives the relation

$$\Lambda = \left(f_{akmd}\right)_{water} \times \text{WPC}\left(r = 1.0 \text{ cm}\right)$$

The values of g(r) and F(r,φ) can be obtained by the following expressions:

$$g(r) = \frac{\dot{D}\left(r, \ \phi = 0\right) G\left(r_0 = 1 \text{ cm}, \ \phi = 0\right)}{\dot{D}\left(r_0 = 1 \text{ cm}, \ \phi = 0\right) G\left(r, \ \phi = 0\right)} \tag{17-17}$$

$$F\left(r, \ \phi\right) = \frac{\dot{D}\left(r, \ \phi\right) G\left(r, \ 0\right)}{\dot{D}\left(r, \ 0\right) G\left(r, \ \phi\right)} \tag{17-18}$$

Values of g(r) and F(r,φ) have been derived from experimentally observed dose distributions for some radioactive seeds.[6,27,28,32]

17.6 DOSIMETRY OF A LINEAR SOURCE

17.6.1 ENCAPSULATED SOURCE IN AIR

We first address the simple situation of the dose delivered by a finite line source situated in air. The symbols for the physical dimensions of a typical sealed linear source, as shown in Figure 17.6a, are the following:

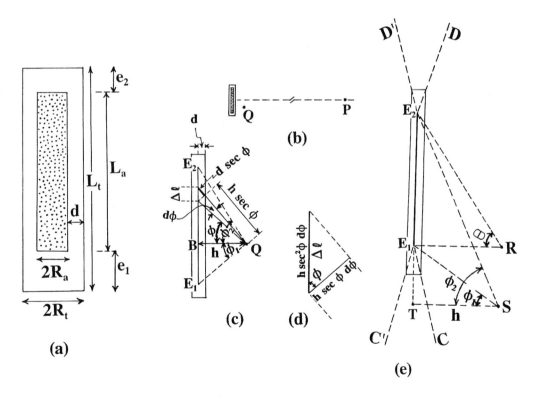

FIGURE 17.6 Encapsulated line source: (a) physical parameters; (b) locations of a distant point P and a proximal point Q with respect to the source; (c) source geometry; (d) an element of the active length of the source; (e) demarcation of different zones around the source.

L_a, length of the inner radioactive region
L_t, total external length of capsule

e_1 and e_2, length of inactive regions at either end

R_a, radius of the inner radioactive region

R_t, radius of the external dimension

$d = (R_t - R_a)$, the thickness of the capsule

Let us consider a linear source having a strength S_{ak} as specified by its air-kerma rate yield. The point P is located in a region perpendicular to the source (Figure 17.6b) and at a distance large compared to the active length, L_a, of the source. For the dosimetry of this point at a large distance from the source, we can regard the source as a point source, and expression (17–11) can be used. Furthermore, all of the rays can be assumed to emerge normal to the source and undergo an attenuation, A_{normal}, in the capsule that is given by

$$A_{normal} = e^{-\mu_{eff}\, d} \qquad (17\text{–}19)$$

where μ_{eff} is an effective attenuation coefficient for the encapsulating material.

For the dosimetry of a point such as Q (Figure 17.6b) in the closer vicinity of the source, we need to recognize the linear spread of the source activity and the emergence of the rays in directions oblique to the source axis. The oblique rays are subject to more than the normal attenuation, A_{normal}, in the capsule. We can consider the linear source as being made up of a series of point sources. We define linear source strength (i.e., the source strength per unit length of the source), ρ_{ak}, as given by

$$\rho_{ak} = \frac{S_{ak}}{L_a \cdot A_{normal}} \qquad (17\text{–}20)$$

In Figure 17.5c, we have simplified the source to be an ideally thin linear source by reducing its active radius to zero. B is a point at the base of the perpendicular from Q to the source. The end points E_1 and E_2 of the active length of the source subtend angles ϕ_1 and ϕ_2, respectively, with line BQ. The elemental source length, $\Delta\ell$, between angles ϕ and $\phi + \Delta\phi$ as shown in Figure 17.6d is given by

$$\Delta\ell = h \sec^2 \phi\, \Delta\phi \qquad (17\text{–}21)$$

Point Q is at a distance of $h \sec \phi$ from this source, and the ray passes through a thickness $d \sec \phi$ of encapsulating material. If we regard the element $\Delta\ell$ as a point source of strength $\rho_{ak}\,\Delta\ell$, the dose rate contributed by it to a small mass of water in air (see Section 11.7.2) at Q, $\left(\Delta\dot{D}_Q\right)_{in\,air}$, is given by

$$\left(\Delta\dot{D}_Q\right)_{in\,air} = \frac{\rho_{ak}\,\Delta\ell\left(f_{akmd}\right)_{water}}{\left(h \sec \phi\right)^2} e^{-\left(\mu_{eff}\, d\right)\sec\phi} \qquad (17\text{–}22)$$

The exponential term allows for the attenuation along the oblique path through the source capsule. Substituting for $\Delta\ell$ and simplifying, we obtain

$$\left(\Delta\dot{D}_Q\right)_{in\,air} = \frac{\rho_{ak}\left(f_{akmd}\right)_{water}}{h} e^{-\left(\mu_{eff}\, d\right)\sec\phi}\, \Delta\phi \qquad (17\text{–}23)$$

The total dose rate, $\left(\dot{D}_Q\right)_{in\,air}$, is obtained by summation from angle ϕ_1 to ϕ_2:

$$\left(\dot{D}_Q\right)_{in\,air} = \frac{\rho_{ak}\left(f_{akmd}\right)_{water}}{h} \int_{-\phi_1}^{\phi_2} e^{-\left(\mu_{eff}\,d\right)\sec\phi}\,d\phi \qquad (17\text{--}24)$$

A limiting case of the above integral results when $\phi_1 = 0$ and the calculation is for a point such as R in Figure 17.6e, which is at the same level as the lower active end of the linear source. In this case, if θ is the total angle subtended by the source at R, the dose rate to water in air at R, $\left(\dot{D}_R\right)_{in\,air}$, is given by

$$\left(\dot{D}_R\right)_{in\,air} = \frac{\rho_{ak}\left(f_{akmd}\right)_{water}}{h} \int_{0}^{\theta} e^{-\left(\mu_{eff}\,d\right)\sec\phi}\,d\phi \qquad (17\text{--}25)$$

Denoting the integral term by $I(\mu_{eff}d, \theta)$, we obtain

$$\left(\dot{D}_R\right)_{in\,air} = \frac{\rho_{ak}\left(f_{akmd}\right)_{water}}{h} I\left(\mu_{eff}\,d, \theta\right) \qquad (17\text{--}26)$$

The integral I is called Sievert's integral and has to be evaluated numerically. Values of this integral for various values of θ and the product $(\mu_{eff}\,d)$ were published by Sievert.[33] The dose rate at point Q in Figure 17.6c can be evaluated if one knows the values of the two integrals $I(\mu_{eff}\,d, \phi_1)$ and $I(\mu_{eff}\,d, \phi_2)$, because expression (17–22) for $\left(\dot{D}_Q\right)_{in\,air}$ can be rewritten as

$$\left(\dot{D}_Q\right)_{in\,air} = \frac{\rho_{ak}\left(f_{akmd}\right)_{water}}{h}\left[I\left(\mu_{eff}\,d, \phi_2\right) + I\left(\mu_{eff}\,d, \phi_1\right)\right] \qquad (17\text{--}27)$$

Similarly, the dose rate at a point such as S in Figure 17.6e, lying beyond the active region of the source, can be derived as the difference of two Sievert integrals for angles ϕ_2 and ϕ_1:

$$\left(\dot{D}_S\right)_{in\,air} = \frac{\rho_{ak}\left(f_{akmd}\right)_{water}}{h}\left[I\left(\mu_{eff}\,d, \phi_2\right) - I\left(\mu_{eff}\,d, \phi_1\right)\right] \qquad (17\text{--}28)$$

In the above expression, the first integral overestimates the dose because the angle ϕ_2 applies to a source length TE$_2$. The second integral corrects this by subtracting the contribution from the nonactive length TE$_1$.

The exponent of the exponential term in the Sievert integral assumes that all of the rays from the source to the point of dose calculation emerge through the cylindrical surface of the capsule. This can be universally valid if the source capsule is of infinite length, extending far beyond its active ends. For actual sources (Figure 17.6e), if the point of calculation falls between lines C and C$'$ (or D and D$'$) in the paraxial end region of the source, some rays will emerge through the end faces of the source. For such points, the Sievert integral will overestimate the attenuation and underestimate the dose. The calculations can be improved if, for rays such as those that emerge through the bottom end of the source, the term $e^{-\left(\mu_{eff}\,d\right)\sec\phi}$ in the integrand of expression (17–24) is replaced by $e^{-\mu e_1}$ to correspond to the attenuation through the bottom end e_1 in Figure 17.6a during the numerical integration.

17.6.2 UNENCAPSULATED SOURCE IN AIR

For a bare source without any encapsulation, $\mu_{eff}\,d = 0$, and the integral I reduces to

$$I\left(\mu_{eff}\,d, \phi\right) = \phi \qquad (17\text{--}29)$$

With $\mu_{\text{eff}}d = 0$, expressions (17–26), (17–27), and (17–28) reduce to the following:

$$\left(\dot{D}_Q\right)_{\text{in air}} = \frac{\rho_{ak}\left(f_{akmd}\right)_{water}}{h}\left[\phi_2 + \phi_1\right] \tag{17–30}$$

$$\left(\dot{D}_S\right)_{\text{in air}} = \frac{\rho_{ak}\left(f_{akmd}\right)_{water}}{h}\left[\phi_2 - \phi_1\right] \tag{17–31}$$

$$\left(\dot{D}_R\right)_{\text{in air}} = \frac{\rho_{ak}\left(f_{akmd}\right)_{water}}{h}\left[\theta\right] \tag{17–32}$$

In Figure 17.6c, if point Q lies on the mid-perpendicular line of the source, ϕ_1 and ϕ_2 will be equal. Under that condition, if the distance h is very short, the angles gradually will approximate their mathematical limits of $\pi/2$ and $-\pi/2$ (i.e., right angles). Then,

$$\left(\dot{D}_Q\right)_{\text{in air}} = \frac{\rho_{ak}\left(f_{akmd}\right)_{water}}{h}\left[\pi/2 - (-\pi/2)\right] = \frac{\pi\rho_{ak}\left(f_{akmd}\right)_{water}}{h} \tag{17–33}$$

Thus, for elongated sources, at distances very close to the source, the air-kerma rate opposite the midregion of the active length of the source and parallel to the source will be uniform, and it will fall off inversely with the distance h. This limiting behavior of inverse distance fall-off may apply in clinical situations in which a very long radioactive wire is used in body cavities such as a bronchus or the esophagus for irradiation of tissues proximal to the wire.

Example 17.2

The dose to the esophagus of a patient who was already irradiated with external beams needs to be boosted by brachytherapy. This is done by intraluminal insertion of a 12 cm long radioactive wire along the esophageal axis. It is known that the spinal cord, which already received 4000 cGy during the external-beam therapy, will be at a distance of 1.0 cm from the wire. What is the maximum dose that can be delivered at a distance of 0.5 cm from the wire without exceeding a total spinal cord tolerance dose of 4500 cGy?

Spinal cord tolerance dose = 4500 cGy.

Dose already delivered (by external beam) = 4000 cGy.

Hence, the dose that can be added in the current treatment is 4500 – 4000 cGy = 500 cGy.

Let us assume (i) that the source is very long compared to the distances of dose calculations and hence the limiting assumption of an inverse distance fall-off can be adopted, and (ii) that no tissue fluence corrections are needed, i.e., WPC = 1.0. The ratio of the dose rates is given by

$$\frac{\text{Dose rate at 0.5 cm}}{\text{Dose rate at 1 cm}} = \frac{1.0 \text{ cm}}{0.5 \text{ cm}} = 2.0$$

We calculated that, at most, 500 cGy can be delivered at 1.0 cm. The dose at 0.5 cm then would be 2×500 cGy = 1000 cGy. (A calculation using the more exact geometric expression of (17–30) gives a dose rate ratio of 2.11 and a maximum deliverable dose of $2.11 \times 500 = 1055$ cGy.)

17.6.3 LINEAR SOURCE IN WATER

Up to now, we have addressed the situation of a linear source in air, ignoring the attenuation and scatter corrections in water. The elemental source $\Delta\ell$ is at a distance h sec ϕ from the point of dose calculation. For calculation of the dose in water, the water perturbation correction (WPC) for this distance, WPC(h sec ϕ), should be incorporated in the integrand of expression (17–24):

$$\left(\dot{D}_{Q}\right)_{\text{in water}} = \frac{\rho_{ak}\left(f_{akmd}\right)_{\text{water}}}{h} \int_{\phi_{1}}^{\phi_{2}} e^{-\left(\mu_{\text{eff}}\, d\right)\sec\phi}\, \text{WPC}\left(h\sec\phi\right)d\phi \qquad (17\text{–}34)$$

17.6.4 DOSE DISTRIBUTION FOR LINEAR SOURCES

Figure 17.7 presents a comparison between calculated and experimentally measured isodose curves for a linear cobalt-60 source.[34] The experimental results were obtained with thermoluminescent dosimeters in a solid tissue-equivalent medium. The agreement between measurement and calculation is good in regions perpendicular to the active length of the source, but there are disagreements in the paraxial end regions of the source. Fortunately, in many clinical situations, structures of dosimetric importance lie in the regions in which the agreement is acceptable. Dose rate tables for linear sources have been published by several authors.[35-38] Table 17.5 provides the dosimetry data for a few typical Cs^{137} sources.

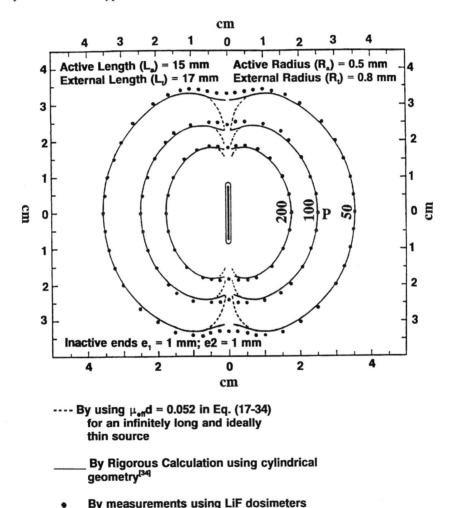

---- **By using $\mu_{\text{eff}}d$ = 0.052 in Eq. (17-34) for an infinitely long and ideally thin source**

_____ **By Rigorous Calculation using cylindrical geometry[34]**

• **By measurements using LiF dosimeters**

FIGURE 17.7   Calculated and experimentally determined isodose curves for a linear cobalt-60 source.

17.6.5 AAPM AND ICWG APPROACH FOR LINEAR SOURCE DOSIMETRY

The geometric factor $G(r,\phi)$ in the ICWG approach (described in Section 17.5.2) applied to a point source. For linear sources, the dosimetry approach of the AAPM Task Group and ICWG

TABLE 17.5
Air-Kerma Yield (cGy cm²) Needed to Deliver 10 cGy in Water at Points in the Vicinity of Cesium Line Sources

Perpendicular Distance from the Source (cm)	Distance from Center of Source Along Source Axis (cm)									
	0.0	0.5	1.0	1.5	2.0	2.5	3.0	3.5	4.0	5.0
Cesium –137; Active Length 1.4 cm; Wall Thickness 1.0 mm Stainless Steel										
0.5	3.393	4.094	8.500	19.50	36.76	60.17	89.96	126.2	169.3	276.8
1.0	10.49	11.91	17.10	27.50	43.58	65.35	93.00	126.6	166.5	266.5
1.5	22.04	23.84	29.64	40.19	56.01	77.22	104.1	136.8	175.5	271.6
2.0	38.28	40.29	46.50	57.37	73.26	94.35	120.9	153.3	191.0	285.7
2.5	59.32	61.47	67.96	79.19	95.23	116.5	142.9	175.1	212.6	306.5
3.0	85.33	87.53	94.23	105.7	122.1	143.4	170.1	202.3	239.7	333.8
3.5	116.3	118.6	125.5	137.1	153.9	175.5	202.3	235.0	272.6	366.3
4.0	152.6	154.9	162.0	173.8	190.5	212.6	239.7	272.6	310.5	403.5
4.5	194.1	196.2	203.5	215.8	232.7	255.1	282.3	316.0	353.6	449.2
5.0	241.3	243.8	250.6	263.6	280.1	302.7	330.7	364.4	403.5	499.5
Cesium-137; Active Length 3.0 cm; Wall Thickness 0.5 mm Stainless Steel										
0.5	5.541	5.681	6.361	9.584	21.19	41.38	68.28	101.5	141.2	241.3
1.0	14.08	14.61	16.65	22.00	33.22	51.53	76.47	107.6	144.9	238.1
1.5	26.48	27.44	30.71	37.49	49.33	67.13	91.22	121.5	157.7	248.0
2.0	43.26	44.57	48.79	56.69	69.28	87.32	111.1	140.9	176.4	266.5
2.5	64.70	66.26	71.21	79.98	93.37	111.8	135.8	165.3	200.6	290.3
3.0	90.99	92.76	98.25	107.7	121.7	140.6	165.0	194.6	230.4	318.9
3.5	122.3	124.2	130.1	140.3	154.9	174.2	199.0	228.9	264.5	353.6
4.0	158.7	160.9	167.3	177.7	193.0	212.6	238.1	268.5	305.2	394.6
4.5	200.6	202.9	209.5	220.4	235.7	256.9	282.3	313.3	350.1	443.6
5.0	248.0	250.6	256.9	268.5	284.6	305.2	332.2	362.6	401.3	492.6
Cesium-137; Active Length 4.5 cm; Wall Thickness 0.5 mm Stainless Steel										
0.5	7.675	7.733	7.944	8.528	10.64	20.25	42.31	73.26	111.3	208.8
1.0	18.04	18.28	19.15	21.19	26.03	36.89	56.37	84.13	119.2	209.5
1.5	31.83	32.35	34.09	37.75	44.67	56.82	75.90	102.2	135.8	222.5
2.0	49.64	50.41	53.06	58.16	66.75	80.16	99.48	125.5	158.0	242.9
2.5	71.78	72.88	76.31	82.57	92.64	107.1	127.1	153.3	185.5	269.5
3.0	98.65	99.90	104.1	111.4	122.5	138.2	143.1	185.5	217.8	301.4
3.5	137.9	131.8	136.6	144.9	157.0	173.4	195.2	221.8	255.1	338.5
4.0	167.3	168.9	174.2	183.1	196.2	213.2	235.7	263.6	297.6	382.0
4.5	209.5	211.3	216.4	226.0	239.7	257.9	281.2	310.5	343.4	384.0
5.0	256.9	258.8	264.5	274.7	289.2	307.9	332.2	360.7	396.8	482.6

Uses conversion 1 cGy/mgh ≈ 71.45 cGy cm² air-kerma for 10 cGy (see Section 17.4.3).

Based on data from Krishnaswamy, V., Radiology, Vol 105, p181-184, 1972.

suggest a modified geometric factor that is based on expressions (17–30) to (17–32).[6,27,28] For example, for point S of Figure 17.6e, based on expression (17–31), it is given by

$$G(r, \phi) = [\phi_2 - \phi_1]/[L_a h] \tag{17–35}$$

17.7 A SIMPLE LINE SOURCE TREATMENT

Table 17.6 is a linear-source dosage table that was originally derived for radium sources. The table gives the equivalent air-kerma yield for delivery of 10 cGy in tissue at different distances from the source along its mid-perpendicular line for sources of different lengths. The sources are assumed to be bare (i.e., unencapsulated). The table is useful for planning of treatments with a single linear source, as illustrated in the following example.

TABLE 17.6
Linear Source Dosage Table: Air-Kerma Yield (cGy cm^2) for Delivery of 10 cGy (in Water)

Active Length	Perpendicular Distance from the Source (cm)						
(cm)	0.5	0.75	1.00	1.50	2.00	2.50	3.00
0.0	2.31	5.09	9.18	20.67	36.71	57.38	82.61
0.5	2.55	5.40	9.33	20.98	36.87	57.62	82.76
1.0	2.93	5.94	9.80	21.37	37.33	58.08	83.45
1.5	3.63	6.63	10.64	22.14	38.33	58.93	84.46
2.0	4.24	7.56	11.80	23.22	39.57	60.16	85.92
2.5	4.94	8.64	12.96	24.68	41.26	61.70	87.70
3.0	5.71	9.64	14.19	26.46	43.04	63.55	89.70
3.5	6.48	10.80	15.66	28.38	44.97	65.79	91.94
4.0	7.25	11.80	16.97	30.23	47.13	68.34	94.25
5.0	8.95	14.11	19.98	34.17	52.06	73.81	99.81
6.0	10.64	16.51	22.91	38.41	57.23	79.83	106.3
7.0	12.26	18.82	25.99	42.65	62.63	86.23	113.4
8.0	13.88	21.13	29.31	47.20	68.41	92.86	120.9
9.0	15.43	23.68	32.47	51.75	74.28	99.65	128.7
10.0	17.05	25.99	35.71	56.38	80.37	106.7	136.8
12.0	20.29	30.93	42.11	65.79	92.25	121.3	153.8
14.0	23.60	35.94	48.67	75.28	104.5	136.4	171.2
16.0	26.92	41.03	55.15	84.84	117.1	151.9	189.1
18.0	30.39	45.97	61.86	94.41	129.8	167.4	207.2
20.0	33.71	51.06	68.41	104.3	142.6	182.9	226.0

Original data giving mgh for 1000 R from Meredith, W.J., Radium Dosage — The Manchester System, Williams & Wilkins, Baltimore, MD, 1967, have been converted as shown in Example 17.1 in text (Section 17.4.3).

Example 17.3

It is desired to treat an obstructive bronchial lesion with local irradiation by insertion of a straight 7 cm long radioactive wire. The plan is to deliver a dose of 2000 cGy at 0.5 cm from the axis of the airway in 48 h. Calculate (i) the source strength required and (ii) the dose delivered in the central region at 1.0 cm from the source.

Let us say that the source strength is S_{ak} and the treatment time is τ.

(i) From Table 17.6, a source of 7 cm active length will deliver 10 cGy at 0.5 cm, if the air-kerma yield $S_{ak} \times \tau$ equals 12.26 cGy cm^2. For delivery of 2000 cGy, the required air-kerma yield is

$$S_{ak} \times \tau = \left[12.26 \text{ cGy cm}^2 / 10 \text{ cGy} \right] \times 2000 \text{ cGy} = 2452 \text{ cGy cm}^2$$

Because $\tau = 48$ h, the source strength S_{ak} needed is

$$S_{ak} = 2452 \text{ cGy cm}^2/48 \text{ h} = 51.1 \text{ cGy cm}^2 \text{ h}^{-1}$$

(ii)   From Table 17.6, we obtain a value of 25.99 cGy cm² for a central point 1 cm away from a 7 cm long source. The dose delivered at 1 cm for 2452 cGy cm² is

$$\left[10 \text{ cGy}/25.99 \text{ cGy cm}^2\right] \times 2452 \text{ cGy cm}^2 = 943 \text{ cGy}$$

Sometimes a string of point sources can be used as a substitute for a linear source. Point sources loaded in a nylon tube can give flexibility for passage through curved airways. The dose distribution possible with multiple point sources spaced 1 cm apart is illustrated in Figure 17.8.

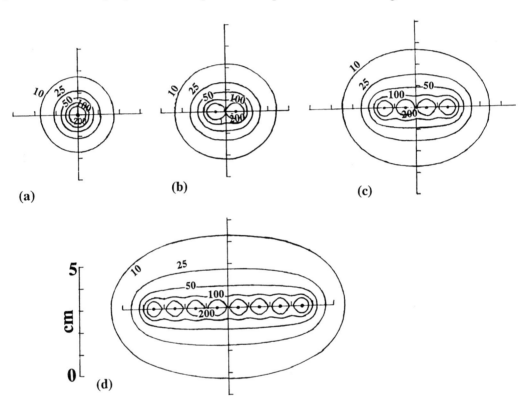

FIGURE 17.8 Radioactive seeds used as dose building blocks: (a) a single seed, (b) two seeds, (c) four seeds, (d) eight seeds. All isodose curves are normalized to 100% in the central region at a distance 5 mm away from the source.

Example 17.4

It is decided to treat the case in the previous example by use of radioactive seeds loaded at 1-cm spacing in a nylon ribbon. The seeds available are of strength 5.8 cGy cm² h⁻¹. Calculate the treatment time, assuming that it is possible to approximate a line source by a series of point sources.

The 7-cm radioactive length needed can be made up of 8 seeds at 1-cm spacing.

The total source strength of 8 seeds = 8 × 5.8 cGy cm² h⁻¹ = 46.4 cGy cm² h⁻¹.

Total cGy cm² of treatment (from Example 17.3) = 2452 cGy cm².

Time of treatment = 2452 cGy cm²/46.4 cGy cm² h⁻¹ = 52.8 h. The treatment time has been changed from the initial plan of 48 h to 52.8 h to accommodate the source strength available for use. It is worthwhile to mention here that only marginal changes in the treatment duration can be accepted. Any major change in the treatment time can have a bearing on the radiobiological response and the treatment outcome.

17.8 FORMING MULTIPLE SOURCE ARRAYS

17.8.1 SOURCES AS DOSE BUILDING BLOCKS

Brachytherapy is a local irradiation technique in which the irradiation takes place just around the sources. We can regard the sources as "dose building blocks." The sources can be arranged to make a geometric pattern to spread the dose delivered and to fashion the dose distribution. Figure 17.8 demonstrates the use of adjacent point sources for producing source arrays that give line source-like dose distributions. In the same manner, several line sources can be used with suitable spacing between them to produce a planar source array. Having several planes of sources can create a volume source array. In clinical situations, the source arrays should be planned and positioned appropriately in relation to the tissues targeted for irradiation.

17.8.2 UNIFORM VS. DIFFERENTIALLY DISTRIBUTED ARRAYS

When sources are spread over an area or volume, the two characteristics of the array that need to be planned are the spatial distribution and the source strength distribution. With regard to spacing of the sources, the practice has been to keep it simple by adopting a uniform spacing between sources. With regard to the distribution of source strengths, two different approaches, a uniform distribution and a differential distribution, have been used.

In the first approach, the sources are such that the total source strength can be spread out uniformly over the area or volume. This can be accomplished by use of either point sources of identical strengths or linear sources of the same linear strengths. Such a uniform source strength distribution is known to result in a nonuniform dose distribution, giving a higher dose in the central regions of the source array than at the periphery.

In the second approach, that of using a differential source strength distribution, the area or volume that is implanted is visualized to be made up of a central "core" zone and a peripheral "rind" zone. The strength of the sources used in the core zone is less than that used in the rind zone; that is, the source strength is located preferentially in the periphery. Such a differential distribution of source strengths in favor of the periphery can produce a more uniform dose. The differences in the dose distributions as obtained by the two approaches are elucidated in a series of examples that follow.

Figures 17.9a and b show orthogonal planar views of a single-plane implant that has five parallel line sources of 6-cm active length with a 1-cm spacing between the sources. All sources are of the same strength. Four different planes, A, B, C, and D, have been selected for examination of the dose distribution. Planes A and B are parallel to the source plane. Plane A contains the sources and plane B is 0.5 cm away from plane A. Planes C and D are perpendicular to the sources. Plane C passes through the central part of the implant and plane D is at 1 cm inward from the ends of the line sources. The isodose distributions shown in Figures 17.9c, d, e, and f are, respectively, applicable to planes A, B, C, and D. The isodose curves are normalized, with the dose received at the center of plane B (which is located 0.5 cm away from the implanted plane) taken as 100%.

The isodose pattern in Figure 17.9c shows high-dose regions of 150% or more. Such high-dose regions appear as discrete volumes surrounding individual sources. The 100% isodose curve covers a contiguous volume that circumscribes adjacent sources. In Figure 17.9e, the dose falls off rapidly with distance from 100% at 0.5 cm to about 60% at 1.0 cm, in the direction perpendicular to the plane of the implant. Figure 17.9d shows that the dose delivered is 100% at the center and falls off to 60–80% at the periphery and in the corners. This is also reflected in Figure 17.9f, which represents the peripheral zone near the source ends.

Figure 17.10 shows the dose distribution in a plane 0.5 cm away from the implanted plane for four possible variations in source arrangements. The source arrays considered are presented in the figure. Figure 17.10a is identical to Figure 17.9d, with the five parallel line sources all having the same strength. In Figure 17.10b, the linear source strengths of the two sources at the periphery are $1\frac{1}{2}$ times that of the three sources in the middle region. This gives a more uniform dose distribution. Doses in the range of 90 to 95% are seen in the lateral edge regions. This configuration of sources

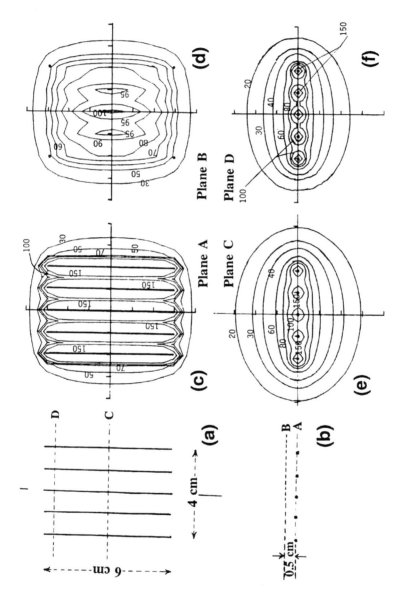

FIGURE 17.9 An array of five parallel linear sources of 6 cm active length, evenly spaced 1 cm apart. All sources are of the same linear source strength. (a) Side view showing planes C and D perpendicular to the sources. (b) End-on view showing plane A containing the sources and plane B 0.5 cm away from it. (c), (d), (e), and (f) give isodose curves in planes A, B, C, and D, respectively. Isodose curves are normalized to 100% at the center of plane B.

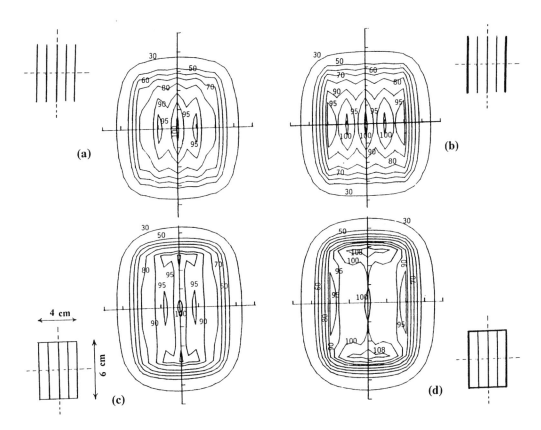

FIGURE 17.10 Isodose distribution in the plane 0.5 cm away from the plane of the implant for four different linear source arrrays occupying a 4 cm wide, 6 cm long area. In (a) and (b), all sources are of the same linear strength. In (c) and (d), the linear strength of the peripheral sources is 1.5 times the linear strength of the inner sources. In (c) and (d), the ends are crossed.

and source strengths is far more uniform than the distribution in Figure 17.10a, but has not improved the doses received in the end regions.

Figure 17.10c shows sources of one uniform source strength, but has two perpendicular line sources added which "cross" the ends. The crossing of the ends removes the fall-off of dose in the end regions, but the low doses in the lateral regions remain. An all-over improvement in dose uniformity is seen in Figure 17.10d, which makes use of both crossed ends and sources of a higher linear source strength in the periphery.

Figure 17.11 illustrates the dose distributions obtained for a two-plane implant that uses linear sources of the same uniform linear strength with uncrossed ends. The isodose curves displayed in Figures 17.11c, d, e, and f are for the four planes identified as A, B, C, and D in Figures 17.11a and b. Figure 17.12 is a two-plane array of the same geometric configuration as in Figure 17.11, but uses peripheral sources that have $1\frac{1}{2}$ times the linear source strength of the central sources.

Figure 17.13 shows a radioactive-seed implant of a spherical volume. The source array as seen in seven different cuts through the sphere is presented in Figures 17.13a to d. The isodose curves are shown for a plane through the center of the sphere bearing the radioactive sources (Figure 17.13f) and for an adjacent parallel plane 0.5 cm away and falling half-way between the source planes (Figure 17.13g). The former shows the high-value isodose curves of 160% encircling 13 implanted seeds. The latter shows the gradual fall-off of the dose from the center (160%) to the periphery (80 to 90%) and only one seed encircled by the 160% isodose curve.

Figure 17.14 is a variation of the same volume implant, but it uses, on the periphery of the sphere, seeds of strength $1\frac{1}{2}$ times that of those at the center, as is illustrated for one central cut in Figure 17.14a. The isodose curves are displayed for a central plane carrying the sources (Figure

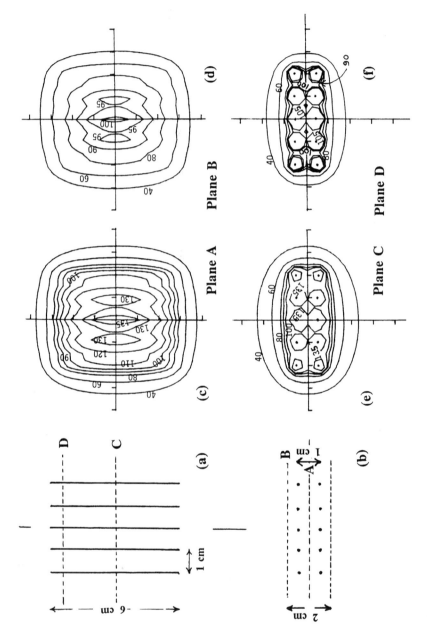

FIGURE 17.11 A two-plane implant having five parallel linear sources of 6 cm active length, evenly spaced 1 cm apart in each plane, with an interplanar separation of 1 cm. All sources are of the same linear source strength. (a) Side view showing planes C and D perpendicular to the sources. (b) End-on view showing plane A midway between the source planes and plane B 0.5 cm away from a source plane. (c), (d), (e), and (f) give isodose curves in planes A, B, C, and D, respectively. Isodose curves are normalized to 100% at the center of plane B.

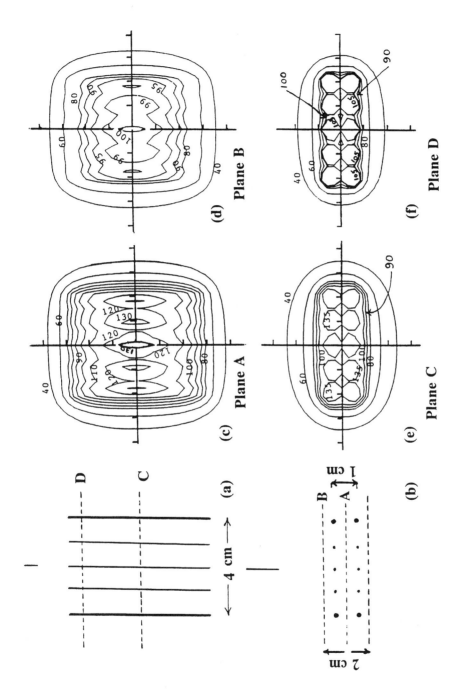

FIGURE 17.12 A two-plane implant consisting of five parallel linear sources of 6 cm active length, evenly spaced 1 cm apart in each plane and with an interplanar separation of 1 cm. The peripheral sources have 1.5 times the linear strength of the inner sources. (a) Side view showing planes C and D perpendicular to the sources. (b) End-on view showing plane A midway between the source planes and plane B 0.5 cm away from a source plane. (c), (d), (e), and (f) give isodose curves in planes A, B, C, and D, respectively. Isodose curves are normalized to 100% at the center of plane B.

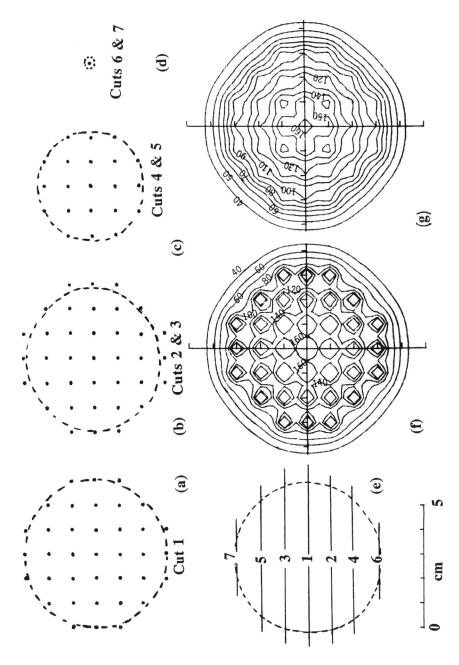

FIGURE 17.13 A near-spherical volume implant of radioactive seeds of uniform strength. (a), (b), (c), and (d) show the array of seeds as visualized in cuts 1–7 through the sphere as indicated in (e). (f) Isodose curves in cut 1 containing the sources, and (g) isodose curves in a plane between cuts 1 and 2. 100% dose has been chosen to be midway between cuts 1 and 2 and between the peripheral sources.

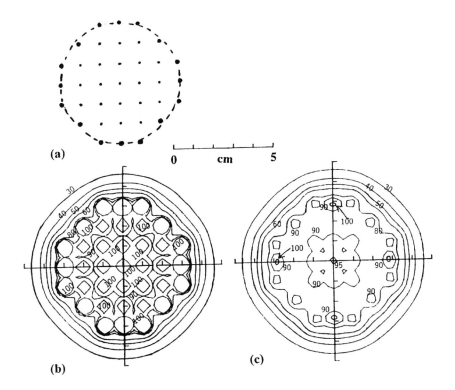

FIGURE 17.14 A near-spherical array of radioactive seeds geometrically identical to that shown in Figure 17.13, but with the strength of the seeds on the surface increased to 3/2 times that of those inside. (a) The array of seeds as seen in cut 1 (see Figure 17.13). (b) Isodose curves in cut 1. (c) Isodose curves between cuts 1 and 2 (see Figure 17.13). 100% dose has been chosen to be midway between cuts 1 and 2 and between the peripheral sources.

17.14b and a plane midway between the source planes (Figure 17.14c). In both of these planes the uniformity of dose delivery is much better than that in Figure 17.13. The fall-off of dose outside the implanted volume is rapid in either case.

Figure 17.15 addresses the situation of a cylindrical mold used for irradiation of the surface of a cylindrical body part. Figures 17.15a and b show twelve linear sources that have been placed at angular intervals of 30° on the surface of a cylindrical plastic applicator of 1 cm thickness. All sources have the same strength. Isodose curves are shown for a mid-plane perpendicular to the sources (Figure 17.15c) and a plane parallel to the sources through the axis of the cylinder (Figure 17.15d). The 100% dose level is assigned to the inner surface of the mold at 1 cm depth from the outer surface. It will be noticed that the middle region of the surface receives a uniform dose, with some fall-off near the source ends. The central region of the body part irradiated receives 80%. As we move along the cylinder axis away from the center, the dose falls off to 60–50%.

For more illustrations of brachytherapy dose distributions, the reader is advised to refer to published atlases.[39,40]

17.9 SYSTEMS FOR BRACHYTHERAPY

17.9.1 WHAT ARE SYSTEMS OR APPROACHES?

Brachytherapy irradiations result in a rather nonuniform dose delivery compared to the uniformity levels possible in external-beam therapy. In any implant, the doses to tissues close to the sources are bound to be very high. The dose falls off with distance from the sources, and the surface of an implanted target volume may receive a lower dose than does its core. Planning of practical treatments in brachytherapy can involve the following three stages:

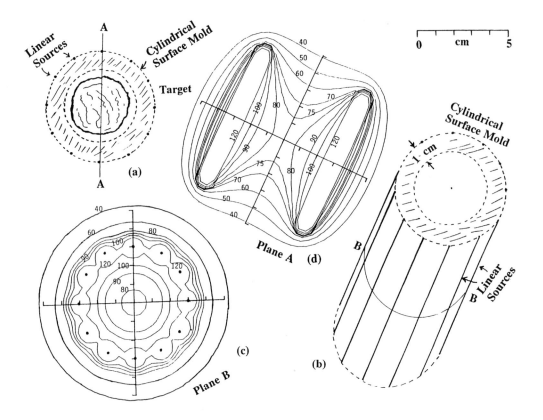

FIGURE 17.15 A linear source array on the surface of a cylindrical mold of 1 cm thickness. (a) Cut view perpendicular to the cylinder axis. (b) Overall view of the mold and the linear sources. (c) Isodose curves in the central plane B, shown in (b), perpendicular to the sources. (d) Isodose curves in plane A, shown in (a), containing the cylindrical axis and passing through a pair of sources. The 100% value is the dose between the sources on the inner surface of the mold.

(a)   Identification and delimiting of the tumor extent and the target volume
(b)   Planning of the source array in terms of the number of sources to be used, their relative strengths, and their positions to produce an acceptable dose distribution
(c)   Assessment of a "reference dose rate" and the duration of treatment for delivery of a stated or prescribed radiation dose

There are different practices for, or approaches to, the above steps. These are also referred to as different brachytherapy systems.

17.9.2 QUIMBY APPROACH

The approach called the "Quimby system" conceived of uniformly distributed arrays of sources of the same strength and provided tables of data for calculation of the reference dose rate for such arrays.[41,42] We already saw, through examples, how a uniform distribution of source strength results in poor uniformity of dose delivery, and how certain nonuniform distributions of source strength result in a more uniform dose delivery. For *planar* source arrays, Quimby adopted the dose delivered at the central point at different distances from the source plane as the reference dose. Figures 17.16a and b illustrate a Quimby-type rectangular planar implant made with evenly spaced line sources of the same linear activity. For *volume* implants, Quimby's tables adopted the minimum dose in the region between the sources on the surface of the implant as the reference dose. This dose is called the minimum peripheral dose (MPD). Tables 17.7 and 17.8 give data for calculation of the reference doses for planar and volume implants by the Quimby approach.

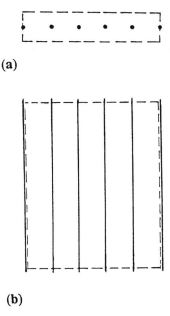

(a)

(b)

FIGURE 17.16 (a) End-on and (b) side views of a Quimby-type single-plane implant. Sources are evenly spaced and are of uniform activity, with the implanted area matching the target cross section as shown by dashed lines.

17.9.3 PARIS APPROACH

The approach called the "Paris system"[43-45] addresses the use of linear radioactive wires of uniform linear strength. Wires of ^{192}Ir are cut to desired lengths and are implanted with a chosen uniform spacing between them. The source ends are left uncrossed. To avoid any underdosing of the end regions of the target volume because of the uncrossed ends, the system specifies that the length of the implanted wires extend beyond the target volume by 10 to 20%. The spacing between the source lines can be flexible, falling in the range of 0.5 to 2.2 cm, with the larger spacing intended for larger volumes and for wires of 10 cm or more in length. An indication of the mean thickness, **t**, of the target volume for a single-plane implant can be derived as 60% of the spacing, **e**, employed between the source lines. This means that if **e** = 1.0 cm, then **t** ≈ 0.6 cm, and if **e** = 1.5 cm, then **t** ≈ 0.9 cm.

Figures 17.17a and b illustrate the relationship of the source array to the target volume and the reference isodose curve in the Paris approach. In the Paris practice, basic dose points (shown by x marks) that are in the central part of the array midway between adjacent source lines are identified. The dose rates at these points are the minimal dose rates in the region between the sources. The numerical average of the dose rates at these points is evaluated and is referred to as the basic dose rate. In the Paris approach, the stated dose and the duration of treatment are based on a reference dose rate that is chosen to be 85% of the basic dose rate. The target volume is, accordingly, the volume covered by the isodose surface for this 85% dose.

In brachytherapy with implanted sources, it is inevitable that the tissues adjoining any source will receive the highest dose. However, these very high doses seem to be well tolerated because the volumes of tissue they cover are not contiguous, but are distributed around the various discrete sources. The basic dose value obtained between two adjacent sources has the significance of representing the maximum dose level at which the isodose volume becomes contiguous to go around both sources. For dose levels that exceed the basic dose, the isodose volumes become discrete volumes that surround the individual sources.

For two-plane or volume implants, the wires are located at corners of either rectangles or equilateral triangles, as shown in Figures 17.17c and d. For these, the dose rates at the central

TABLE 17.7
Dosage Table for Single-Plane Array of Uniformly Distributed Sources:
Air-kerma Yield (cGy cm²) to Deliver 10 cGy in Water

Distance (cm)	Circular Areas Diameter (cm)					
	1.0	**2.0**	**3.0**	**4.0**	**5.0**	**6.0**
0.5	3.40	5.79	7.95	13.1	16.9	23.1
1.0	10.5	13.6	17.0	23.1	28.5	35.0
1.5	21.8	25.0	30.9	36.7	43.4	52.5
2.0	38.3	41.8	46.8	54.0	61.3	70.8
2.5	56.7	61.3	66.7	73.7	89.1	97.6
3.0	84.1	88.7	94.1	101.9	110.5	120.7

Distance (cm)	Square Areas Side of Square (cm)					
	1.0	**2.0**	**3.0**	**4.0**	**5.0**	**6.0**
0.5	3.55	6.17	8.87	15.2	19.3	27.0
1.0	10.9	14.5	18.4	25.2	31.2	3.49
1.5	22.8	26.6	32.0	39.4	46.3	56.7
2.0	38.6	44.0	49.7	57.6	66.0	77.2
2.5	56.3	61.3	69.1	77.9	88.0	105.7
3.0	84.1	88.7	98.0	107.3	117.3	128.9

Distance (cm)	Rectangular Areas Length of Sides (cm)					
	1 × 1.5	**2 × 3**	**3 × 4**	**4 × 6**	**6 × 9**	**8 × 12**
0.5	3.94	7.95	11.0	22.1	44.0	73.7
1.0	11.4	16.5	21.1	32.9	56.0	85.6
1.5	23.0	28.5	36.0	48.1	72.9	104.6
2.0	39.0	45.5	55.2	67.1	95.7	128.9
2.5	55.6	64.8	76.4	88.0	117.3	154.3
3.0	85.6	91.8	103.2	117.3	148.9	192.9

Uses the conversion 1 mgh for 1000 R ≈ 7.716 × 10⁻² cGy cm² air kerma yield for 10 cGy (see Section 17.4.3). Reference points for dosage are at different distances perpendicular to the source plane opposite the center of the source array.

Based on data from Glasser, O., Quimby, E.H., Taylor, L., and Weatherwax, J.L., Physical Foundations of Radiology, Paul Hoeber, New York, 1952.

points (as indicated by crosses) within the triangles or rectangles in the midplane of the implant need to be evaluated and averaged to yield the basic dose rate.

17.9.4 APPROACH OF MEMORIAL HOSPITAL IN NEW YORK

The approach to the design of source arrays and evaluation of the dose delivered as developed at Memorial Hospital, New York, is referred to as the New York or Memorial system. This system adopts the use of sources of uniform activity in a uniform spacing. Laughlin et al.,[46] in 1963, published dosage tables for planar and volume implants of seeds of uniform strength spaced 1 cm apart. For single-plane implants, their reference dose was the minimum peripheral dose, defined as the dose at a point opposite the corner of the implanted area in a plane 0.5 cm away from the plane of the implant. For volume implants, they defined a minimum peripheral dose (MPD), a centerline peripheral dose (CPD), and a maximum reference dose. MPD represented the dose obtained half-way between adjacent seeds near a corner of an array. CPD referred to the dose half-

TABLE 17.8
Volume Implant Dosage Table: Quimby System —
Air-Kerma Yield to Deliver 10 cGy Minimum Peripheral Dose

Volume (cm³)	Air-Kerma Yield (cGy cm²)	Diameter of Sphere (cm)	Air-Kerma Yield (cGy cm²)
5	15.4	1.0	3.09
10	24.7	1.5	7.72
15	30.1	2.0	13.9
20	34.0	2.5	21.6
30	41.7	3.0	30.1
40	47.8	3.5	36.7
60	57.9	4.0	44.4
80	67.1	4.5	52.1
100	77.2	5.0	61.0
125	86.4	6.0	82.6
150	96.5	7.0	108.0
175	107.3		
200	115.7		
250	129.6		
300	138.9		

Uses the conversion 1 mgh for 1000 R ≈ 7.716×10^{-2} cGy cm² air-kerma yield for 10 cGy (see Section 17.4.3).

Based on data from Glasser, O., Quimby, E.H., Taylor, L.S., and Weatherwax, J.L., *Physical Foundations of Radiology*, 2nd Edition, Paul B. Hoeber, New York, 1952.

way between adjacent seeds in the central region of the surface of an array. The maximum reference dose was the dose obtained between adjacent seeds in the central core of the implant.

The dosage tables for planar and volume implants as derived by the Memorial group are modified and presented in Tables 17.9 and 17.10, respectively. Revised tables for planar implants have been published more recently by Anderson et al.[47] for the New York system. These data, presented in Table 17.11, apply to an array of parallel nylon ribbons carrying radioactive seeds spaced 1 cm apart. The point for the reference dose has been defined to be the point lying midway between the two edge ribbons at 1.5 seed spacings inward along the ribbons from the source ends.

For permanent volume implants of ^{125}I seeds, the New York approach is based on the average dimensions (rather than the volume) of the target region to be implanted. The system specifies the total initial source strength to be implanted[48-50] as a function of the average dimension. This method is called the dimension-averaging method. It results in delivery of increasing doses to increasing volumes.[51] Nomograms for planning the number of seeds and the strength of seeds by the New York approach have been published.[52,53]

17.9.5 MANCHESTER APPROACH OF PATERSON AND PARKER

Paterson and Parker[54-56] evolved very sophisticated and comprehensive source distribution rules and dosage tables for brachytherapy practice. In their approach, which is called the Manchester system, they considered arrays of different possible geometries and provided guidelines for the spacings between the sources, the source strengths to be used, and dosage tables for calculation of the treatment time.[54-57] A spacing of 1 cm between sources for a single-plane implant was suggested. They recommended a nonuniform distribution of source strengths to obtain improved dose uniformity. The principle was to concentrate the source strengths more in the peripheral regions of the array than at the center. For example, they recommended that, for a rectangular array (see Figure 17.18a and b), if ρ is the linear source strength of four line sources forming the periphery, the linear source strength for the sources in the central region should be 2ρ/3. If there were only one

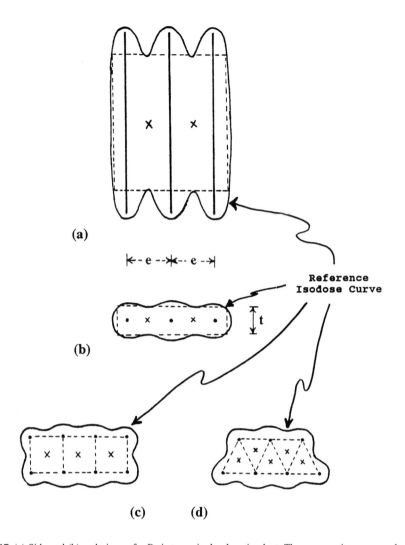

FIGURE 17.17 (a) Side and (b) end views of a Paris-type single-plane implant. The source wires are evenly spaced and are of equal linear strength. The implanted area is 20% larger than the target cross section marked by the dashed lines. (c) A rectangular configuration of source wires in a two-plane implant. (d) A triangular configuration of source wires. Cross marks, x, indicate the reference points where the basic doses are evaluated. Dots mark the source locations in (b), (c), and (d). The reference isodose curve, taken to be 85% of the basic dose, is shown in each plane.

central line, the recommended linear source strength would be $\rho/2$. Such nonuniform loading reduced the disparity between the central dose and the peripheral dose. This also demanded the use of sources of different strengths at the center and at the periphery. Thus, a complicated inventory of sources consisting of varying linear strengths was needed. (This is unlike the philosophy in the Paris and Quimby systems of using sources of uniform linear strength to keep the inventory simple, even if it does not give the best possible uniformity of dose distribution.) The reference dose in the Manchester system is an effective minimum dose called net minimum dose (NMD), defined to be 10% higher than the actual minimum dose. Tables 17.12, 17.13, and 17.14 are dosage tables for surface molds, single-plane implants, and volume implants when the sources are arranged according to the Manchester distribution rules.

An overview of the Manchester system can enrich our understanding of the physics of brachytherapy. Many insights provided by the Manchester system are useful for the day-to-day practice of brachytherapy, even if the system may not be fully adhered to. For this reason, in Section 17.10,

TABLE 17.9
Planar Implant Dosage Table: Air-Kerma Yield to Deliver 10 cGy to Designated
Reference Points for Planar Point Source Arrays

| | Reference Point | | |
Area (cm²)	Peripheral Point (cGy cm²)	Central Point (cGy cm²)	Ratio of central to Peripheral Dose
1	6.84	6.05	1.13
2	8.36	6.77	1.23
3	9.94	7.71	1.29
4	11.9	8.93	1.33
5	13.6	9.94	1.37
6	15.2	11.0	1.39
7	17.0	12.0	1.42
8	18.4	12.8	1.44
9	20.2	13.9	1.45
10	21.6	14.7	1.47
12	24.6	16.4	1.50
14	27.4	18.0	1.52
16	30.2	19.6	1.54
18	32.7	21.0	1.56
20	35.2	22.4	1.57
25	41.1	25.5	1.61
30	46.8	28.7	1.63
35	52.9	31.8	1.66
40	58.5	34.9	1.68
45	64.3	38.0	1.69
50	70.1	41.0	1.71

Note: Modified Memorial System. The sources are of uniform strength spaced 1 cm apart. The peripheral and the central reference points lie in a plane 5 mm away from the source plane opposite the interspace between corner sources and the central sources, respectively. Values are based on data from Laughlin, J.S., Siler, W.M., Holodney, E.I. et al., Am. J. Roentgenol., Vol 89, p470-490, 1963. Uses a conversion 1 mgh for 1000 rad $\approx 7.205 \times 10^{-2}$ cGy cm² for 10 cGy (see Section 17.4.3).

we provide a brief review of the distribution rules of the Manchester system, recommending to the reader References 54 and 57 for a more detailed study.

17.9.6 PITFALLS OF MIXING SYSTEMS OR APPROACHES

Apart from the systems discussed above, various other approaches have been outlined (for example, References 58 to 64) for planning the source arrays and determining the treatment time. It is to be noted that the relationship of the source arrays with respect to the target volume, the nonuniformity of the dose distribution accepted for treatment, and the basis of the stated dose are all subject to variation, based on the system or approach used. Some articles have compared the differences in these respects between various approaches.[65-69]

It is worth reiterating that the doses prescribed and delivered in brachytherapy are based on past clinical experience. Much caution should be exercised before one assumes that clinical results obtained with doses stated for any one system of practice can be adopted *in toto* for a practice that follows another system. It would be better to follow the same system or approach in planning, monitoring, and administration of the current treatment as was used for past treatments on which a prescription is based. This also means that the clinical results reported as having been obtained with stated doses in one institution practicing one particular system cannot be compared with the doses and results in another institution practicing another system, without taking into account the

TABLE 17.10
Volume Implant Dosage Table: Air-Kerma Yield (cGy cm²) to Deliver
10 cGy in Water at Selected Reference Points

Volume (cm³)	cGy cm² to Deliver 10 Gy			Central Dose Expressed as Multiple of	
	At Corner of Surface[a]	At Center of Surface[b]	At Center of Array[c]	Corner Surface Dose	Central Surface Dose
1	6.84	6.84	6.05	1.13	1.13
5	13.3	11.9	10.4	1.27	1.14
10	18.3	15.4	13.3	1.37	1.16
15	23.2	18.9	16.2	1.43	1.17
20	27.2	21.7	18.4	1.48	1.18
25	31.2	24.4	20.5	1.52	1.19
30	34.0	26.4	22.0	1.55	1.20
40	40.3	30.5	25.2	1.60	1.21
50	46.1	34.4	28.1	1.64	1.23
60	51.8	39.2	31.0	1.67	1.24
80	62.3	45.0	36.0	1.73	1.25
100	72.0	51.5	40.7	1.77	1.27
120	81.4	57.6	45.0	1.81	1.28
140	89.3	63.0	49.0	1.83	1.29
160	98.3	68.6	53.0	1.86	1.30
180	106.3	73.5	56.6	1.88	1.30
200	113.5	78.5	59.8	1.90	1.31
250	132.6	90.1	68.1	1.95	1.32
300	149.9	100.9	75.6	1.98	1.34
350	166.4	111.7	83.2	2.00	1.34
400	183.0	121.8	90.4	2.20	1.35

Note: Modified Memorial System. Arrays are made of point sources of uniform strength spaced 1 cm apart.

[a] At a point between seeds at the corner of the surface of the array.
[b] At a point between seeds on the central region of the surface of the array.
[c] At a point between seeds in the central region of the array of sources.

Based on data from Laughlin, J.S., Siler, W.M., Holodny, E.I. et al., Am. J. Roentgenol., Vol 89, p470-490, 1963. Uses a conversion 1 mgh for 1000 rad ≈ 7.205×10^{-2} cGy cm² air-kerma yield for 10 cGy (see Section 17.4.3).

differences in the systems. Through interinstitutional and international study groups, the radiation oncology community should develop a universal system for the practice of brachytherapy that becomes acceptable to all institutions in the future.

It is also worthwhile to mention that the data tables for radium should be used with caution for planning of treatment with other radioisotope sources. This is because the dose rate depends not only on the air-kerma rate, but also on the values of $(f_{akmd})_{water}$ and WPC(r), both of which can vary for different sources. Fortunately, the variations of $(f_{akmd})_{water}$ and WPC(r) are not too significant among [226]Ra, ^{60}Co, ^{137}Cs, ^{192}Ir, and [198]Au, because all emit photons of sufficiently high energies. However, for ^{125}I and [103]Pd sources, which emit low-energy photons, only data tables especially generated for them should be used.

TABLE 17.11
Planar Implant Dosage Table for Iridium-192 Seeds: Air-Kerma Yield to
Deliver 10 cGy at the Reference Point

Area (cm²)	Air-Kerma Yield for 10 cGy (cGy cm²)
10	17.2
20	28.7
30	38.7
40	48.8
50	58.1
60	66.7
80	83.9
100	100.4
120	116.2
140	131.9
160	147.1
180	162.1
200	176.4
250	211.6
300	246.1
350	278.0
400	311.4

Note: Values derived from mgh for 1000 cGy from Anderson, L., Hilaris, B.S., and Wagner, L.K., Endocurietherapy/Hyperthermic Oncology, Vol 1, p9-15, 1985, assuming that 1 mg Raeq of iridium-192 yields 7.174 CGy cm² h⁻¹ air-kerma. Sources are in nylon ribbons implanted in parallel lines with 1 cm of interseed and interribbon spacing. The reference point is in a plane 5 mm away from the source plane and is removed from the corner seed of the array by 5 mm perpendicular to the ribbons and 15 mm along the ribbons.

17.10 MANCHESTER (PATERSON AND PARKER) DISTRIBUTION RULES

17.10.1 SURFACE APPLICATIONS

In surface applications, the sources are placed on top of a mold of thickness h placed on the surface area to be treated, which can be of any shape (circular, rectangular, or irregular). Paterson and Parker recommended ways of distributing the radioactive material to obtain ±10% uniformity of dose in the treated area. The reference dose was selected to be 10% above the minimum dose observed in the treated area. For rectangles, the low doses in the corner regions were disregarded. Thus, the reference dose became much like a single representative dose, valid within ±10%, stated for the entire area. Table 17.12 gives "area tables," which list the air-kerma yield that corresponds to delivery of a 10-cGy reference dose, when Paterson and Parker's distribution rules are followed. The data in the table are applicable to both circular and rectangular areas, if the source arrays conform to the recommended distribution rules.

Circular Areas: Distribution Rules

Let us assume that the treated area is a circle of diameter D and h is the distance between the source plane and the target plane. For very small circles with D < 3 h, the rule recommends that the radioactive material be placed uniformly around the periphery of the circle to provide ±10%

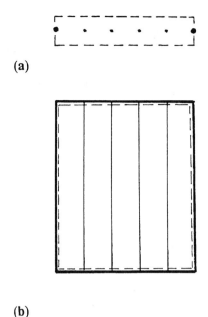

(a)

(b)

FIGURE 17.18 (a) End and (b) side views of a Manchester-type single-plane implant. Sources are distributed along the periphery and evenly in the central region, with the linear strength higher in the periphery. The implanted area matches the target cross section indicated by the dashed lines.

uniformity of dose in the treated area (Figure 17.19a). For $3 < D/h < 6$, the recommendation is to have, in addition to the peripheral circle, a central source having 5% of the total radioactive strength (Figure 17.19b). For still larger D/h values, two concentric circles of sources and a center source are recommended (Figure 17.19c), with the center source having 3% of the total radioactive strength. The distribution of the radioactive strength between the inner circle and the outer circle is to be a function of D/h, as given in Table 17.15.

Rectangular Areas: Distribution Rules

For rectangular areas, the approach illustrated in Figure 17.20 is to be followed. For areas of small width, the periphery alone is lined with radioactive sources. As the width increases, any underdosing of the central region of the target volume is avoided by addition of lines parallel to the long side of the rectangle at a spacing not exceeding 2h (where h is the distance between the source and target planes.) If L is the length and W the width of the rectangle, for $W < 2h$, only the peripheral sources are needed (Figure 17.20a). If W exceeds 2h, a central line source is added (Figure 17.20b). If W exceeds 4h, a second, parallel line source is added (Figure 17.20c). Every additional increment of W by 2h warrants addition of a line. If the linear source strength for the peripheral sources is ρ, a single added line should have a linear source strength of $\rho/2$. If there are multiple added lines, the recommended linear source strength for them is $2\rho/3$.

Areas of Irregular Shape: Distribution Rules

Any irregular shape to be treated can usually be approximated by either a circle or a rectangle. If such an approximation is not possible, the irregularly shaped periphery should first be lined with radioactive sources. Then, either the approach of using rings and a center source, as for circular areas, or the approach of using peripheral sources with added lines, as for rectangular areas, can be adopted.

TABLE 17.12

Dosage Table for Planar Molds with Source Arrays Conforming to the Manchester System: Air-Kerma Yield (cGy cm²) for Delivering 10 cGy to Water

Area (cm²)	Treatment Distance (cm)					
	0.5	1.0	1.5	2.0	3.0	5.0
1	5.25	13.19	—	—	—	—
2	7.48	16.43	28.93	46.14	92.30	240.48
3	9.26	19.06				
4	10.88	21.45	35.64	53.85	100.68	250.20
5	12.42	23.61				
6	13.66	25.69	41.35	60.31	108.40	259.22
8	15.89	29.63	46.21	50.91	115.73	267.86
10	18.13	33.41	50.53	71.21	122.67	276.20
15	23.30	42.12	60.87	83.55	138.21	295.79
20	28.39	49.45	70.21	94.51	152.68	314.77
30	37.80	61.33	88.11	114.72	178.99	349.80
40	46.52	72.06	103.84	133.62	202.13	381.28
50	54.39	82.70	117.42	151.06	184.93	410.98
60	61.72	93.04	129.77	168.19	243.79	438.98
80	75.68	113.41	151.68	197.66	282.14	489.90
100	89.11	132.39	172.66	222.96	317.86	536.60
150	148.46	177.68	225.30	277.97	—	—
200	145.04	217.56	274.65	330.82	—	—
300	192.49	289.08	367.23	434.35	—	—
400	237.62	356.43	450.56	529.56	—	—

Values have been derived from original data from Meredith, W.J., *Radium Dosage — The Manchester System*, Williams & Wilkins, Baltimore, MD, 1967, assuming that 1 mgh for 1000 R ≈ 7.716×10^{-2} cGy cm² air-kerma yield for 10 cGy. See Example 17.1 in text.

17.10.2 SINGLE-PLANE IMPLANTS

Single-plane implants are utilized for treating a slab of target volume having a cross section that matches the area covered by the sources and a thickness extending up to 0.5 cm from the source plane to either of its sides. The same distribution rules as proposed for surface applications can be adopted for implants, with the reference dose rate also maintained to be the net minimum dose in the plane 0.5 cm away. This means that the spacing between adjacent lines in a rectangular array cannot exceed $2 \times h = 2 \times 0.5$ cm = 1 cm.

The distribution rules for implants have also been presented in another form in terms of the way in which the total source strength can be divided between the periphery and the central region of the implant. The recommendation presented in Table 17.16 is useful for planning of treatments with radioactive seeds. Table 17.14 gives the dosage data for Manchester-type single-plane implants.

Thus far, we have assumed that it is always possible to line up the radioactive material along the periphery of the area to be treated. With some implants, this is not possible. For example, in the case of a rectangular tongue implant, the far side of the tongue may not be accessible for implanting, and thus the far side of the rectangle may remain uncrossed. In the Manchester system, the dose fall-off caused by an uncrossed end is presumed to cause the effective area treated to be 10% smaller than the implanted area. Therefore, if crossing an end is not possible in a practical situation, the length of the implant should extend 10% beyond the area that needs to be treated.

TABLE 17.13
Single-Plane Implant Dosage Table (Manchester System):
Air-Kerma Yield (cGy cm²) for Delivering 10 cGy to Water

Area (cm²)	cGy cm² for 10 cGy
0	2.31
2	7.48
3	9.26
4	10.88
5	12.42
6	13.66
8	15.89
10	18.13
15	23.26
20	28.39
30	37.80
40	46.52
50	54.39
60	61.72
80	75.68
100	89.11
150	118.4
200	145.0
300	192.5
400	237.6

Values are derived from original data from Meredith, W.J., Radium Dosage — The Manchester System, Williams & Wilkins, Baltimore, MD, 1967, assuming 1 mgh for 1000 R $\approx$ 7.716 × 10⁻² cGy cm² air-kerma yield for 10 cGy. See Example 17.1 in text.

17.10.3 TWO-PLANE IMPLANTS

The distribution rules for single-plane implants are also recommended for two-plane implants. The data for two-plane implants are obtained by multiplication of the data in Table 17.13 for single-plane implants by the two-plane correction factors given in Table 17.17. Together with the correction factor, the reference dose is the net minimum dose in the plane 0.5 cm outward from either implanted plane (and not between the planes).

17.10.4 VOLUME IMPLANTS

In a volume implant, the sources are implanted to cover an entire volume of tissue to be irradiated. An attempt can be made to encompass the tumor volume by one of several simple geometric shapes, such as a cylinder, cube, sphere, or ellipsoid. Paterson and Parker visualized any volume as consisting of two components, a rind and a core. The rind for the sphere is the surface or shell. For a cylinder, the rind consists of the curved surface and the two ends. For a cube, it is made up of the six faces. In all of these cases, the core is the whole volume enclosed within the surface. The amount of radioactivity implanted in the rind and the core should bear a suggested ratio. For this purpose, it is recommended that the total amount be divided into eight parts and then allocated as follows for the different shapes of the volumes implanted:

(a) Cylinder

      Belt, four parts
      Core, two parts

TABLE 17.14
Volume Implant Dosage Table (Manchester System):
Air-Kerma Yield for 10 cGy Reference Dose to Water

Volume (cm³)	(cGy cm²) for 10 cGy
1	2.63
2	4.17
3	5.47
4	6.63
5	7.69
10	12.2
15	16.0
20	19.4
25	22.5
30	25.4
40	30.8
50	35.7
60	40.3
70	44.7
80	48.8
90	52.8
100	56.7
125	64.4
150	74.3
200	90.0
250	104
300	118
350	131
400	143

Values are derived from data from Table E in Meredith, W.J., Radium Dosage — The Manchester System, Williams & Wilkins, Baltimore, MD, 1967. Uses a conversion 1 mgh for 1000 R ≈ 7.716×10^{-2} cGy cm² air-kerma yield for 10 cGy. See Example 17.1 in text.

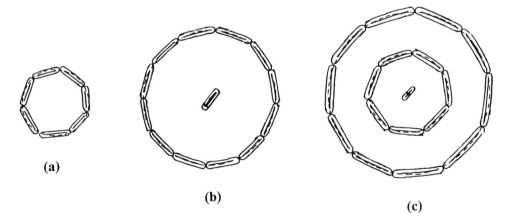

FIGURE 17.19 (a) Small circle with sources forming the periphery. (b) A larger circle with peripheral sources and a central source. (c) A still larger circle with pheripheral sources, a central source, and an inner ring of sources.

TABLE 17.15
Circular Areas: Source Strength Distribution

D/h	<3	>3<6	>6<7.5	>7.5<10	>10
Peripheral circle	100%	95%	80%	75%	70%
Center spot	0%	5%	3%	3%	3%
Inner circle	0%	0%	17%	22%	27%

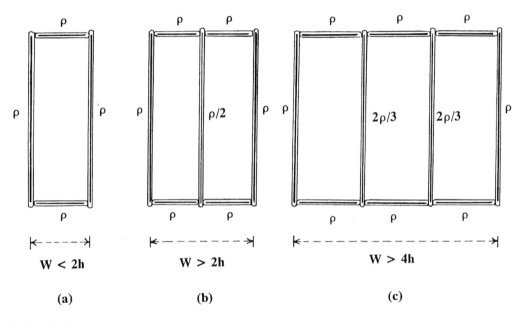

(a)   (b)   (c)

FIGURE 17.20 Rectangular arrays of area W × L; h is the distance between the source plane and the target plane. (a) A peripheral rectangle to be used when W < 2h. (b) Rectangle with one added line, to be used when 2h < W < 4h. (c) Rectangle with two added lines, to be used when W > 4h.

TABLE 17.16
Planar Implants: Distribution Rules

Area	<25 cm²	25–100 cm²	>100 cm²
Peripheral fraction of total source strength	2/3	1/2	1/3

TABLE 17.17
Two-Plane Separation Factors

Separation (cm)	Factor
1.5	1.25
2.0	1.4
2.5	1.5

The data for single-plane implant in Table 17.14 are to be increased by this factor. The specified dose is on planes at 0.5 cm away from either implanted plane, and not on the plane between them.

Each end, one part

(b) Sphere

Shell, six parts
Core, two parts

(c) Cube

Each side, one part
Each end, one part
Core, two parts

All of the above distributions adopt a surface-to-core ratio of 6:2 of radioactive material. The recommendation is to use sources at not more than 1.0- to 1.5-cm spacing and to spread them out as evenly as possible over the surfaces and within the volume.

Paterson and Parker provided a volume dosage table (Table 17.14) for dosage evaluations when their distribution rules are adopted. The stated reference dose is the "net minimum dose," which is defined to be 10% higher than the absolute minimum dose in the effective volume. The tabulated data apply directly to all shapes if the three dimensions, length, width, and height, are approximately equal for the volume implanted. However, if the volume is elongated, the source strength to be used should be increased by the elongation factors given in Table 17.18, according to the ratio of the longest to the shortest dimension.

TABLE 17.18
Elongation Correction Factors for Volumes

Longest Dimension ÷ Shortest Dimension	Correction Factor[a]
1.5	1.036
2	1.073
2.5	1.111
3	1.150

[a] Recommended multiplicative factor to increase the air-kerma yield to reference dose ratio in Manchester system.[57]

17.11 PLANNING AND IMPLEMENTING A PRACTICAL CASE

17.11.1 A SAMPLE TARGET VOLUME

Let us say that a breast lesion having a cross-sectional area of 4.5 cm × 4.5 cm and a thickness of 0.8 cm is to be implanted. For covering of the entire lesion with some margins, a volume having a cross section of 5.0 cm × 5.0 cm and a thickness of 1 cm is designated as the target volume. The plan is to deliver a dose of 2000 cGy in 40 h.

17.11.2 PLANNING THE GEOMETRY OF THE ARRAY

We can treat the lesion by a single-plane implant. Our plan is to use nylon ribbons carrying ^{192}Ir seeds at 1-cm spacing, with an inter-ribbon spacing of 1 cm, and to leave the ribbon ends uncrossed. We decide to follow the Paterson and Parker distribution rules. The rules state that any uncrossed end can cause a 10% reduction in the area treated. Hence, the active length of the implanted ribbons should extend beyond the intended target area by 10% if any end is left uncrossed. Thus, for covering a 5-cm length, an active length of 6 cm should be used. Figures 17.21a and b show the views of a proposed array of radioactive seeds in two mutually perpendicular planes. Six nylon ribbons are spaced at 1-cm intervals, covering a width of 5 cm. Each ribbon carries seven radioactive seeds, with 1-cm spacing between seeds to give an active length of 6 cm.

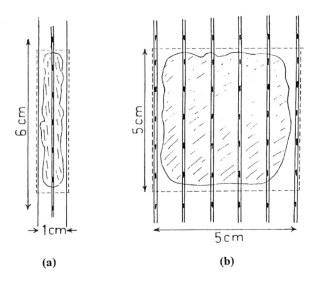

(a) **(b)**

FIGURE 17.21 (a) End and (b) side views of a single planar array of radioactive ^{192}Ir seeds in a nylon ribbon for treatment of a target volume having a 5 cm × 5 cm cross section.

17.11.3 DETERMINING THE SOURCE STRENGTHS

In this case, we have the following information:

Length of implanted area = 6 cm
Width of implanted area = 5 cm
Length of target area = 5 cm (6 cm reduced by 2 × 10% for 2 uncrossed ends)
Width of the target area = 5 cm
Target area = 5 cm × 5 cm = 25 cm^2

From the Paterson and Parker single-plane implant dosage table (Table 17.13), it is noted that a total air-kerma of 33.1 cGy cm^2 can deliver a dose of 10 cGy. Accordingly, for a total of 2000 cGy to be delivered by the implant, the total air-kerma needed will be

$$\left(33.1 \text{ cGy cm}^2/10 \text{ cGy}\right) \times 2000 \text{ cGy} = 6620 \text{ cGy cm}^2$$

If this is to be delivered in a 40-h period, the total source strength to be employed will be

$$6620 \text{ cGy cm}^2/40 \text{ h} = 165.5 \text{ cGy cm}^2 \text{ h}^{-1}$$

The Paterson and Parker rules recommend the use of linear source strengths of ρ and of $2\rho/3$ in the peripheral and central source lines, respectively. This means that, if seeds of strength S_{ak} are used in the two peripheral ribbons, seeds of strength $2S_{ak}/3$ should be used in the four inner ribbons. Hence, the total strength of all seeds is

$$S_{ak} \times 7 \text{ seeds} \times 2 \text{ peripheral ribbons}$$
$$+ \left(2 S_{ak}/3\right) \times 7 \text{ seeds} \times 4 \text{ inner ribbons} = 165.5 \text{ cGy cm}^2 \text{ h}^{-1}$$

i.e., $\qquad 32.7\,S_{ak} = 165.5 \text{ cGy cm}^2 \text{ h}^{-1}$

or $\qquad S_{ak} = 5.06 \text{ cGy cm}^2 \text{ h}^{-1} \text{ and } \left(2\,S_{ak}/3\right) = 3.37 \text{ cGy cm}^2 \text{ h}^{-1}$

This means that seeds of strengths 5.06 cGy cm² h⁻¹ and 3.37 cGy cm² h⁻¹ should be used in the peripheral and inner ribbons, respectively.

17.11.4 PROCURING THE SOURCES

The above sources are to be procured from a vendor. Let us say that, on contact with the vendor, it is found that these exact source strengths are not available, but seeds of 4.8 cGy cm² h⁻¹ and 2.9 cGy cm² h⁻¹ can be obtained as the closest approximations. If the available sources are used, the total source strength in the implant will be

$$4.8 \text{ cGy cm}^2 \text{ h}^{-1} \times 7 \text{ seeds} \times 2 \text{ peripheral ribbons}$$
$$+\,2.9 \text{ cGy cm}^2 \text{ h}^{-1} \times 7 \text{ seeds} \times 4 \text{ inner ribbons} = 148.4 \text{ cGy cm}^2 \text{ h}^{-1}$$

Because we have deviated from the distribution rules only marginally, we continue to use the information (derived in Section 17.11.3 based on data of Table 17.13) that 6620 cGy cm² can deliver a dose of 2000 cGy. Accordingly, the revised treatment time and dose rate will be

$$6620 \text{ cGy cm}^2 / 148.4 \text{ cGy cm}^2 \text{ h}^{-1} = 44.6 \text{ h}$$

and

$$\text{Dose rate} = 2000 \text{ cGy} / 44.6 \text{ h} \approx 45 \text{ cGy h}^{-1}$$

This value can be reascertained or fine-tuned on the basis of dosimetry calculations done with the aid of computers, after the plan is implemented on the patient.

17.11.5 IMPLANTING THE SOURCES

The treatment dose rate calculated above can be applied if, and only if, the spatial relationship between the sources as obtained in the patient conforms exactly to the planned array. In actual implants, such exact conformity may not be achieved. The spacings between the source ribbons can turn out to be uneven or nonparallel for practical reasons such as the need to avoid piercing of blood vessels, mechanical difficulties of passage, or inconvenient access. In the current-day practice of afterloading radiotherapy, it is usual to implant tubes or catheters first. The catheters can be loaded with dummy sources (nonradioactive sources that simulate the real sources) and radiographed. The radiotherapy simulator, with its isocentric rotation, can be used for radiography. The resulting radiographs showing the dummy seeds in the catheters can be used for judging the location of the target volume with respect to the catheters and the possible source positions. The number of seeds to be loaded in the different catheters can be altered or revised if needed. Detailed calculations can be done by computer in multiple planes through the implant and isodose curves plotted. Examination of the dose distribution can help to decide the actual treatment time. The afterloading catheters can then be loaded with radioactive sources according to the treatment plan. The sources are left in the patient for a predetermined period of irradiation.

17.11.6 RADIOGRAPHIC LOCALIZATION OF SOURCES

The aim of radiographic localization is to determine geometrically the spatial coordinates of the sources and any other identifiable point in the radiograph with respect to a reference origin. In the language of coordinate geometry, we would like to be able to decide the three-dimensional rectangular Cartesian coordinates (x, y, z) of any identifiable point in the radiograph. Because any radiograph is two-dimensional, it is necessary to have more than one radiograph to obtain the three-dimensional data sought. We will discuss here two common methods, tube-shift radiography and orthogonal radiography, for localization of implanted sources. Localization by orthogonal projections is known to provide better accuracy than do stereo projections.[70]

Tube Shift Radiographic Localization

In this method, illustrated in Figure 17.22, a single film is exposed twice. A radio-opaque marker M has been placed on the patient support table and is maintained in a fixed geometry with respect to the patient. First, the film is exposed with the X-ray source at position S_1. Then either the X-ray source or the patient is moved so as to have the X-rays emerge from position S_2 relative to the patient, and another exposure is made. In the figure, the film is parallel to the (x,z) plane and is perpendicular to the y axis. The system of coordinates has its origin on the central ray for the first exposure at the level of the table top. The projection of a point P(x, y, z) on the film moves from P_1 to P_2 by a distance Δx_1 in the x direction. The displacements of point P_1 from the origin along the x and z directions are x_1 and z_1, respectively. The image of marker M has moved from M_1 to M_2 on the film. If SFD and STD are source-to-film distance and source-to-table-top distance, respectively, the following geometric relations hold true:

$$\frac{M_1 M_2}{S_1 S_2} = \frac{\text{vertical distance from film to table}}{\text{vertical distance from source to table}} = \frac{SFD - STD}{STD} = \frac{SFD}{STD} - 1$$

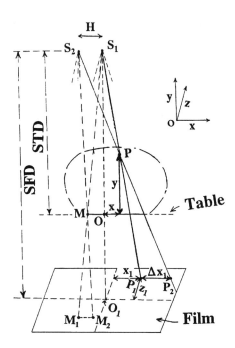

FIGURE 17.22 Illustration of the principle of single-film stereo radiography for localization of sources in an implant (see text for definition of symbols).

Hence,

$$STD = \frac{S_1 S_2 \cdot SFD}{S_1 S_2 + M_1 M_2}$$

$$x = \frac{x_1 (STD - y)}{SFD}; \quad z = \frac{z_1 (STD - y)}{SFD}$$

$$\frac{\Delta x_1}{S_1 S_2} = \frac{\text{vertical distance from P to film}}{\text{vertical distance from source to P}} = \frac{SFD - STD + y}{STD - y}$$

Hence,

$$y = \frac{\left[\Delta x_1 \cdot \text{STD} - S_1 S_2 (\text{SFD} - \text{STD})\right]}{\left[\Delta x_1 + S_1 S_2\right]}$$

If y << STD, the following approximations are possible for x and z:

$$x = x_1 (\text{STD/SFD}) \quad \text{and} \quad z = z_1 (\text{STD/SFD})$$

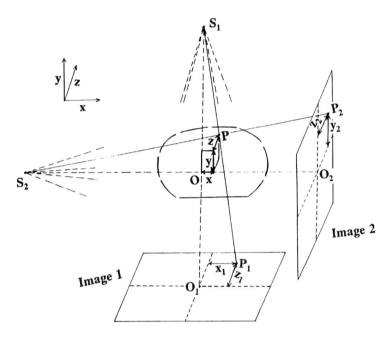

FIGURE 17.23 Illustration of the principle of orthogonal radiography for localization of sources in an implant (see text for definition of symbols).

Orthogonal Radiographic Localization

Figure 17.23 illustrates the principle of using orthogonal radiographic projections for three-dimensional localization of a point object in a patient. Two successive radiographs are taken as isocentric projections in mutually perpendicular directions, usually the front-to-back (AP) and right-to-left (lateral) projections. These can be obtained with the help of a radiotherapy treatment simulator. Ideally, there should be no motion of the patient between the two projections. The point P may represent a surgical clip, a point source, the end point of a line source, a bony landmark, or any other site that is uniquely identifiable in both radiographs. In Figure 17.23, the two positions of the X-ray source are S_1 and S_2. The central rays of the two projections strike the two radiographic images at points O_1 and O_2. The rectangular Cartesian coordinates of point P are (x,y,z) with respect to an origin O selected to be at the intersection of the central rays $S_1 O_1$ and $S_2 O_2$. The x and y directions have been chosen to be parallel to $S_2 O_2$ and $S_1 O_1$. Image 1 is perpendicular to the y axis, and image 2 is perpendicular to the x axis. P_1 and P_2 are the observed images of point P in the two radiographs. It is noted that P_1 is at position (x_1, z_1) in image 1 and P_2 is at position (y_2, z_2) in image 2. The following simple geometric relationships hold:

$$x_1 = \frac{x \cdot S_1 O_1}{S_1 O - y'} \qquad z_1 = \frac{z \cdot S_1 O_1}{S_1 O - y}$$

$$y_2 = \frac{y \cdot S_2 O_2}{S_2 O + x} \qquad z_2 = \frac{z \cdot S_2 O_2}{S_2 O + x}$$

In many practical situations, because the distances $S_1 O$ and $S_2 O$ are large (80 to 100 cm) compared to x, y, and z, the following approximations can be used:

$$x_1 = (MF_1) \cdot x \qquad z_1 = (MF_1) \cdot z$$

$$y_2 = (MF_2) \cdot y \qquad z_2 = (MF_2) \cdot z$$

where MF_1 and MF_2 are the magnification factors for the two images, given by

$$MF_1 = \frac{S_1 O_1}{S_1 O} \quad \text{and} \quad MF_2 = \frac{S_2 O_2}{S_2 O}$$

The values of the magnification factors can be determined as above if the relevant distances are known. Alternatively and more commonly, the location of the central ray and the magnification factor can both be inferred from the projection of a graduated cross hair in the therapy simulator. Furthermore, the fact that both images give information about the z coordinate (that is, z_1 and z_2) is useful for checking the mutual agreement between the two projections. In practice, some discrepancies in the z values as derived from the two radiographs can occur for several reasons, which include incorrect knowledge of the magnification factors, nonorthogonality, nonisocentricity, and patient motion.

17.11.7 ORTHOGONAL RECONSTRUCTION — A PRACTICAL CASE

The implant that we planned in Section 17.11.1 is now to be carried out on a patient. Empty nylon tubes or catheters are first implanted in the patient, and these can be loaded with radioactive sources after the radiographic projections have been obtained. In our example, the catheters used have one end closed and the other end open for loading of the sources. Six such catheters have been implanted in the patient in such a way that the closed ends are toward the medial side and the open ends are toward the right side of the chest wall. Figures 17.24a and b show the orthogonal (AP and lateral) radiographs obtained after each catheter has been loaded with a string of 12 dummy seeds at 1-cm spacing, imitating the real sources. It is possible to determine the number of seeds that any catheter can accommodate by carefully observing how many dummy seeds go inside the patient's body during the insertion of the dummy string. The rest of the dummy seeds remain in the part of the catheter outside the patient's body, in air. In this example, by such observation as well as by radiography, it is inferred that, if the six catheters were each loaded with seven seeds, the coverage of the target volume would be adequate.

Figures 17.25a and b are line tracings of the salient features in the orthogonal radiographs of Figure 17.24. They show the positions of the seeds to be loaded and the cross hair scale from the simulator indicating the magnification. The AP and lateral projections have been so positioned that the z coordinates of different seeds match after allowance is made for the difference in magnification between the two images. It can be observed that the positions of the cross hair scales representing the z = 0 level do not match exactly. This indicates apparent patient motion in the z (i.e., head-to-foot) direction between the two radiographs. This systematic error has been identified, and the z = 0 level in Figure 17.25b has been redefined to match the z = 0 level of Figure 17.25a.

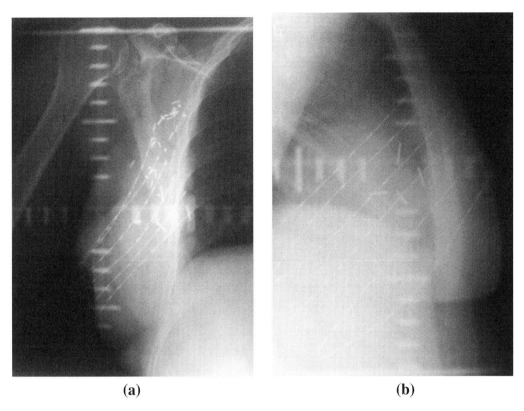

FIGURE 17.24 Orthogonal (a) front-to-back (AP) and (b) left-to-right (lateral) projections of the catheters of a breast implant loaded with imitation seeds, as obtained with a radiotherapy simulator.

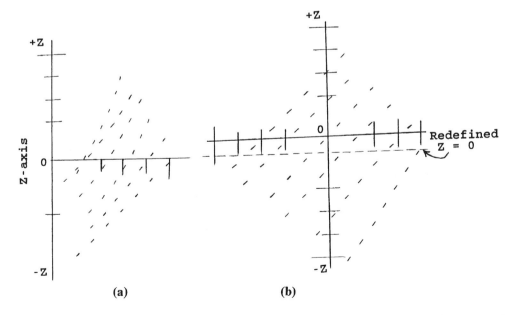

FIGURE 17.25 Line tracings of the orthogonal radiographs of Figure 17.24, showing the positions of the seeds to be loaded and the cross hair image from the simulator.

17.11.8 DOSIMETRY USING COMPUTER AND INTERPRETATION

The (x_1, z_1) and (y_2, z_2) coordinates of the different seeds from the two images (in Figure 17.25) are input to a computer, along with the information that the two peripheral catheters are loaded with seeds of 4.8 cGy cm² h⁻¹ and the four central catheters with seeds of 2.9 cGy cm² h⁻¹, as has been planned. Here we use a computer program that offers the facility to transform the coordinate information, perform the dose calculations, and plot the dose distribution, in any plane through the implant. Figure 17.26 displays the isodose rate curves (in units of cGy h⁻¹) in two mutually perpendicular planes through the middle of the implant. These two planes have been chosen to be approximately perpendicular and parallel to the source ribbons.

The interpretation of these isodose curves requires both scientific and artistic intuition. It will be noticed that there are isodose curves of high denominations that encircle the apparent source positions. The source positions thus inferred have been identified by cross marks. We recall the convention that a single-plane implant treats a target of thickness of 1.0 cm extending up to 0.5 cm on either side of the source plane. Hence, the broken lines have been drawn on both sides of the source plane at 0.5 cm from it. In Figure 17.26a, the isodose rate curve for 40 cGy h⁻¹ follows the dashed lines most closely, although a part of it falls within and some outside the dashed lines.

The next isodose rate levels plotted are for 50 cGy h⁻¹ and 30 cGy h⁻¹. If we disregard the end regions of the implant and use visual interpolation, the surface dose rate appears to lie within 40 ± 5 cGy h⁻¹. This number should be compared with the 45 cGy h⁻¹ that we estimated in Section 17.11.4 by using the area dosage tables. In this clinical example, the spacing between the catheters turned out to be uneven. The spacing is more than 1.0 cm on one side of the implant, less than 1.0 cm on the other side, and close to the intended 1.0 cm in the middle. The increased spacing results in a low dose at point **A** on the surface. At point **B**, the reduced spacing results in an increased dose rate.

We loaded the catheters with seeds of unequal strengths in the above case. However, let us say instead that the total strength of 148.4 cGy cm² h⁻¹ used above is divided equally among the 42 seeds and that all catheters are loaded with seeds of identical strength of 3.53 cGy cm² h⁻¹. The dose distributions then change to those shown in Figures 17.27a and b for the same two planes through the implant. The reader is advised to compare the isodose pattern in Figure 17.27 with that in Figure 17.26 to understand the differences that result from the use of nonuniform and uniform source strengths.

Example 17.5

Use the isodose rate curves of Figure 17.27a (i) to estimate the mean basic dose rate and (ii) to calculate the treatment time to deliver 2000 cGy if 85% of the mean basic dose rate is chosen as the reference dose rate.

By definition, the basic dose rate is the dose rate obtained at a point half-way between adjacent source lines in the central region of the implant. In Figure 17.27a, there are six catheters and five interspaces between them. If we adopt steps of 5 cGy h⁻¹ for interpolation between the isodose curves, observation of the dose distribution in the five interspaces between the six source strings suggests that the dose rates at the midway points are 40, 45, 55, 60, and 75 cGy h⁻¹. Averaging these, the

$$\text{Mean basic dose rate} = (40 + 45 + 55 + 60 + 75)/5 \text{ cGy h}^{-1}$$

$$= 55 \text{ cGy h}^{-1}$$

$$85\% \text{ of mean basic dose rate} = 55 \times 0.85 \approx 47 \text{ cGy h}^{-1}$$

$$\text{Treatment time to deliver 2000 cGy} = 2000/47 \approx 42.5 \text{ h}$$

The above example resembles the dosimetry in the Paris system, although the Paris system addresses the use of continuous radioactive wires rather than seeds with spacings.

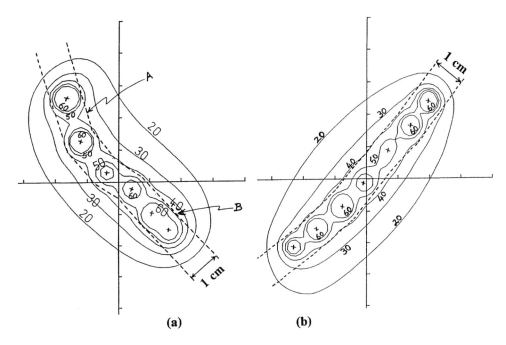

FIGURE 17.26 Isodose rate curves in two central planes (a and b) in perpendicular directions through the breast implant, as obtained by computer dosimetry for nonuniform loading. The two outer catheters are loaded with sources having 4.8 cGy cm^2 h^{-1}. The inner catheters carry sources of 2.9 cGy cm^2 h^{-1}. The cross (x) marks are inferred positions of source ribbons.

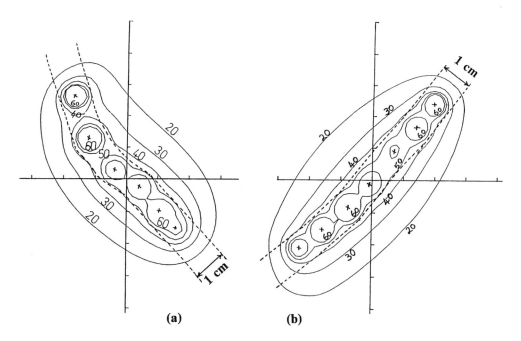

FIGURE 17.27 Isodose rate curves in two central planes (a and b) in perpendicular directions through the breast implant, as obtained by computer dosimetry for uniform loading. All sources have a strength of 3.53 cGy cm^2 h^{-1}. The cross (x) marks are inferred positions of source ribbons.

17.12 PERMANENT IMPLANTS

In permanent implants, the implanted sources are left in the patient to irradiate a lesion until they fully decay. The dose rate gradually decreases from a high value at the beginning of treatment to a negligible level in the natural radioactive decay process. The time of treatment is not a parameter controlled by the user, but is governed by the half-life of the source. The selection of the strength of the source for implantation thus becomes an important parameter for assuring the delivery of the preplanned dose. Most permanent implants are seed implants consisting of sources of 2 to 3 mm length. An interseed spacing of 1.0 cm or 0.5 cm can be adopted. Paying detailed attention to the number of planes to be implanted and the areas to be covered can help one to know in advance the size of the volume and the number of seeds that will be needed. ^{222}Rn, ^{198}Au, ^{125}I, and ^{103}Pd have been used for permanent implants.

Example 17.6

A spherical volume (as illustrated in Figure 17.13) having a diameter of 7 cm is to be permanently implanted with seeds of radioactive gold, ^{198}Au. Calculate the initial source strength needed to deliver a total of 6000 cGy minimum peripheral dose. (Use an array of seeds with 1-cm spacing and the data in Table 17.10.)

First, we need to visualize the successive planes at 1-cm spacing throughout the volume to be implanted as filled with seeds spaced 1 cm apart. This has already been done in Figure 17.13. The total number of seeds spread over seven planes is 155. The volume of sphere of radius (7.0 cm/2) = 3.5 cm is

$$V = (4/3)\pi(3.5)^3 \approx 180 \text{ cm}^3$$

We assume that the data in Table 17.10 for radium can be used for ^{198}Au. (For ^{125}I and ^{103}Pd sources, which emit very low-energy photons, only data tables generated especially for them should be used.) From this table, the total air-kerma strength needed to deliver 10 cGy MPD for a volume of 180 cm^3 is 107.3 cGy cm^2. For 6000 cGy, we need

$$107.3 \text{ cGy cm}^2 \times \frac{6000 \text{ cGy}}{10 \text{ cGy}} = 64380 \text{ cGy cm}^2$$

^{198}Au decays with a half-life $T_h = 2.7$ d. Hence the effective duration of the treatment given is the mean life, T_m:

$$T_m = 1.44 \ T_h = 1.44 \times 2.7 \text{ d} \times 24 \text{ h/d} = 93.3 \text{ h}$$

The total initial source strength needed $= \dfrac{64380 \text{ cGy cm}^2}{93.3 \text{ h}} \approx 690 \text{ cGy cm}^2 \text{ h}^{-1}$

The needed intitial source strength per seed is

$$S_{ak} = \frac{690 \text{ cGy cm}^2 \text{ h}^{-1}}{155 \text{ seeds}} \approx 4.45 \text{ cGy cm}^2 \text{ h}^{-1}/\text{seed}$$

17.13 INTRACAVITARY IRRADIATION

17.13.1 VAGINAL CYLINDER

Insertion of a plastic cylindrical applicator inside the vaginal canal and loading of the cylinder axis with a series of line sources in tandem is a commonly used intracavitary irradiation technique.

Several cylinders of different diameters and lengths can be kept in stock, and the size that best fits a particular patient can be selected for use. The cylinder helps to keep the tissues irradiated at a fixed geometry with respect to the sources. It also displaces the tissues away from the sources and thereby avoids regions of very rapid dose fall-off in the immediate proximity of the sources. The sources can first be loaded in a nylon tube, and that tube can be afterloaded into the applicator.

Figures 17.28a and b illustrate the dose distributions obtained around a vaginal cylinder loaded with sources in two different arrangements. In both distributions, the 100% dose has been normalized to lie at the surface of the central part of the applicator. In Figure 17.28a, three linear sources of identical active length (2 cm) and linear strength are used. In Figure 17.28b, a dumb-bell-type source loading has been used, with a central source of 4 cm active length and two end sources of 1 cm active length. The end sources have a linear strength about three times that of the central source. Such a "dumb-bell" arrangement gives isodose curves that are nearly parallel to the surface of the applicator, indicating a uniform delivery of surface dose. The volume covered by the isodose curves is larger than that obtained with the use of uniform linear activity.

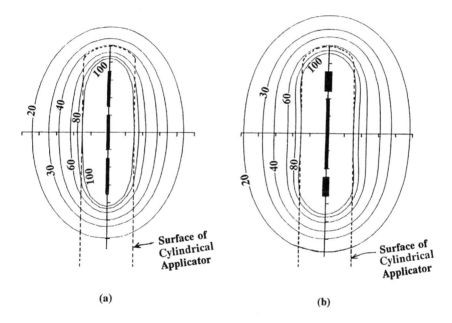

(a)   **(b)**

FIGURE 17.28 Dose distributions for a vaginal cylinder loaded with linear sources along the cylinder axis (a) for three linear sources of identical length and source strength; (b) for a nonuniform "dumb-bell"-type loading that uses a linear strength ratio of 3.3:1 between end sources and the central source. The 100% level is the dose on the surface of the cylinder in the central region.

17.13.2 PAIRS OF COLPOSTATS

In a different type of vaginal irradiation, a pair of applicators (called colpostats) is inserted to occupy the vaginal fornices. The source-carrying part of the applicator is specially designed to keep the irradiated tissue surface at a distance from the source and to make it conform to the shape of a cylinder or ovoid (a volume of oval cross section). For example, the applicators may have an external cylindrical surface of 3.0 cm length and a diameter of 2.0 cm. By addition of plastic caps of 2.5 mm or 5 mm thickness, the external diameter can be increased to 2.5 cm or 3.0 cm. Each applicator may be loaded with a linear source of about 1.4 cm active length and 2.0 cm external length. This size comes from the experience of using radium sources of similar dimensions in the past. In afterloading designs, a long access handle may be provided through which the linear source, which is held at the tip of a wire, can be inserted into the colpostat and removed. Some colpostats have been designed to incorporate lead shields in an appropriate manner to provide a 15% to 20%

reduction in dose in the direction of radiosensitive normal organs, including the bladder and rectum.[71-73]

The isodose distribution for a pair of applicators with 2.0 cm external diameter is shown in Figure 17.29a. Figure 17.29b shows the distribution when caps of 0.5 cm thickness are added. It is necessary in such treatments not to exceed the tolerance of the normal tissues touching the surface of the applicators. For this purpose, the dose rate can be monitored at a point such as **V** on the vaginal cuff. It is obvious that, if one is to obtain the same dose rate at point **V**, the source strength to be used without caps will be less than that to be used when the caps are affixed. It was estimated that sources of 40 cGy cm^2 h^{-1} and 85 cGy cm^2 h^{-1} can deliver a dose of 1000 cGy in about 24 h at **V** in the two situations of Figures 17.29a and b, respectively.

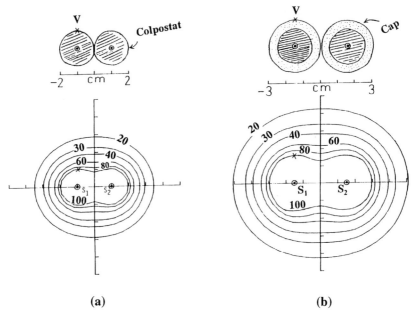

(a)   **(b)**

FIGURE 17.29 Pairs of colpostats in the vaginal apex. (a) Small pair without caps, and (b) large pair with caps. The 100% dose is on the surface at point V.

17.13.3 IRRADIATIONS OF UTERINE CERVIX

Figure 17.30 shows the long-established irradiation technique used for treatment of cancer of the cervix.[72-74] The cervix is the site where the uterine canal meets the vaginal canal. The cancer is known to originate at the cervix and invade the parametrium. A typical source arrangement that consists of a series of line sources, S_1, S_2, and S_3, in tandem along the uterine canal and a pair of colpostats in the vaginal canal is shown. Such intracavitary irradiation methods deliver an enormously high dose to the cancerous sites adjoining the sources. No accurate quantitative dosimetry is possible at these sites. However, the clinically established norms with respect to the source strengths to be used at these locations should be observed. It is usual that the bottom end of the lowest source, S_3, in the uterine canal is positioned so as to be at the cervix, where it delivers a high dose.

In the Manchester system,[57,74] a reference point, called point **A**, is chosen for dosimetry purposes. Point **A**, shown in Figure 17.30, is meant to signify a cancerous site that needs to be irradiated, but that is also in a region of limited radiation tolerance. In this region, called the paracervical triangle, a major blood vessel to the uterus crosses the ureter on its route from the kidneys to the bladder. For clinical dosimetry purposes, the position of point A has often been defined in geometric terms (rather than in anatomic terms) to be a point 2 cm lateral to the uterine canal and 2 cm above the level of the cervix and vaginal vault.

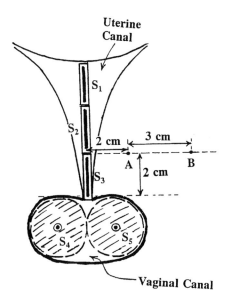

FIGURE 17.30 Source arrangement used for intracavitary irradiation of cancer of the cervix. The uterine canal carries sources S_1, S_2, and S_3. A pair of vaginal colpostats carry sources S_4 and S_5. Points A and B are reference points for dosage control (see text).

Point **B** is another reference point, chosen to represent the lymph nodes near the pelvic wall. It is defined to be at the same level as point **A**, but 5 cm away from the uterine canal. Many physicians prescribe the dose as stated at point **A**, and they calculate the dose rate there to determine the treatment duration. The dose at point **B** can be useful for deciding whether the dose to the pelvic nodes is adequate or will need to be boosted by an external beam.

The anatomy of the patient may determine the number of sources that can be lined up in the uterine canal and the size of the colpostats that the vagina can accommodate. In the Manchester system, different combinations of source strengths and source arrangements have been recommended not only for maintaining a constant dose rate at point **A**, but also for keeping a balance between the dose to the vaginal mucosa and that to point **A**.

In afterloading techniques, a long intrauterine tube is first inserted and positioned along with the afterloadable vaginal colpostats. The sources are inserted after it is ascertained that the applicators have been positioned acceptably. Dummy sources simulating the real ones can first be inserted and radiographs obtained with radio-opaque contrast medium in the bladder and rectum to indicate their locations, because the bladder and rectum are known to be radiosensitive organs and their tolerance doses can limit the duration of intracavitary irradiation.

Figures 17.31a and b illustrate schematically the coronal and sagittal views of such an intrauterine application. The following reference points have been identified in the figures for dosimetric control:

Points A_L, A_R — Point A on the left and right sides of the uterine canal
Points B_L, B_R — Point B on the left and right sides of the uterine canal
Point S — A reference point for the sigmoid colon
Point R — A reference point for the rectum
Point U — A reference point for the urinary bladder

In Figure 17.31, the reference points **S**, **R**, and **U** are chosen at positions in close proximity to the radioactive sources. ICRU Report 38 provides many guidelines for dosimetry in intracavitary irradiation for gynecologic applications.[75]

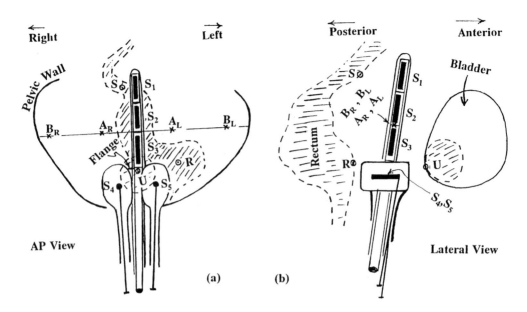

FIGURE 17.31 Projections of a typical intracavitary insertion for treatment of cervical cancer, showing the locations of the various reference points and the contrast-delineated outlines of bladder and rectum. (a) AP view, (b) lateral view.

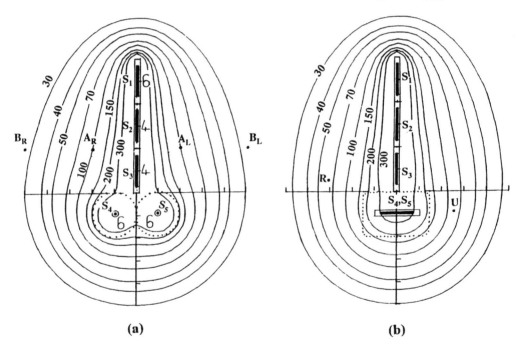

FIGURE 17.32 Isodose curves in two perpendicular planes (a) and (b) for a typical intracavitary insertion. Sources S_1, S_2, S_3, S_4, and S_5 have relative source strengths of 6, 4, 4, 6, and 6, respectively. The 100% dose is taken to be the dose received at point A.

The dose distributions obtained in two perpendicular planes for a typical cervical cancer insertion are shown in Figures 17.32a and b. The two planes correspond to the midcoronal and midsagittal planes through the cervix. The orientations of the tubes in the vaginal colpostats are such that the isodose curves are narrower in the sagittal plane (thus sparing the bladder and rectum) than in the coronal plane (to encompass the usual route of spread of the disease).

Use of only a single line of sources along the uterine canal, such as in Figure 17.32, produces a rapid fall-off of dose from the uterine wall. Cancerous lesions of the body of the uterus may need delivery of a substantial dose to tissues extending to 1.0–2.0 cm from the uterine axis. The dose distribution becomes broader if the uterine cavity is packed with multiple sources. This is referred to as Heyman packing.[76]

REFERENCES

1. Quimby, E.H., Fifty years of radium, Am. J. Roentgenol., Vol 60, p723-730, 1948.
2. Martin, C.L., and Martin, J.A., Low Intensity Radium Therapy, Little, Brown, Boston, 1959.
3. Wood, V.A. (Ed.), A collection of radium leak test articles, U.S. Dept. Health, Education and Welfare, MORP-68-1, Rockville, MD, March 1968.
4. International Atomic Energy Agency (IAEA), Physical Aspects of Radioisotope Brachytherapy, Technical Report Series No. 75, International Atomic Energy Agency, Vienna, 1967.
5. Trott, N.G. (Ed.), Radionuclides in Brachytherapy, Radium and After, Br. J. Radiol., Suppl. 21, British Institute of Radiology, London, 1988.
6. Nath, R., New directions in radionuclide sources for brachytherapy, Semin. Radiat. Oncol., Vol 3, p279-289, 1993.
7. Hospital Physicists' Association, Guidance on Testing of Sealed Sources of Radioisotopes for Leakage and Surface Contamination, HPA Report Series No. 1, Hospital Physicists' Association, London, U.K., 1970.
8. International Organisation for Standardisation (ISO), Sealed Radioactive Sources — Leak Test Methods, Technical Report Series 4862, International Organisation for Standardisation, Geneva, Switzerland, 1979.
9. Lommartzsch, P.K., Beta irradiation of choroidal melanoma with ^{106}Ru, ^{106}Rh applicators, Arch. Ophthalmol., Vol 101, p713-717, 1983.
10. Freidel, H.L., Thomas, C.I., and Krohmer, J.S., An evaluation of the clinical use of a ^{90}Sr beta ray applicator with a review of the underlying principles, Am. J. Roentgenol., Vol 71, p25-39, 1954.
11. Sinclair, W.K., and Trott, N.G., The construction and measurement of beta-ray applicators for use in ophthalmology, Br. J. Radiol., Vol 29, p15-23, 1956.
12. Supe, S.J., and Cunningham, J.R., A physical study of a strontium-90 beta-ray applicator, Am. J. Roentgenol., Vol 89, p570-574, 1963.
13. Henschke, U.K., Hilaris, B.S., and Mahan, G.D., Afterloading in interstitial and intracavitary radiotherapy, Am. J. Roentgenol., Vol. 90, p386-395, 1963.
14. Paine, C.H., Modern afterloading methods for interstitial radiotherapy, Clin. Radiol., Vol 23, p263-272, 1972.
15. Hillaris, B.S. (Ed.), Afterloading, 20 Years of Experience 1955-1975, Proceedings of the II International Symposium on Radiation Therapy, American Institute of Physics, Memorial Sloan-Kettering Cancer Center, New York, 1975.
16. Syed, A.M., and Feber, B.S., Technique of afterloading interstitial implants, Radiol. Clin., Vol 46, p458-475, 1977.
17. Syed, A.M., Nisar, S., and Feber, B.S., Techniques of afterloading interstitial implants, in Renaissance of Interstitial Brachytherapy, Proceedings of the 12th Annual San Francisco Cancer Symposium, California, 1977, Frontiers of Radiation Therapy Oncology, Vol 12, Vaeth, J.M. (Ed.), S. Karger, Basel, 1978, p119-135.
18. Delclos, L., Afterloading methods for interstitial gamma-ray therapy, Chapter 1, in Textbook of Radiotherapy, Fletcher, G.H. (Ed.), Lea & Febiger, Philadelphia, 1980, p84-92.
19. Almond, P.R., Remote afterloading, Chapter 8, in Advances in Radiotherapy Treatment Planning, Wright, A.E., and Boyer, A.L. (Eds.), American Institute of Physics, New York, 1983, p601-619.
20. Delclos, L., Afterloading interstitial irradiation techniques, Chapter 11, p123-154, in Levitt and Tapley's Technological Basis of Radiation Therapy: Practical Clinical Applications, Levitt, S.L., Khan, F.M., and Potish, R.A. (Eds.), Lea & Febiger, Philadelphia, 1992.
21. Williamson, J.F., and Nath, R., Clinical implementation of Task Group 32 recommendations on brachytherapy source strength specification, Med. Phys., Vol 18, p439-448, 1991.
22. American Association of Physicists in Medicine, AAPM Report 21, Specification of Brachytherapy Source Strength, Report of Task Group 32, American Institute of Physics, New York, 1987.
23. Williamson, J.F., Khan, F.M., Sharma, S.C., and Fullerton, G.D., Methods for routine calibration of brachytherapy sources, Radiology, Vol 142, p511-515, 1982.
24. Williamson, J.F., Morin, R.L., and Khan, F.M., Dose calibrator response to brachytherapy sources: A Monte Carlo and analytic evaluation, Med. Phys., Vol 10, p135-140, 1983.
25. Gibb, R., and Massey, J.B., Radium dosage; SI units and the Manchester system, Br. J. Radiol., Vol 53, p1100-1101, 1980.

26. Meisberger, L.L., Keller, R.J., and Shalek, R.J., The effective attenuation in water of the gamma rays of gold-198, iridium-192, cesium-137, radium-226 and cobalt-60, Radiology, Vol 90, p953-957, 1968.

27. Meli, J.A., Anderson, L.L., and Weaver, K.A., Dose distibution, p21-34, in Interstitial Brachytherapy, Physical, Biological and Clinical Considerations, Interstitial Collaborative Working Group, Raven Press, New York, 1990.

28. Nath, R., Anderson, L.L., Luxton, G., Weaver, K.A., Williamson, J.F., and Meigooni, A.S., Dosimetry of interstitial brachytherapy sources: Recommendations of the AAPM Radiotherapy Committee, Task Group No. 43, Med. Phys., Vol 22, p 209-234, 1995.

29. Weaver, K.A., Anderson, L.L., and Meli, J.A., Source characteristics, p3-13 in Interstitial Brachytherapy, Physical, Biological and Clinical Considerations, Interstitial Collaborative Working Group, Raven Press, New York, 1990.

30. Ling, C.C., Gromadzki, Z.C., Rustgi, S.N., and Cundiff, J.H., Directional dependence of radiation fluence from ^{192}Ir and ^{198}Au sources, Radiology, Vol 146, p791-792, 1983.

31. Meigooni, A.S., Sabnis, S., and Nath, R., Dosimetry of palladium-103 brachytherapy sources for permanent implants, Endocurietherapy/Hyperthermic Oncology, Vol 6, p107-117, 1990.

32. Meigooni, A.S., and Nath, R., A comparison of radial dose functions for ^{103}Pd, ^{125}I, ^{145}Sm, ^{241}Am, ^{169}Yb, ^{192}Ir, and ^{137}Cs brachytherapy sources, Int. J. Radiat. Oncol. Biol. Phys., Vol 22, p1125-1130, 1992.

33. Sievert, R.M., Eine Methode zur Messung von Roentgen-, Radium- und Ultrastrahlung; uber die Anwendbarkeit derselben in der Physik und in der Medizin, Acta Radiol. (Suppl. XIV), 1932.

34. Jayaraman, S., and Iyer, P.S., Dose distributions in paraxial regions of Cs-137 and Co-60 line sources, p327-333, in Proceedings of Symposium on Biomedical Dosimetry, International Atomic Energy Agency, Vienna, Austria, 1975.

35. Quimby, E.H., Dosage tables for linear radium sources, Radiology, Vol 43, p572-577, 1944.

36. Young, M.E.J., and Batho, H.F., Dose tables for linear radium sources calculated by an electronic computer, Br. J. Radiol., Vol 37, p38-44, 1964.

37. Krishnaswamy, V., Dose distribution about ^{137}Cs sources in tissue, Radiology, Vol 105, p181-184, 1972.

38. Breitman, K.E., Dose rate tables for clinical ^{137}Cs sources sheathed in platinum, Br. J. Radiol., Vol 47, p657-664, 1974.

39. Stovall, M., Lanzl, L.H., and Moos, W.S., Atlas of Radiation Dose Distribution, Brachytherapy Isodose Charts, Vol IV, Sealed Radium Sources, International Atomic Energy Agency, Vienna, Austria, 1972.

40. Hilaris, B.S., Nori, D., and Anderson, L.L., Atlas of Brachytherapy, MacMillan, New York, 1988.

41. Quimby, E.H., and Castro, V., The calculation of dosage in interstitial radium therapy, Am. J. Roentgenol., Vol 70, p739-749, 1953.

42. Quimby, E.H., and Goodwin, P.N., Dosage calculations with radioactive materials, Chapter 13, in Physical Foundations of Radiology, 4th Ed., Harper & Row, New York, 1970.

43. Pierquin, B., Dutreix, A., Paine, C.H., Chassagne, D., Marinello, G., and Ash, D., The Paris system in interstitial radiation therapy, Acta Radiol. (Oncol. Radiat. Phys. Biol.), Vol 17, p33-48, 1978.

44. Dutreix, A., and Marinello, G., The Paris system, p25-42, in Modern Brachytherapy, Pierquin, B., Wilson, J.F., and Chassagne, D. (Eds.), Masson Publishers, New York, 1987.

45. Pierquin, B., Chassagne, D.J., Chahbazian, D.J., and Wilson, J.F., Dosimetry, Chapter 5, in Brachytherapy, Pierquin, B. (Ed.), W. H. Green, St. Louis, Missouri, 1978.

46. Laughlin, J.S., Siler, W.M., Holodny, E.J., and Ritter, F.W., A dose description system for interstitial radiation therapy, Am. J. Roentgenol., Vol 89, p470-490, 1963.

47. Anderson, L.L., Wagner, L.K., and Schuer, T.H., Memorial methods of dose calculation for Ir-192, p1-7, in Modern Interstitial and Intracavitary Radiation Cancer Management, George, F. III (Ed.), Masson, New York, 1981.

48. Henschke, U.K., and Ceve, P., Dimension averaging: A simple method for dosimetry of interstitial implants, Radiat. Biol. Ther., Vol 9, p187-198, 1968.

49. Anderson, L.L., Kuan, H.M., and Ding, I.Y., Clinical dosimetry with I-125, p9-15, in Modern Interstitial and Intracavitary Radiation Cancer Management, George, F. III (Ed.), Masson, New York, 1981.

50. Anderson, L.L., and Osian, A.D., Brachytherapy optimization and evaluation, Endocurietherapy/Hyperthermic Oncology, Vol 2, pS25-S31, 1986.

51. Rao, U.V.G., Kan, P.T., and Howells, R., Interstitial volume implants with I-125 seeds, Int. J. Radiat. Oncol. Biol. Phys., Vol 7, p431-438, 1981.

52. Anderson, L.L., Hilaris, B.S., and Wagner, L.K., A nomograph for planar implant planning, Endocurietherapy/Hyperthermic Oncology, Vol 1, p9-15, 1985.

53. Anderson, L.L., Spacing nomograph for interstitial implants of I-125 seeds, Med. Phys., Vol 3, p48-51, 1976.

54. Paterson, R., and Parker, H.M., A dosage system for gamma-ray therapy. I, Br. J. Radiol., Vol 7, p592-632, 1934; reprinted Br. J. Radiol., Vol 68, No. 808, pH60-100, April 1995.

55. Paterson, R., and Parker, H.M., Dosage system for interstitial radium therapy, Br. J. Radiol., Vol 11, p252-266, 1938.

56. Parker, H.M., A dosage system for interstitial radium therapy. II. Physical aspects, Br. J. Radiol., Vol 11, p313-340, 1938.

57. Meredith, W.J. (Ed.), Radium Dosage — Manchester System, 2nd Ed., E & S Livingstone, Edinburgh, 1967.

58. Wu, A., Zwicker, R.D., and Sternick, E.S., Tumor dose specification of I-125 seed implants, Med. Phys., Vol 12, p27-31, 1985.

59. Busch, M., Dosage in interstitial therapy with gamma emitters, Strahlentherapie, Vol 153, p589-593, 1977.

60. Kwan, D., Kagan, A.R., Wollin, M. et al., A simple volume iridium implant dosimetry system, Endocurietherapy/Hyperthermic Oncology, Vol 3, p183-191, 1987.
61. Casebow, M.P., Dosimetry tables for standard iridium-192 wire implants, Br. J. Radiol., Vol 57, p515-518, 1984.
62. Neblett, D.L., Syed, N., and Puthawala, A.A., An interstitial implant technique evaluated by contiguous volume analysis, Endocurietherapy/Hyperthermic Oncology, Vol 1, p213-222, 1985.
63. Olch, A., Kagan, A.R., Wollin, M. et al., A simple volume iridium implant dosimetry system, Endocurietherapy/Hyperthermic Oncology, Vol 3, p183-191, 1987.
64. Murphy, D.J., and Doss, L.L., Small computer algorithms for comparing therapeutic performances of single-plane iridium implants, Med. Phys., Vol 11, p193-196, 1984.
65. Olch, A., Kagan, A.R., Wollin, M. et al., Multi-institutional survey of techniques in volume iridium implants, Endocurietherapy/Hyperthermic Oncology, Vol 2, p193-197, 1986.
66. Gillin, M.T., Kline, R.W., Wilson, J.F., and Cox, J.D., Single and double plane implants: Comparison of the Manchester system with the Paris system, Int. J. Radiat. Oncol. Biol. Phys., Vol 10, p921-925, 1984.
67. Paul, J.M., Koch, R.F., Philip, P.C., and Khan, F.R., Uniformity of dose distribution in interstitial implants, Endocurietherapy/Hyperthermic Oncology, Vol 2, p107-118, 1986.
68. Dutreix, A., Can we compare systems for interstitial therapy?, Radiother. Oncol., Vol 13, p127-135, 1988.
69. Paul, J.M., Koch, R.F., and Philip, P.C., Uniform analysis of dose distribution in interstitial brachytherapy and dosimetry systems, Radiother. Oncol., Vol 13, p105-125, 1988.
70. Sharma, S.H., Williamson, J.F., and Cytacki, E., Dosimetric analysis of stereo and orthogonal reconstruction of interstitial implants, Int. J. Radiat. Oncol. Biol. Phys., Vol 8, p1803-1805, 1982.
71. Fletcher, G.H., Shalek, R.J., and Cole, A., Cervical radium applicators with screening in the direction of bladder and rectum, Radiology, Vol 60, p77-84, 1953.
72. Fletcher, G.H., Hamberger, A.D., Wharton, J.T., Rutledge, F.N., and Delclos, L., Female pelvis, Chapter 11, p720-808, in Textbook of Radiotherapy, Fletcher, G.H. (Ed.), 3rd Ed., Lea & Febiger, Philadelphia, 1980.
73. Delclos, L., Gynecologic cancers: Pelvic examination and treatment planning, Chapter 11, p193-227, in Technological Basis of Radiation Therapy: Practical Clinical Applications, Levitt, S.L., and Tapley, N. duV. (Eds.), Lea & Febiger, Philadelphia, 1984.
74. Todd, M., and Meredith, W.J., Treatment of cancer of the cervix uteri — a revised Manchester method, Br. J. Radiol., Vol 26, p252-257, 1953.
75. ICRU, Dose and Volume Specification for Reporting Intracavitary Therapy in Gynecology, Report 38, International Commission on Radiation Units and Measurements, Bethesda, MD, 1985.
76. Heyman, J., Reuterwall, O., and Benner, S., The Radiumhemmet experience with radiotherapy of corpus of the uterus, Acta Radiol., Vol 22, p11-98, 1941.

ADDITIONAL READING

1. Anderson, L.L. et al. (Eds.), Interstitial Brachytherapy: Physical, Biological and Clinical Considerations, Interstitial Collaborative Working Group, Raven Press, New York, 1990.
2. Pierquin, B., Chassagne, D., Chahbazian, D.J., and Wilson, J.F., Brachytherapy, W.H. Green, St. Louis, Missouri, 1978.
3. Dutreix, A., Marinello, G., and Wambersie, A., Dosimetrie en Curietherapie, Masson, Paris, 1982.
4. Glasgow, G., Physics of brachytherapy, Chapter 10, p213-251, in Principles and Practice of Radiation Oncology, Perez, C.A., and Brady, L.W. (Eds.), J.B. Lippincott, Philadelphia, 1987.
5. Meredith, W.J. (Ed.), Radium Dosage — Manchester System, 2nd Ed., E & S Livingstone, Edinburgh, 1967.
6. George, F. III (Ed.), Modern Interstitial and Intracavitary Radiation Cancer Management, Masson, New York, 1981.
7. Hilaris, B.S., Nori, D., and Anderson, L.L., Atlas of Brachytherapy, MacMillan, New York, 1988.
8. Hilaris, B.S. (Ed.), Handbook of Interstitial Brachytherapy, Publishing Sciences Group, Acton, Massachussetts, 1975.
9. International Atomic Energy Agency (IAEA), Physical Aspects of Radioisotope Brachytherapy, Technical Report Series No. 75, International Atomic Energy Agency, Vienna, 1967.
10. Shearer, D.R. (Ed.), Recent Advances in Brachytherapy Physics, Proceedings of a Workshop of the American Association of Physicists in Medicine, American Institute of Physics, New York, 1979.
11. Trott, N.G. (Ed.), Radionuclides in Brachytherapy, Radium and After, Br. J. Radiology, Supplement 21, British Institute of Radiology, London, U.K., 1988.
12. Harrison, L.B. (Guest Ed.) and Tepper, J.E. (Ed.), Brachytherapy, Semin. Radiat. Oncol., Vol 3, No. 4, 1993.
13. Aird, E.G.A., Jones, C.H., Joslin, C.A.F., Klevenhagen, S.C., Rossiter, M.J., Welsh, A.D., Wilkinson, J.M., Woods, M.J., and Wright, S.J., Recommendations for brachytherapy dosimetry, Report of a joint BIR/IPSM working party, British Institute of Radiology, London, 1993.

Chapter 18

RADIATION SAFETY STANDARDS

18.1 INTRODUCTION

Ionizing radiation is a beneficial agent that contributes to improved health care. However, unnecessary exposure to ionizing radiation can be harmful[1,2] and should be avoided. Because penetrating radiations cannot be contained entirely, some irradiation of staff members, visitors, and the public is bound to occur incidental to any use of radiation. All radiation work should be carried out in a preplanned and controlled manner so that the exposure to the workers and persons in and near sites of radiation use is kept as low as reasonably achievable (ALARA) and does not exceed the recommended limits. In the U.S., guidelines to ensure the radiation safety of radiation and non-radiation workers and members of the public are provided by the National Council on Radiation Protection and Measurements (NCRP).[3] Recommendations are also provided by the International Commission on Radiation Protection (ICRP)[4,5] and by the International Atomic Energy Agency.[6] In some geographic regions, governmental regulatory agencies formulate the safety limits for radiation exposure and mandate that radiation users adhere to them. A radiotherapy department should plan and conduct its activities in such a manner that the safety recommendations (or regulations) are followed.

Scientific committees that are engaged in the process of setting guidelines for safe use of radiation face a rather formidable job. Whereas radiation damage is readily observable at high doses, at low dose levels the harm done is not easily discerned. The radiation risk (i.e., the probability of an adverse effect) at low dose levels needs to be estimated based on effects observed at high dose levels. The estimation process is laborious and is subject to many assumptions and uncertainties. This task involves the following steps: (i) consolidating all available epidemiologic data on populations exposed to radiation; (ii) comparing these with the epidemiologic information on an unexposed control population; (iii) observing any increased incidence of adverse effects in the exposed population compared to controls; (iv) assessing the radiation dose, received by the exposed population, to which an excess incidence can be attributed; (v) establishing a relationship between the radiation dose and excess risk; (vi) identifying the excess risk that society is willing to accept (as judged from the risks due to causes other than radiation that society is known to tolerate); and (vii) using that insight to identify the level of radiation exposure that can be recommended as acceptable, commensurate with the benefit that the radiation use offers to society.

Assessments of radiation risk have been made and reported on by several committees.[7-12] The risk evaluation is an ongoing process in which advantage is taken of all the latest information and the models of analysis available to the scientific community. Accordingly, the recommendations on dose limits have also undergone several revisions over the years.[13]

It is our purpose in this chapter to describe the harmful effects of exposure to low levels of ionizing radiation, the various uncertainties of correlating the dose with the risk of damage, and the philosophy of radiation safety, and to outline the most recent recommendations on dose limits for safe use of ionizing radiations. This presentation mainly covers the 1993 recommendations of the NCRP.[3] The discussion also touches on the 1991 recommendations of the ICRP[4,5] wherever appropriate.

18.2 HARMFUL EFFECTS OF RADIATION

18.2.1 ACUTE RADIATION SYNDROME

By "acute irradiation" we mean a single, large, one-time, whole-body irradiation. Partial-body irradiation, as done in radiotherapy of malignant conditions, is not considered here. The acute radiation syndrome is dependent on the dose received and on the time that has elapsed after irradiation. At dose levels of less than 25 cGy, no detectable acute effects occur. At doses up to 100 cGy, nausea and lack of appetite may result in a few people. Additionally, some reduction in counts of red and white blood cells, blood platelets, and lymphocytes can be observed on careful scrutiny. At 300 to 600 cGy, severe bone marrow damage can result, leading to serious hematologic symptoms, sometimes to irreversible gastrointestinal symptoms of nausea and diarrhea, and to epilation. Fatalities may occur. At doses higher than 600 cGy, damage to the central nervous system can set in. It has been assessed that an acute whole-body dose of 300 cGy of gamma rays delivered to a human population can result in the death of 50% of the population within 30 days after the irradiation.[14] This dose is referred to as lethal dose for 50% in 30 days (LD$_{50/30}$).

18.2.2 STOCHASTIC EFFECTS AND DETERMINISTIC EFFECTS

In one method of classification, radiation effects are classified as stochastic effects or deterministic effects. Stochastic effects are effects that occur in a random manner. Let us say that a large group of people is exposed to a given dose. Over a period of time, we can expect to see excess cancers in them compared to the incidence in the normal population. This excess number of cancers (i.e., radiation-induced cancers) will increase with the size of the exposed population and with the dose received. It is impossible to foretell who among those irradiated will suffer a radiation-induced cancer. Furthermore, neither can the severity of the disease to be suffered by anyone be predicted. Hence, cancer induction by radiation is a stochastic effect.

Deterministic effects, on the other hand, are predictable events, usually with a known threshold dose above which the effect is known to happen. Acute irradiation to high doses has many demonstrable dose thresholds for deterministic effects. Examples of these effects are eye lens opacification (cataract), blood changes, and reddening of the skin. For stochastic effects, *the probability of occurrence* increases with dose, whereas for deterministic effects *the severity of the effect* increases with dose.

18.2.3 SOMATIC AND GENETIC EFFECTS

In another method of classification, radiation effects can be categorized as somatic or genetic. Somatic effects refer to the harm that exposed individuals suffer during their lifetime. Radiation-induced cancers, opacification of the eye lens, sterility, and life shortening are examples of somatic effects. Genetic effects are radiation-induced mutations to an individual's genes and DNA, which can contribute to the birth of defective descendants. Genetic effects show up in the progeny of those irradiated and may include stillbirths, major congenital defects, alteration of the sex ratio, impaired physical development at an early age, and childhood cancers.[10,11,15] Exposure of a human embryo to radiation in the uterus has been interpreted to cause stunted growth, mental retardation, and carcinogenic effects.[16]

18.3 EVALUATION OF DOSE FOR RADIATION PROTECTION

18.3.1 INADEQUACY OF DOSE AS AN INDEX OF HARM

In radiation protection, we try to keep within limits the harm that can result from radiation exposure. Operationally, all radiation work should be carried out in such a way that the radiation exposure to the staff and to the general public is well below recommended safe limits. For evaluation of the degree of safety and for checking of compliance with regulations, such recommendations on safe limits of exposure should be stated as numerical limits of an evaluable quantity. This quantity needs to be evaluated in such a way that it would act as a measure of the radiation risk.[17] Hence, it should allow for as many factors that influence the radiation harm as can be identified and accounted for.

Although a numerical assessment of the radiation dose (which is the radiation energy absorbed per unit mass) is the first major step for evaluating the damage, it is not sufficient by itself to serve as an index of harm for radiation protection purposes. For example, it is known that the risk varies for different types of radiation at the same dose. Furthermore, the risk differs depending upon whether the whole body, a part of the body, or only an individual organ is irradiated. The stochastic risk and the radiosensitivity of the different body organs differ also. Thus, it is necessary to derive an index that can be correlated with the harm that can result to an individual or population from a radiation dose. Equivalent dose and effective dose are such indices, formulated by the ICRP and the NCRP. The dose-limiting recommendations for safe use of ionizing radiation are stated in terms of these indices.

18.3.2 MICROSCOPIC ENERGY DEPOSITION

It is known from biological experiments that different types of radiations (such as gamma rays, neutrons, and alpha particles) produce different degrees of biological damage for an identical dose.[18] Thus, for radiation protection purposes, it is necessary to give some consideration or weight to the kind of radiation to which a person is exposed, in addition to the radiation dose. In Chapter 11, we defined the radiation dose as the energy absorbed per unit mass of the substance irradiated. Dose is a macroscopic quantity and averages the energy absorbed over a mass consisting of an aggregate of cells. If the mass is subdivided into its component microscopic cells and the energy absorbed in the individual cells is observed, then, because of statistical variations, there will be differences in the energy absorbed by individual cells. Among three adjacent cells, one might have been traversed by one ionizing particle, the second might have been spared, and the third traversed by two particles. Accordingly, the three cells might suffer damage of different degrees, such as undergoing partial damage, no damage, or irrevokable damage.

The pattern of microscopic energy deposition varies for different types of radiation, such as X-rays, alpha particles, or neutrons. Therefore, equal doses of different radiations can produce unequal degrees of biological damage. The physical parameter of linear energy transfer (LET), discussed in Chapter 6, influences the effectiveness of different radiations for the same radiation dose delivered. As a charged particle traverses a medium, it leaves a trail of ions along its own track and along the tracks of the secondary electrons that it sets in motion. The linear density of ionization (i.e., the number of ions per unit path length) is a function of the LET. In Chapter 6 (Figures 6.8a and b), we illustrated schematically the trails of ions along low- and high-LET tracks, respectively.

In Figures 18.1a and b, we show a macroscopic square-shaped area irradiated by low-LET and high-LET radiations, respectively. The total number of ionizing events in the two squares is the same, although the ionization densities along the tracks are different. Three cells, numbered 1, 2, and 3, have been identified. If, say, a minimum of two ionizing events within a cell is needed to cause permanent damage to its functioning, only cell 2 is killed with low LET in Figure 18.1a. However, both cells 1 and 2 are killed in Figure 18.1b for high LET. Thus, the probability of permanent damage increases with LET.

18.3.3 RELATIVE BIOLOGICAL EFFECTIVENESS (RBE)

The relative biological effectiveness (RBE) is defined to serve as a measure of the biological effectiveness of any test radiation with respect to a reference radiation. If a dose D_g, given with a chosen type of radiation, produces a particular biological effect, and the same biological effect is produced by dose D_{ref} of a reference radiation, the RBE of the chosen radiation is given by the ratio

$$RBE = \left(D_{ref}/D_g\right) \tag{18–1}$$

The reference radiation traditionally has been chosen as low-energy X-rays.

It will be noticed that no particular biological effect or endpoint is specified in the above definition of RBE. Because of this, it turns out that RBE is not a unique value for any given radiation. For example, the ratio may differ for skin erythema and for soft-tissue necrosis. It can also depend on the biological system chosen. Cells irradiated *in vitro* show a sensitivity different from that of cells *in vivo*. There are many other variables, such as dose rate, fractionation,

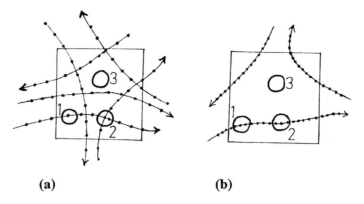

(a)   **(b)**

FIGURE 18.1   A square volume of tissue with three distinct cells (identified as 1, 2, and 3) is traversed by ionizing tracks. Dots along tracks represent ionizing events. (a) Irradiation by six low-LET tracks and (b) irradiation by three high-LET tracks having twice the linear ionization density of those in (a). The total number of ionizing events within the square is the same in (a) and (b).

temperature, oxygenation, spatial dose distribution, and volume of the sample, on which the RBE can depend. Table 18.1 gives the observed RBE values at minimal doses (denoted by RBE_M based on Table 4.1 of Reference 3) for fission neutrons and different biological endpoints. The lack of uniqueness of the RBE disqualifies it from serving as a ratio that can be applied to the dose as a weighting factor for different radiations for radiation protection purposes.

TABLE 18.1

Summary of RBE_M Values for Fission Neutrons vs. Gamma Rays[a]

Biological Endpoint	Range of Values of RBE_M
Chromosome aberrations, human lymphocytes in culture	34–53
Oncogenic transformation	3–80
Specific locus mutations in mice	5–70
Mutation endpoints in plant systems	2–100
Life shortening in mice	10–46
Tumor induction in mice	16–59

[a] RBE_M is the limiting value of the relative biological effectiveness (RBE) at minimal dose levels.

Table adapted from NCRP REPORT 116, 1993.[3]

18.3.4 QUALITY FACTOR AND DOSE EQUIVALENT

In another approach to allowing for variations in the biological impact of different radiations for the same dose, the ICRU[19] defined the concepts of quality factor (denoted by Q) and dose equivalent (designated by H). The quality factor Q is a dimensionless weighting factor that is related to the physical parameter LET. This is unlike the RBE, which has a reference to a biological endpoint in its definition. The dose equivalent H is the dose delivered, D, times the quality factor, Q, recommended for the radiation; i.e.,

$$H = D \cdot Q \tag{18--2}$$

For distinguishing the dose equivalent from the dose, the dose equivalent is expressed in units of rem (an acronym for roentgen equivalent man) when the dose D is in rad. When D is expressed in Gy, the dose equivalent will be in sieverts (Sv).

Although Q is not related to any particular biological endpoint, the purpose in its use was to make it applicable to carcinogenic and mutagenic effects from the radiation protection point of view. Special consideration has been given to chromosome aberrations in human lymphocytes.

The values assigned to Q have undergone several revisions. Values of Q as a function of energy are given in the 1986 ICRU report for photons, neutrons, and alpha particles. The Q values for neutrons are known to change rapidly with neutron energy. Table 18.2 presents the quality factors as a function of LET as accepted by the NCRP[3] and ICRP.[4]

TABLE 18.2
Quality Factor-LET Relationships

LET$_\infty$ in Water (keV μm^{-1})	$\overline{Q}$ (LET$_\infty$)[a]
<10	1
10 to 100	0.32 LET$_\infty$−2.2
>100	300 (LET$_\infty$)$^{-0.5}$

[a] $\overline{Q}$ should be rounded off to the nearest whole number and LET$_\infty$ expressed in keV μm^{-1}.

Table adapted from NCRP Report 116, 1993.[3]

In general, a total dose D may be delivered with the LET spread over a spectrum of values. Let L denote the linear energy transfer (LET) (described in Volume 1, Chapter 6, Section 6.3.5). If D(L)dL is the dose in an LET interval L to L + dL and Q(L) is the corresponding quality factor, the effective quality factor $\overline{Q}$ can be evaluated by

$$\overline{Q} = \frac{1}{D}\int_0^\infty Q(L)\,D(L)\,dL \qquad (18\text{--}3)$$

18.3.5 WEIGHTING FACTORS FOR DIFFERENT RADIATIONS

The wide range of the observed RBE values at low doses prompted the question whether the detail and precision implied in the formal relationship of Q to LET can be valid for radiation protection purposes. The ICRP considered this issue in 1991 and suggested the use of a radiation weighting factor, W_R, rather than the quality factor $\overline{Q}$, to account for the biological effectiveness of different radiations at the same dose. Table 18.3 gives the radiation weighting factors as adapted by the NCRP (which closely follows the values recommended by the ICRP) for different radiations. The basis for these values is the observed RBE at low doses for biological endpoints of concern for radiation protection. For radiation types not included in Table 18.3, the ICRP and NCRP suggest that the value of W_R can be the same as the value of $\overline{Q}$ calculated from expression (18–3).

18.3.6 EQUIVALENT DOSE

If a tissue or organ, T, receives an average dose, $D_{T,R}$, due to radiation, R, having a recommended weighting factor W_R, the equivalent dose, $H_{T,R}$, is evaluated by multiplication of $D_{T,R}$ by W_R. That is,

$$H_{T,R} = D_{T,R} \cdot W_R \qquad (18\text{--}4)$$

Equivalent dose and dose equivalent have different connotations. Dose equivalent is based on the absorbed dose at a *point* in tissue weighted by the quality factor Q, which, in turn, is related to the LET distribution at that point. Equivalent dose, on the other hand, uses not the point dose, but the average absorbed dose in the organ and weights it by the radiation weighting factor W_R.

If an organ T is irradiated by several types of radiation, the average organ dose, $D_{T,R}$, due to each radiation type R should first be evaluated. Then these averages should be multiplied by the

TABLE 18.3
Radiation Weighting Factors, W_R

Type and Energy	W_R
X- and gamma rays, electrons,[a] positrons, muons	1
Neutrons, energy <10 keV	5
>10–100 keV	10
>100 keV–2 MeV	20
>2–20 MeV	10
> 20 MeV	5
Protons other than recoil protons, energy >2 MeV	2[b]
Alpha particles, fission fragments, nonrelativistic heavy nuclei	20

Note: All values apply to radiation incident on the body or, if internal sources, emitted from the source.

[a] Excluding Auger electrons emitted from nuclei bound to DNA.
[b] For body irradiated by protons of >100 MeV energy, W_R of unity applies.

Adapted from NCRP Report 116, 1993.[3]

respective radiation weighting factors, W_R, which will yield the equivalent doses, $H_{T,R}$, from each component. These equivalent doses should be summed up to give the total equivalent dose, H_T, to the organ. That is,

$$H_T = \sum_R D_{T,R} \cdot W_R \qquad (18\text{–}5)$$

The following example illustrates this.

Example 18.1

A person receives 0.02 Gy (2 rad), 0.032 Gy (3.2 rad), and 0.015 Gy (1.5 rad) from X-rays, thermal neutrons, and alpha particles. Use the radiation weighting factors in Table 18.3 to evaluate the equivalent dose.

Radiation	Dose ($D_{T,R}$)	W_R (From Table 18.3)	Equivalent Dose $H_{T,R} = D_{T,R} \cdot W_R$
X-rays	0.02 Gy	1	0.02 Sv
Thermal neutrons	0.032 Gy	5	0.16 Sv
Alphas	0.015 Gy	20	0.30 Sv
Total	0.067 Gy (6.7 rad)		0.48 Sv (48 rem)

Total equivalent dose is 0.48 Sv (48 rem).

Example 18.2

In the surroundings of a nuclear reactor, a person receives doses of 0.01 Gy from gamma radiation and 0.005 Gy from neutrons. The neutron energy is unknown. Estimate the equivalent dose in the best- and worst-case situations.

Total equivalent dose = equivalent dose from gammas + equivalent dose from neutrons

For the gamma component, $W_R = 1$. For the neutrons, in the best-case situation, we assume that the neutrons are all of low energy, with $W_R = 5$. Then

$$\text{Total equivalent dose} = 0.01 \text{ Gy} \times 1 + 0.005 \text{ Gy} \times 5 = 0.035 \text{ Sv}$$

In the worst-case situation, all of the neutron dose is from fast neutrons having $W_R = 20$. Then

$$\text{Total equivalent dose} = 0.01 \text{ Gy} \times 1 + 0.005 \text{ Gy} \times 20 = 0.11 \text{ Sv}$$

18.3.7 WEIGHTING FACTORS FOR DIFFERENT BODY TISSUES

Tissues or organs vary in their sensitivity to stochastic detriment, especially radiation-induced cancer.[20,21] The ICRP, in 1977, considered making an allowance for this variation by using tissue weighting factors, W_T, for different organs in the body.[22] Table 18.4 gives the W_T values recently adopted by the NCRP[3,21] (as recommended by the ICRP[4,5]) for 12 specific organs. W_T represents the proportionate detriment (stochastic) to a tissue T when the whole body is irradiated to an equivalent dose H_T. It will be noticed that the sum of W_T (for the 12 specified organs and the remainder) adds up to 1. The value of W_T specified for "remainder" in Table 18.4 should be used in the way recommended in the footnote of the table.

TABLE 18.4

Tissue Weighting Factors (W_T) for Different Tissues and Organs

Organs	Skin	Bladder Breast Liver Esophagus Thyroid Remainder[a,b]	Bone marrow Colon Lung Stomach	Gonads
	Bone surface			
W_T	0.01	0.05	0.12	0.20

[a] Remainder includes adrenals, brain, small intestine, large intestine, kidney, muscle, pancreas, spleen, thymus, and uterus as a group. It may also include any other tissues or organs selectively irradiated.

[b] If, in an exceptional case, one of the remainder tissues receives an equivalent dose greater than the highest dose to any of the 12 organs specifically identified in the table, a W_T of 0.025 is to be used for that tissue, together with a W_T of 0.025 applied to the average equivalent dose received by the other remainder tissues.

Table adapted from NCRP Report 116, 1993.[3]

18.3.8 EFFECTIVE DOSE

The effective dose, E, is the sum of the weighted equivalent doses for all irradiated tissues and organs. It is designed to serve as a single measure of effective detriment and is given by

$$E = \sum_T H_T W_T = \sum_T W_T \sum_R D_{T,R} \cdot W_R \qquad (18-6)$$

Example 18.3

The film badge reading indicates that a staff member was exposed to low-energy X-rays and received a skin dose of 5.5 mGy and an average dose of 1.1 mGy to deep-seated organs. The gonads were completely shielded. Calculate the effective dose.

We tabulate the dose received, radiation weighting factor, equivalent dose, organ weighting factor, and effective dose to each individual organ, as shown below:

Organ(*)	Dose Received $D_{T,R}$ (mGy)	Radiation Weighting Factor W_R	Equivalent Dose $D_{T,R} W_R$ (mSv)	Organ(*) Weighting Factor W_T	Effective Dose $D_{T,R} W_R W_T$ (mSv)
Bone surface	1.1	1.0	1.1	0.01	0.011
Skin	5.5	1.0	5.5	0.01	0.055
Bladder	1.1	1.0	1.1	0.05	0.055
Breast	1.1	1.0	1.1	0.05	0.055
Liver	1.1	1.0	1.1	0.05	0.055
Esophagus	1.1	1.0	1.1	0.05	0.055
Thyroid	1.1	1.0	1.1	0.05	0.055
Remainder	1.1	1.0	1.1	0.05	0.055
Bone marrow	1.1	1.0	1.1	0.12	0.132
Colon	1.1	1.0	1.1	0.12	0.132
Lung	1.1	1.0	1.1	0.12	0.132
Stomach	1.1	1.0	1.1	0.12	0.132
Gonad	0.0	1.0	1.1	0.20	0.000

* As listed in Table 18.4

Total of column 5, $\Sigma W_T = 1.0$.
Total of column 6, $\Sigma D_{T,R} W_R W_T = 0.924$ mSv.

Thus, effective dose = 0.92 mSv (92 mrem).

18.4 UNCERTAINTIES IN RADIATION RISK ASSESSMENT

18.4.1 PROBLEM OF SAMPLE SIZE

In protecting radiation workers and the general public from exposures incidental to practical applications of radiation, we are concerned about the consequences of chronic low-level irradiations. To interpret the radiation risk for a human population, we need to rely on epidemiologic data on human populations exposed to radiation. The single largest group of exposed individuals from which much of our understanding has come is that of the survivors of the atomic bomb explosions in Japan.

The study of the effects of radiation on human populations is not easily accomplished. For a better understanding of this complex task, the reader is referred to the comprehensive reviews on this subject presented by a committee of experts.[8,9] This section is restricted to a brief overview.

Almost all of the effects caused by radiation also occur from causes other than radiation. Basically, such a study needs two groups of people, one exposed to radiation and the other unexposed. The epidemiologic studies on the two populations should reveal an excess of defects, damage, or cancers in the irradiated compared to the unirradiated group. Thus, we are looking for "excess effects" observable and attributable to radiation.

To distinguish the excess incidence from the normal background level of incidence in a statistically reliable manner, one needs large sample sizes. For example, let us say that about 250,000 solid cancers (excluding leukemia and bone cancers) are known to occur normally in a million persons and it is suspected that about 6,000 excess cancers of the same kind may be caused by a single exposure to 0.1 Gy (10 rad). For the comparison of the cancer incidence in an exposed group with that in an unexposed group to be statistically reliable, the exposed and unexposed groups should each consist of 60,000 people. However, it would be unethical to expose a human population only for the purpose of understanding the radiation risk.

Many radiation effects are demonstrable in animals. Animal experiments, in which large samples can be employed, are a possible option. However, experience has shown that not all radiation effects observed in animals can be proved in human subjects. Hence, epidemiologic studies have to be carried out with the limited sample sizes of already exposed human populations. It is a challenge to identify large groups of people who were incidentally exposed to radiation. Another problem is that, within a given group of people, one would need to allow for other factors such as smoking, alcoholism, sex, age, etc., that modify the effects of radiation. These further divide the existing sample size into smaller subsets. Furthermore, because low-level radiation effects occur over periods of several decades after irradiation, irradiated populations should be observed for many years.

18.4.2 IMPERFECT KNOWLEDGE OF RADIATION DOSE

Because radioepidemiologic studies are retrospective studies on populations incidentally or accidentally irradiated, there is great difficulty in estimating the doses they received. In this text, we have discussed methods for delivering a predetermined radiation dose in radiotherapy. We know that delivery of a therapeutic dose is not achieved unless many parameters of irradiation are known exactly and a system for dose calculation together with appropriate data tables is established. If the dose determination can be so difficult to achieve in a situation where controlled delivery of radiation is the intent, it becomes a challenging task to calculate the dose received in a situation where delivery of dose was not the intent, but was incidental. For example, the doses received by the survivors of the atomic bomb explosions in Japan have been revised and reassessed on an ongoing basis.[23-27] Accordingly, the risk estimates have also changed.

18.4.3 DOSE-RESPONSE PROJECTION

The radiation hazard with which we are most concerned in setting radiation safety limits for radiation workers is radiation-induced cancer, although genetic effects are not to be ignored. Radioepidemiologic studies have detected excess cancers in various groups of exposed populations.

One of the major questions confronted during the estimation of radiation risk is, how can one extrapolate the excess cancer incidence observed in a population exposed acutely to high doses and infer the possible rate of cancer induction at the low levels of exposure that are encountered in occupational situations? That is, what is the mathematical function that can relate the cancer incidence rate to the dose D? Mathematically, this function can have the general form

$$F(D) = \left(\alpha_0 + \alpha_1 D + \alpha_2 D^2\right) \exp\left(-\beta_1 D - \beta_2 D^2\right) \tag{18-7}$$

where α_0, α_1, α_2, β_1, and β_2 are empirical parameters. The above expression is referred to as a linear-quadratic model with cell killing and has the graphic form shown in Figure 18.2a. At very high doses, the curve shows a reduction in cancer incidence. This is attributable to the exponential term which indicates that cells, when given high radiation doses, lose the capacity to become cancerous. Two simplified versions of the above general expression are the linear quadratic model and the linear model, which have the following forms:

$$F(D) = \alpha D + \beta D^2 \tag{18-8}$$

and
$$F(D) = \alpha D \tag{18-9}$$

The latter model gives higher risks at low doses compared to the former when the effects observed at high doses are extrapolated to low doses, as is shown graphically in Figure 18.2b.

18.4.4 LIFETIME RISK PROJECTION

Cancer incidence rates vary with the age of the exposed population. The delivery of a radiation dose can cause an excess risk of cancer as a complex function of age at exposure and time after exposure. The radioepidemiologic analysis can be based on two different models of projecting the risk over the lifetime of an exposed population.[8,11] These are absolute-risk and relative-risk models, as illustrated in Figure 18.3, in which curve 1 represents the normal rate of cancer incidence for a given population as a function of age. When a radiation dose, D, is received by the population at

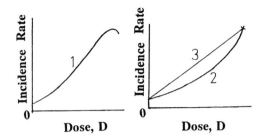

FIGURE 18.2   Models of dose vs. cancer incidence. Curve 1: linear quadratic model with cell killing; curve 2: linear quadratic model; curve 3: linear model.

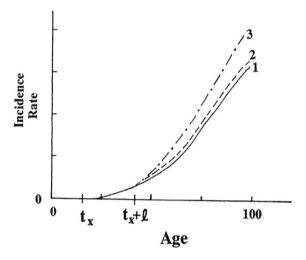

FIGURE 18.3   Projection of cancer incidence rate for an irradiated population. Curve 1 applies to a normal, unexposed population. Curves 2 and 3 represent absolute-risk and relative-risk models of lifetime risk projection, respectively. The radiation dose is received at age t_X, and ℓ is the latency period for cancer induction after irradiation.

age t_X, the cancer incidence changes to curve 2 or 3 depending on the model of lifetime risk projection employed. Curve 2 applies for the absolute-risk model (also called additive-risk projection model). Curve 3 applies for the relative-risk model (also called multiplicative-risk projection model). Both curves show no observable number of excess cancers above the normal level for a latency period of ℓ years after age t_X. After that, curve 2 shows an excess risk that seems like an addition, [say, $F_A(D)$], over the normal risk (curve 1). The excess risk shown by curve 3 appears as a multiplier [say, $F_R(D)$] of the normal risk (curve 1).

In a given population, there is a baseline rate of cancer incidence, $\lambda_0(t)$, at age t. In general, a radiation exposure to dose D(t) at age t may change the cancer incidence rate to $\lambda[T,D(t)]$ at an observation age T. Then, in the two models, the expressions for $\lambda[T,D(t)]$ are

$$\text{Absolute risk: } \lambda\big[T,D(t)\big] = \lambda_0(t) + F_A\big[D(t)\big] \tag{18–10}$$

$$\text{Relative risk: } \lambda\big[T,D(t)\big] = \lambda_0(t)\,F_R\big[D(t)\big] \tag{18–11}$$

For protracted exposures occurring over a lifetime, we can assume, in a simple model, that each increment of exposure contributes independently to the excess cancer rate. Then the excess cancer rate, $\Delta\lambda[T,D]$, that can represent the total lifetime risk when a radiation dose D(t) is received at age t is

$$\Delta\lambda[T,D] = \int_0^T \left\{ \lambda[T,D(t)] - \lambda_0(t) \right\} dt \qquad (18\text{--}12)$$

In the absolute-risk hypothesis, the excess risk attributed to dose D is independent of the existing normal cancer risk. All populations, irrespective of their age, ethnic origin, or nationality, are assumed to have the same excess risk from dose D. However, in the relative-risk model, the excess cancers will be more numerous in the population that has a higher rate of normal cancer incidence, because the radiation dose plays the role of a catalyst that aggravates the already existing risk. For the relative-risk model, the expression for $\Delta\lambda[T,D]$ becomes

$$\Delta\lambda[T,D] = \int_0^T \left\{ F_R[D(t)] - 1 \right\} \lambda_0(t) \, dt \qquad (18\text{--}13)$$

To interpret the total risk to an actual living population for a given radiation exposure, one can employ standard life table techniques[28] by using the mortality and cancer incidence data applicable to that population. The fate of a population of a million newborn infants may be followed over a period of 100 years. For persons exposed to radiation at different ages, the probability of radiation-induced cancer at various time intervals can be evaluated after allowance is made for a latency period for cancer induction subsequent to the irradiation.

Our understanding of the subject of lifetime carcinogenic risk is gradually progressing. At this time, it seems that the absolute-risk model may apply to the incidence of leukemia and the relative-risk hypothesis to the induction of solid cancers.

18.4.5 DOSE AND DOSE RATE EFFECTIVENESS FACTOR (DDREF)

The doses and dose rates at which persons are exposed incidental to the use of ionizing radiations are much lower than the high dose rates at which the populations used in epidemiologic studies were exposed. Hence, the risk factors evaluated in epidemiologic studies should be lowered by a dose and dose rate effectiveness factor (DDREF). (As an analogue, the damage caused by throwing of a heavy bowling ball cannot be matched by throws of hundreds of ping pong balls one at a time, even if all of their masses together equal the heavy mass of the bowling ball.) Based on experimental information and information on human subjects, the ICRP and the NCRP have adopted a DDREF of 2.0 in their recent reports.[2,3]

18.4.6 ASSESSED RADIATION RISK

For radiation protection purposes, the ICRP estimated total detriment by adding to the risk of fatal cancer the risks of nonfatal cancers and severe genetic effects. The nominal values of the risk factors (as assessed by the ICRP and adopted by the NCRP) are given in Table 18.5 for an adult working population and a population of all ages, including children. The W_T values in Table 18.4 are based on the relative contributions of different body parts to the total detriment.

TABLE 18.5
Nominal Probability Coefficients for Stochastic Effects

Exposed Population	Detriment (10^{-2} Sv^{-1})			
	Fatal Cancers	Nonfatal Cancers	Severe Genetic Effects	Total Detriment
Adult workers	4.0	0.8	0.8	5.6
Whole population	5.0	1.0	1.3	7.3

Table adapted from NCRP Report 116 (1993).[3]

18.5 RADIATION SAFETY PHILOSOPHY

18.5.1 NATURAL BACKGROUND RADIATION

In the development of a radiation protection philosophy for safe use of ionizing radiation, it is appropriate to keep in mind the fact that the manmade radiation sources used in radiologic applications are not the only cause of radiation exposure of the population. We do not live in a radiation-free world. A natural radiation background exists[29] and contributes to the equivalent doses listed in Table 18.6. This background consists in part of radiation coming from radioactive materials that are naturally present in the earth and in commonly used building materials. Such terrestrial emission depends on the constituents of the terrain and varies from place to place. To this is added the radiation from outer space, called cosmic rays. The intensity of cosmic radiation is observed to vary with altitude and latitude. Cosmic ray-produced radionuclides (mainly ^{3}H, ^{14}C, ^{7}Be, and ^{22}Na) contribute the cosmogenic component in Table 18.6. In addition to the terrestrial and cosmic radiations, the human body contains radioactive atoms assimilated by ingestion and inhalation. A long-lived naturally occurring radionuclide, ^{40}K, is also a significant contributor. A small radiation component is added by the fall-out from atomic weapons testing, the effluents from nuclear power plants, consumer products such as smoke detectors and watches with luminous dials that use radioactive materials, tobacco products, etc. Aircraft flying at high altitudes expose the passengers to cosmic ray intensities higher than those on the surface of the earth. During a transcontinental flight at a 12 km altitude, passengers can receive a dose equivalent of 25 µSv (2.5 mrem) to the whole body.[30]

TABLE 18.6
Background Radiation Dose (Received by Body Soft Tissues)

Component	Total Dose Equivalent[a] Rate (mSv/year)
Cosmic rays	0.27
Cosmogenic	0.01
Terrestrial	0.28
Human body	0.35
Total	0.91

[a] Average values for U.S. population.[29]

18.5.2 MEDICAL EXPOSURES

Medical exposures are exposures of patients for medical diagnosis or therapy. The medical procedures are carried out only when a physician prescribes them with the intention of providing a medical benefit to the exposed individual. Under such conditions, it is considered that the benefit from the radiation outweighs any risk. However, accumulation of medical exposures can gradually add to the genetic risk and stochastic risk to the population as a whole. Especially in order to control the genetic risk to progeny, all diagnostic medical procedures should be done in such a manner that the patient exposures remain optimally low without compromising the diagnostic reliability. All technologic advances should be applied for the purpose of reducing the exposure to patients and staff. Instances of procedures involving repeat radiation exposure (after a missed diagnosis) should be minimized.

18.5.3 RISK VS. BENEFIT PHILOSOPHY

The NCRP and ICRP provide recommendations on dose limits. For a more complete study of the subject, readers are referred to the original references[3-5] from which the safe exposure limits presented here were obtained.

As a matter of basic principle, no intentional exposure to radiation should occur unless there are benefits to be accrued either to an individual or to society. Any activity involving radiation should be planned and conducted in such a way that the exposures to individuals are optimally low, taking into consideration the economic and cost aspects.[31-33] This principle of optimization is called ALARA, as mentioned in the introduction to this chapter.

The aims in radiation protection are (i) to avoid the occurrence of deterministic effects and (ii) to limit the risk of stochastic effects. The control of deterministic effects is relatively straightforward; it should merely be ensured that, during the lifetime of an individual, the threshold doses above which these effects are known to occur are not exceeded. However, setting guidelines for the safe use of radiation to control the stochastic effects is not as straightforward. Derivation of the dose limits for restricting the stochastic detriment should be based on the perception of society regarding what can be considered an acceptable risk. A first step can be to look at the risks other than radiation which currently exist in society and which society perceives as acceptable.

In the implementation of a radiation safety program, the exposed populations are viewed as belonging to two distinct groups, radiation workers and the general public. The former are persons who are gainfully employed in an occupation that is related to a radiation application. The latter are those who themselves are not radiation workers, but who may work near or may visit a locale where radiation work is carried out. Whereas, for the former, working with radiation helps them to have an income and earn a livelihood, the latter have no such gain from radiation. Thus, it is appropriate to stipulate that the benefit-to-risk ratio for a certain level of radiation exposure is greater for the radiation workers than for the general public. Accordingly, the maximum exposure limits also should be set at different levels for the two groups.

The NCRP and ICRP have adopted an approach in which, first, the maximum exposure limits for radiation workers are set based on radiation risk estimates. Then the limits for the general public are set to be a fraction of those accepted for radiation workers.

Any occupation can have some associated risk. Let us say that the incidence of a radiation-induced cancer in a radiation worker is comparable to the occurrence of a fatal accident in any conventional industry. It is reasonable to stipulate that the chance for a radiation-induced cancer in a radiation worker should not be greater than that for a fatal incident to occur in (what NCRP refers to as) safe industries.

Although making such comparisons with other industries can place the acceptability of radiation risk in an overall perspective, there can be many areas of uncertainty. For example, in addition to fatal accidents, the other industries have incidents of nonfatal injuries with substantial morbidity. However, with the passage of time, initiation of safer practices in other industries can result in improved safety. In the same way, the detection and treatment of cancer are improving. It is also important to mention that cancer (whether caused by radiation or otherwise) apparently tends to be a disease of old age, whereas accidental death in industry has no such age bias. Consequently, the average number of livable years lost due to cancer and that due to an industrial accident are different at the ages of about 15 years and 40 years, respectively. Overall, a combination of observed effects and judgment needs to be employed for recommending the maximum limits of exposure acceptable for radiation workers.

18.6 SAFETY OF RADIATION WORKERS

18.6.1 LIMITS FOR ADULT WORKERS

The current annual maximum dose limits for radiation workers are based on comparison of the fatal accident risk in safe industries with the assumed risk of radiation-induced fatal cancers, a fraction of the nonfatal cancers, and severe genetic effects. The annual rate of accidental deaths in industries is about 0.2 to 5 per year per 10,000 workers.[17,34] Accordingly, in a worst-case situation, the total lifetime risk for an individual who works for 50 years in an unsafe industry is

$$(5/\text{year}) \times (50 \text{ years})(1/10,000) = 2.5 \times 10^{-2}$$

The dose limits to a radiation worker should be set such that the risk assessed for a radiation worker in a worst-case situation of his or her being exposed at the maximum suggested limit, year after year, throughout a working career, is nearly the same as the above number.

Radiation protection recommendations are intended for controlling both the annual risk and the cumulative risk to radiation workers. The NCRP and ICRP recommend that the occupational effective dose be limited to 50 mSv per year. The NCRP recommends that the accumulated effective dose not exceed the numerical limit given by 10 mSv multiplied by the individual's age, which implies a rate of 10 mSv per year. (The ICRP recommends a cumulative effective dose limit of 100 mSv in 5 years, which implies a rate of 20 mSv per year.) These limits apply to adult workers above the age of 18 years and are not intended to include exposures either for medical reasons or from natural background.

Many industries considered to be safe and not using radiation have fatal accident rates of one in 10,000 persons or less. Hence, it is only appropriate that industries which make use of radiation use it in such a way that the actual levels of exposures to individual workers stay well below the suggested maximum limits. The NCRP recommends that all new radiation facilities and practices be designed to limit the annual equivalent doses to individuals to a fraction of 10 mSv per year, so that the 5-year cumulative dose will also be well below the 50 mSv limit.

To control the deterministic effects, the NCRP observes that recommendations are required only for the crystalline lens of the eye, for the skin, and for the hands and feet. These limits (which are identical to the ICRP limits) for radiation workers are

Lens of the eye, 150 mSv/year
Skin, hands, and feet, 500 mSv/year

These limits recommended for stochastic risk are deemed to be adequate also for avoiding all possible deterministic effects. Table 18.7A summarizes the radiation safety limits for occupationally exposed populations.

TABLE 18.7A

Recommended Upper Limits of Exposure for Radiation Protection of Radiation Workers

Ref.	Based on Stochastic Effects[a]	Based on Deterministic Effects[b]	Embryo-fetus[b]
NCRP-116[3]	50 mSv annually and 10 mSv × age in years cumulative	150 mSv annually to lens of the eye and 500 mSv annually to skin, hands, and feet	0.5 mSv per month once pregnancy is known
ICRP-60[4,5]	50 mSv annually and 100 mSv in 5 years cumulative	150 mSv annually to lens of the eye and 500 mSv annually to skin, hands, and feet	2 mSv to woman's abdomen once pregnancy is known

[a] Stated in terms of effective dose.
[b] Stated in terms of equivalent dose.

18.6.2 LIMITS FOR EMBRYO OR FETUS

For pregnant radiation workers, the NCRP recommends a monthly equivalent dose limit of 0.5 mSv to the embryo or fetus (excluding medical and natural background radiation) once the pregnancy is known.

18.6.3 LIMITS FOR WORKERS UNDER AGE 18

Persons under the age of 18 years may occasionally be exposed to radiation during their education or training. In such situations, their work should be carried out with a high assurance of safety so that the following limits are met (excluding medical and natural background exposures):

Annual (whole-body) effective dose, 1 mSv/year

Lens of the eye, 15 mSv

Skin, hands, and feet, 50 mSv

18.6.4 PERSONNEL MONITORING

All personnel who are occupationally exposed to radiation should wear a radiation monitoring device for measurement of the radiation exposures which they receive. The monitor should be worn continuously and evaluated at regular intervals. The measuring device should be of an appropriate type to be sensitive to the type of radiation to which the personnel are exposed and should cover the anticipated range of exposures. Photographic films, thermoluminescent dosimeters, and pocket ionization chambers are common detectors used for personnel monitoring purposes. Film badges provide a permanent record of the exposure, but are less accurate than are thermoluminescent dosimeters. Pocket chambers can give instant information on the exposure received and can offer an advantage when an immediate reading is necessary. The main measuring device is worn on the chest and is called a chest badge. It is meant to give an indication of the body dose. In addition, wrist badges and finger badges can be used during procedures (such as handling of sealed sources in brachytherapy) that can cause a high exposure to the wrist or finger.

Personnel monitoring is done with the purpose of ensuring that all operations are done to maintain ALARA. The radiation safety officer (RSO) of the institution is the person entrusted with the responsibilty of overseeing radiation safety on an ongoing basis. The RSO reports to the Radiation Safety Committee (RSC) of the institution. The RSC may typically be composed of radiation physicists, safety specialists, administrators, and representatives from different departments that use radiation. The RSO reviews the personnel exposures periodically to report to the RSC on the status of safety. Any instance of high exposure to personnel can prompt the RSO and the RSC to discuss or investigate the case. This may result in the initiation of remedial steps either to improve the situation or to avoid a recurrence in the future. The details of the personnel monitoring program in an institution, such as the types of badges to be worn, the sites of monitoring, the frequency of evaluation of personnel exposure, and the levels of exposures that can be considered as acceptable ALARA are all policy decisions to be made by the RSO and RSC based on the guidelines recommended by the NCRP and ICRP.

18.7 SAFETY OF THE GENERAL PUBLIC

For the protection of nonoccupationally exposed individuals and members of the public against stochastic effects in contexts of continuous (or frequent) radiation exposure, an annual effective dose of 1 mSv is recommended by the NCRP and also by the ICRP. This is 10% of the limit recommended for occupationally exposed persons. In addition, for situations that involve infrequent annual exposures, the NCRP suggests that a higher limit of 5 mSv may be observed, provided that such exposures are suffered only by "a small group of people" and also not repeatedly by any one particular group. (The ICRP allows the annual limit of 1 mSv to be exceeded, if necessary, provided the average over 5 years does not exceed 1 mSv.)

Based on deterministic effects, the NCRP recommends an annual equivalent dose limit of 50 mSv to the lens of the eye, the skin, and the extremities, whereas the ICRP recommends an annual limit of 15 mSv for the lens of the eye and 50 mSv for skin and extremities. Table 18.7B summarizes the radiation safety limits for the nonoccupational population and the general public.

TABLE 18.7B
Recommended Upper Limits of Exposure for Radiation Protection of General Public

Ref.	Based on Stochastic Effects[a]	Based on Deterministic Effects[b]
NCRP-116[3]	1 mSv annually for continuous exposure and 5 mSv annually for infrequent exposure, cumulative	50 mSv annually to lens of eye, skin, and extremities
ICRP-60[4,5]	1 mSv annually and, if needed, higher values, provided that the annual average over 5 years does not exceed 1 mSv	15 mSv annually to lens of the eye and 50 mSv annually to skin, hands, and feet

[a]   Stated in terms of effective dose.
[b]   Stated in terms of equivalent dose.

REFERENCES

1. ICRP, International Commission on Radiological Protection, Risks associated with ionizing radiations, Ann. ICRP, Vol 22, No. 1, Pergamon, New York, 1991.
2. ICRP, International Commission on Radiological Protection, Non-stochastic effects of radiation, ICRP Publication 41, Pergamon, Oxford, 1984.
3. NCRP, National Council on Radiation Protection and Measurements, Limitations of exposure to ionizing radiation, NCRP Report 116, National Council on Radiation Protection and Measurements, Bethesda, Maryland, 1993.
4. ICRP, International Commission on Radiological Protection, Recommendations of the ICRP, ICRP-60, Ann. ICRP, Vol 21, No. 1-3, Pergamon, Oxford, 1991.
5. ICRP, International Commission on Radiological Protection, Recommendations of the International Commission on Radiological Protection: Users' Edition, Pergamon, Oxford, 1992.
6. IAEA, International Atomic Energy Agency, Recommendations for the safe use and regulation of radiation sources in industry, medicine, research, and teaching, IAEA Safety Series No. 102, International Atomic Energy Agency, Vienna, Austria, 1990.
7. Thompson, D., Mabuchi, K., Ron, E. et al., Solid Tumor Incidence in Atomic Bomb Survivors, 1958-87, RERF Technical Report 5-92, Radiation Effects Research Foundation, Hiroshima, Japan, 1992.
8. NRC, National Research Council, Committee on Biological Effects of Ionizing Radiation, BEIR V, Health effects of exposure to low levels of ionizing radiations, National Academy Press, Washington, D.C., 1990.
9. UNSCEAR, United Nations Scientific Committee on the Effects of Atomic Radiation, Sources, Effects, and Risks of Ionising Radiation, Report to the U.N. General Assembly, with annexes, United Nations Publication, New York, 1988.
10. UNSCEAR, United Nations Scientific Committee on the Effects of Atomic Radiation, Genetic and Somatic Effects of Ionising Radiation, Report to the U.N. General Assembly, with annexes, United Nations Publication, New York, 1986.
11. NRC, National Research Council, Committee on Biological Effects of Ionizing Radiation, BEIR III, The effects on population exposure to low levels of ionizing radiations, National Academy Press, Washington, D.C., 1980.
12. UNSCEAR, United Nations Scientific Committee on the Effects of Atomic Radiation, Sources, Effects of Ionising Radiation, Report to the U.N. General Assembly, with annexes, United Nations Publication, New York, 1977.
13. Kocher, D.C., Perspective on the historical development of radiation standards, Health Phys., Vol 61, p519-527, 1991.
14. Lushbaugh, C.C., Reflections on some recent progress in human radiobiology, p277-314, in Advances in Radiation Biology, Augenstein, L.G., Mason, R., and Zelle, M. (Eds.), Academic Press, New York, 1969.
15. Mole, R.H., Consequence of pre-natal radiation exposure for post-natal development: A review, Int. J. Radiat. Biol., Vol 42, p1-12, 1982.
16. Neal, J.V., Update on the genetic effects of ionizing radiation (Commentary), JAMA, Vol 266, p698-701, 1991.
17. ICRP, International Commission on Radiological Protection, Quantitative bases for developing a unified index of harm, ICRP Publication 45, Ann. ICRP, Vol 20 (1), 1985, Pergamon, Elmsford, New York.
18. NCRP, National Council on Radiation Protection and Measurements, Relative biological effectiveness of radiations of different quality, NCRP Report 104, National Council on Radiation Protection and Measurements, Bethesda, Maryland, 1990.
19. ICRU, International Commission on Radiological Units and Measurements, The quality factor in radiation protection, ICRU Report 40, International Commission on Radiological Units and Measurements, Bethesda, Maryland, 1986.

20. Land, C.E., and Sinclair, W.K., The relative contribution of different organ sites to the total cancer mortality associated with low dose radiation exposure, p31-57, in Risks Associated with Ionizing Radiations, Ann. ICRP, Vol 22 (1), 1991.
21. NCRP, National Council on Radiation Protection and Measurements, Evaluation of risk estimates for radiation protection purposes, NCRP Report 115, National Council on Radiation Protection and Measurements, Bethesda, Maryland, 1993.
22. ICRP, International Commission on Radiological Protection, Recommendations of the ICRP, ICRP Publication 26, Ann. ICRP, Vol 1, No.3, 1977, Pergamon, Oxford.
23. Auxier, J.A., Ichiban, Technical Information Center, Energy Research and Development Administration, TID-27080, National Technical Information Service, U.S. Dept. of Commerce, Springfield, VA, 1977.
24. Milton, R., and Shohoji, T., Tentative 1965 radiation dose estimation for atomic bomb survivors, Hiroshima and Nagasaki, 1968, ABCC TR 1-68, Hiroshima, Japan, 1968.
25. NRC, National Research Council, An assessment of the new dosimetry for A-bomb survivors, Panel on the reassessment of A-bomb dosimetry, Ellett, W.H. (Ed.), National Academy Press, Washington, D.C., 1987.
26. RERF, Radiation Effects Research Foundation, U.S.-Japan Joint Reassessment of Atomic Bomb Radiation Dosimetry in Hiroshima and Nagasaki — Final Report, Vol 1, Radiation Effects Research Foundation, Hiroshima, Japan, 1987.
27. RERF, Radiation Effects Research Foundation, U.S.-Japan Joint Reassessment of Atomic Bomb Radiation Dosimetry in Hiroshima and Nagasaki — Final Report, Vol 2, Radiation Effects Research Foundation, Hiroshima, Japan, 1988.
28. Bunger, B.M., Cook, J.R., and Barrick, M.K., Life table methodology for evaluating radiation risk: An application based on occupational exposures, Health Phys., Vol 40, p439-455, 1971.
29. NCRP, National Council on Radiation Protection and Measurements, Exposure to population in the US and Canada from natural background radiation, NCRP Report 94, Table 9.3, p142, National Council on Radiation Protection and Measurements, Bethesda, Maryland, 1987.
30. Barish, R.J., Health physics concerns in commercial aviation, Health Phys., Vol 59, p199-204, 1990.
31. ICRP, International Commission on Radiation Protection, Cost benefit analysis in the optimization of radiation protection, ICRP Publication 37, Ann. ICRP, Vol 10 (2/3), 1983, Pergamon, Elmsford, New York.
32. ICRP, International Commission on Radiation Protection, Optimization and decision making in radiological protection, ICRP Publication 55, Ann. ICRP, Vol 20 (1), 1989, Pergamon, Elmsford, New York.
33. NCRP, National Council on Radiation Protection and Measurements, Implementation of the principle of as low as reasonably achievable (ALARA) for medical and dental personnel, NCRP Report 107, National Council on Radiation Protection and Measurements, Bethesda, Maryland, 1990.
34. NSC, National Safety Council, Accident facts, 1992 ed., National Safety Council, Chicago, Illinois.

ADDITIONAL READING

1. Kondo, S., Health Effects of Low-level Radiation, Medical Physics Publishing, Madison, Wisconsin, 1993.
2. Bond, V., When is Dose Not A Dose?, Lauriston S. Taylor Lecture Series #15, National Council on Radiation Protection and Measurements, Bethesda, Maryland, 1992.
3. Wilson, R., and Crouch, E.A.C., Risk/Benefit Analysis, Ballinger Publ. Co., Cambridge, Massachusetts, 1982.
4. Pochin, E.E., A Perspective on Risk, in Health and Risk Analysis, Proceedings of the Third Oak Ridge National Laboratory's Life Sciences Symposium, Franklin Institute Press, Philadelphia, 1981.
5. Upton, A.C., Albert, R.E., Burns, F., and Shore, R.E. (Eds.), Radiation Carcinogenesis, Elsevier, New York, 1986.
6. Sherer, E., Streffer, C., and Trott, K.R. (Eds.), Radiation Exposure and Occupational Risks, Springer-Verlag, Berlin, 1990.
7. Hall, E.J., Radiobiology for the Radiologist, Harper & Row, Philadelphia, 1978.
8. Jayaraman, S., Lanzl, L.H., Agarwal, S.K., and Chung-Bin, A., An analysis of risk versus benefit in mammography, Appl. Radiol., Vol 15, p45-52, 1986.

Chapter 19

RADIATION SAFETY IN EXTERNAL-BEAM THERAPY

19.1 INTRODUCTION

In Chapter 18, we discussed the harmful effects of radiation and the need to conduct the activities involving radiation so as to keep the radiation dose to workers and the general public within recommended limits. In this chapter, we discuss the major factors that need to be considered in the design and building of any external-beam radiation therapy facility.

The International Commission on Radiological Protection (ICRP) and the National Council on Radiation Protection and Measurements (NCRP) are recognized as authorities on the subject of radiation safety. The 1993 guidelines of the NCRP for limiting the exposure of persons (reviewed in Chapter 18) are adopted for the numerical examples in this chapter. It usually takes a few years before the recommendations of scientific bodies such as the NCRP become assimilated in the binding laws of the regional health-regulatory agencies. At the time of this writing, the 1993 NCRP recommendations had been released a few months earlier.[1] There is some ongoing controversy in the scientific community as to whether the dose limits recently recommended by the NCRP and ICRP are based on hypotheses that overestimate the radiation risk and hence are too restrictive.[2-5] Although it is not our purpose in this text to discuss such controversies, it is appropriate to draw attention to the following important facts:

(a) Radiation risk assessments and recommended dose limits have changed with time,[6] and they can be expected to change in the future. For example, the NCRP published a report, No. 91, entitled "Recommendations on Limits for Exposure to Ionizing Radiation," in 1987.[7] In 1991, the ICRP revised its past recommendations and published new guidelines for radiation safety based on newer data and analysis.[8] In 1993, the NCRP followed, replacing its 1987 report in its entirety with a new report, No. 116, entitled "Limitation of Exposure to Ionizing Radiation."[1]

(b) NCRP guidelines are only recommendations and are not legally binding. Although many governments may adopt the NCRP guidelines, there can be variations. Only the rules and regulations formulated by local governments carry the force of law. For purposes of safe design of any facility, the rules and regulations promulgated by the local authorities are binding. Furthermore, any emerging trends or expected changes in the future should be taken into account. Dose limits adopted by a facility should be "as low as reasonably achievable" (ALARA).[9]

19.2 TIME, DISTANCE, AND SHIELDING

Time, *distance*, and *shielding* are the three basic parameters that affect the radiation dose received from a radiation source. A proper mixture of the values of these three parameters is necessary if the exposure of persons involved in the uses of radiation is to be kept at acceptably low levels.

Considering *time*, the shorter the time required for a procedure, the lower will be the dose to which the worker is exposed. That is, if the other two parameters, distance and shielding, remain unchanged, the dose received by a worker will be directly proportional to the time he remains in the radiation field. Thus, it is important for the worker to carry out procedures with dispatch.

The second parameter is the *distance* between the radiation source and the worker. If the physical size of the source is small compared to this distance, the dose to the worker will be inversely proportional to the square of the distance.

The third parameter, *shielding*, refers to the interposition of an attenuating barrier between the source and the worker, with the purpose of reducing the exposure to the worker. Usually, shielding is used in situations where improvement in time and distance alone cannot provide the necessary degree of safety. Sometimes, shielding is added for the purpose of ALARA.

Safe operation of an external-beam therapy machine is possible only when it is installed in a well-shielded treatment room. Several references give detailed presentations of the shielding and design considerations for external-beam therapy facilities.[10-14]

19.3 APPROACH TO SHIELDING DESIGN OF A BEAM-THERAPY FACILITY

19.3.1 SELECTION OF ACCEPTABLE WEEKLY EQUIVALENT DOSE LIMITS (P)

In order to estimate the shielding to be provided by a protective barrier, one must decide on a maximum weekly dose, P, that is acceptable to the occupants behind the barrier. From Tables 18.7 A and B, we extract the following annual and cumulative radiation limits recommended by the NCRP for radiation protection purposes:

(a) A limit of 50 mSv per year for radiation workers, with a cumulative limit of 10 mSv multiplied by the age of the person in years
(b) 1 mSv annually for nonradiation workers and the general public if they are likely to be continuously exposed, and 5 mSv annually if the exposure is infrequent

NCRP Report No. 116,[1] in addition, states the following: "The 50 mSv annual limit should be utilized only to provide flexibility required for existing facilities and practices. The NCRP recommends that all new facilities and the introduction of all new practices should be designed to limit annual exposures to individuals to a fraction of 10 mSv per year limit implied by the cumulative dose limit by occupation."

In this chapter, based on (a) and (b) above, we use a limit of 10 mSv per year for areas occupied by radiation workers and of 1 mSv for the other areas where nonradiation workers of the staff, the public, or patients can be present. The high-radiation areas where the radiation workers function are to be controlled to allow only minimum access to nonradiation workers or the public. Such areas are referred to as controlled areas. If we use an organ weighting factor, W_T, of 1.0 (for whole-body irradiation) and a radiation weighting factor, W_R, of 1.0 (for photons), the limits stated above result in approximate P values of 200 µGy/week and 20 µGy/week for the controlled and noncontrolled areas, respectively.

19.3.2 RADIATION COMPONENTS

In the design of the shielding of an external-beam therapy facility, it is important, first, to recognize that (as shown in Figure 19.1) there are three major radiation components, primary photons, scattered photons, and leakage photons, against which the persons have to be protected. The primary component refers to the photons of the direct beam irradiating the patient. The scattered component consists of photons scattered from the patient and the walls of the treatment room. The leakage radiation refers to the photons from the source that emerge by penetrating the source-head shielding. In addition to these, for high-energy machines (above 10 MV), protection against photoneutrons and neutron capture gamma rays should also be taken into account.[12,15]

19.3.3 RECOMMENDED LEAKAGE LEVELS

Radiation is emitted from the target within the source head in all directions. The shielding design of the source head should take this fact into account and should be such as to limit the radiation intensity in all directions other than the direction of the useful beam. For accelerators, the leakage ceases when the beam current is turned off. For machines that use radioisotope sources,

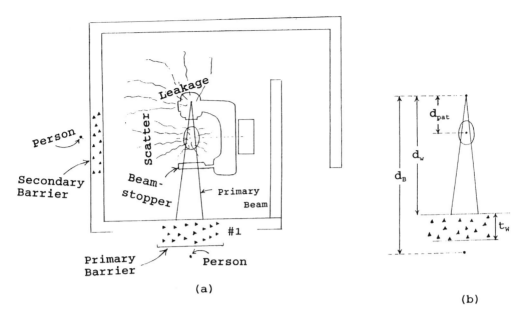

FIGURE 19.1 Diagram showing (a) the primary, leakage, and scattered radiation components, primary barrier, secondary barrier, and beam stopper, and (b) the different distances involved in the shielding evaluation.

leakage radiation emerges from the source heads at all times and irradiates the staff even when the source is in the "OFF" position.

For radiation safety purposes, allowable leakage limits have been given most recently in NCRP Report 102.[16] For X-ray equipment, NCRP Report 102 divides the source housing assemblies into three categories based upon the energy of the X-rays. The NCRP recommends that the equipment manufacturer construct the source housing to meet the following upper limits for leakage:

(1) For X-ray production at tube potentials from 5 kV to 50 kV, the leakage kerma rate at any position 5 centimeters from the assembly shall not exceed 0.1 cGy in any one hour.

(2) For X-ray production at tube potentials greater than 50 kV and less than 500 kV, the leakage kerma rate measured at a distance of one meter from the source in any direction shall not exceed 1 cGy in any one hour. ... In addition, these assemblies shall limit the kerma rate at a distance of 5 cm from the surface of the assembly to 30 cGy in any one hour.

(3) For X-ray and electron beam equipment operated above 500 kV, the assembly <u>shall</u> be designed so that the following conditions are fulfilled for the regions outside the useful beam.

(i) The absorbed dose rate due to leakage radiation. ... at any point outside the maximum sized useful beam, but within a circular plane of radius 2 m which is perpendicular to and centered on the central axis of the useful beam at the normal treatment distance, <u>shall</u> not exceed 0.2 percent of the absorbed dose rate to tissue on the central axis at the treatment distance.(The leakage radiation shall be measured with the useful beam blocked by an absorber capable of reducing the useful beam intensity to 0.1 percent of its normal value.

(ii) Except for the area defined above, the absorbed dose rate in tissue (excluding that from neutrons) at 1 m from the electron path between the source and the target or the electron window <u>shall</u> not exceed 0.5 percent of the absorbed dose rate in tissue on the central axis of the beam at the normal treatment distance.

For therapy source heads using gamma sealed sources, the leakage limits are stated for both the "off" and "on" conditions of the source as follows:

(1) The housing <u>shall</u> be so constructed that at 1 m from the source in the OFF condition, the maximum and average leakage kerma rates through the housing shall not exceed 100 μGy h^{-1} and 20 μGy h^{-1}, respectively. In the design of the housing, consideration should also be given to reducing the surface kerma rate for small diameter housings to less than 2 mGy h^{-1} at 5 cm from surface. (See NCRP Report No. 102 for details as to where measurements are to be made for determining the maximum and average leakage rates.)

(2) The housing shall be so constructed that at 1 m from the source in the ON position the housing leakage kerma rate <u>shall</u> not exceed 0.1 percent of the useful beam kerma rate at one meter. For sources with useful beam kerma rate of less than 10 Gy h^{-1} at 1 m the housing leakage kerma rate <u>shall not</u> exceed 1 cGy h^{-1} at 1 m from the source in the ON position. For both cases the limits apply when the beam is completely intercepted by the collimation or an equivalent barrier. These limits do not apply to housings designed exclusively for whole body irradiations.

19.3.4 SHIELDING DATA

Shielding calculations are meant to give an estimate of acceptable barrier transmissions. A tenth-value thickness (TVT) is the thickness of a barrier that attenuates the radiation to one tenth of its intensity, in the same manner as a half-value thickness (HVT) provides attenuation to one half. TVT and HVT are related as

$$TVT \approx 3.32 \; HVT$$

A barrier thickness X that can give a barrier transmission B is related to the TVT by

$$10^{-X/TVT} = B$$

i.e., $$X = n\,(TVT), \; \text{where} \; n = -\log_{10}(B)$$

The value n gives the number of TVTs needed for the barrier. For non-monoenergetic beams, the TVT and HVT can change due to the effect of beam hardening (see Chapter 8, Section 8.6.3). However, after some degree of initial hardening, a steady value called equilibrium TVT (designated TVT$_e$) is reached.

Scatter and leakage together are referred to as secondary radiations. Unlike the primary beam, the secondaries have no specific direction. Because the primary beam is very intense and is also highly penetrating, the barriers needed for protection against the primary beam are usually very thick. Thus, a wall that is designed to protect against the primary beam is generally also adequate to protect against the secondary radiation. If a wall is exposed only to secondary radiations, a secondary protective barrier will suffice there. By the proper choice of the orientation of the therapy equipment during installation, irradiation of high-occupancy areas by the primary beam can be avoided and the shielding cost reduced. The leaking X-radiation, which has been hardened by the heavy shielding of the source head, is of higher average energy than is the primary. The scattered radiation, on the other hand, is less penetrating than the primary radiation. The energy and penetration of the scattered radiation are a function of the angle of scatter. Here TVT$_e$s for primary, scattered, and leakage radiations are designated by (TVT$_e$)$_P$, (TVT$_e$)$_S$, and (TVT$_e$)$_L$, respectively.

Data on the transmission of broad X-ray beams of different energies in various shielding materials have been published. The (TVT$_e$)$_P$ values given in Table 19.1 and the (TVT$_e$)$_S$ in Table 19.2 will be used for shielding evaluations in this chapter. We also assume that (TVT$_e$)$_L$ $\approx$ (TVT$_e$)$_P$. Concrete of density 2.35 g cm^{-3} is the most commonly used shielding material for the walls. The

TABLE 19.1
Tenth-Value Thickness, $(TVT_e)_P$, of Attenuation for Broad Primary Photon Beams of Different Energies and Materials

Beam	Concrete[a] (cm)	Barite[b] (cm)	Steel[c] (cm)	Lead[d] (cm)
0.25-MV X-rays	9	—	—	0.22
0.5-MV X-rays	14	—	—	—
^{137}Cs (0.66-MeV gamma rays)	15.7	—	5.3	2.1
1.0 MV X-rays	20	—	—	3.0
^{60}Co ($\approx$1.25-MeV gamma rays)	24	17	7.0	4.0
4 MV X-rays	29	20	8.5	5.3
6 MV X-rays	34	25	10	5.6
10 MV X-rays	39	29	11	5.6
20 MV X-rays	45	34	11	5.6

Note: Values compiled by the authors from references listed in the text.

[a] Density 2.35 g cm^{-3}.
[b] Density 3.2 g cm^{-3}.
[c] Density 7.8 g cm^{-3}.
[d] Density 11.35 g cm^{-3}

TABLE 19.2
Tenth-Value Thickness, $(TVT_e)_S$, of Attenuation for Scattered Radiations

Primary Beam	Angle of Scatter	Concrete[a] (cm)	Lead[b] (cm)
^{137}Cs	30°	15.7	1.8
(0.660-MeV	45°	14.6	1.5
gamma rays)	60°	13.3	1.3
	90°	12.3	0.7
	135°	11.3	0.4
^{60}Co	30°	21	3.4
($\approx$1.25-MeV	60°	19	2.5
gamma rays)	90°	16	1.5
4-MV X-rays	90°	17	—
6-MV X-rays	30°	26	—
	60°	21	—
	90°	18	—

Note: Values were compiled by the authors from references listed in the text. Useful for shielding calculations only.

[a] Density 2.35 g cm^{-3}.
[b] Density 11.35 g cm^{-3}.

density of any proposed shielding material should be ascertained by measurement of a sample. The TVTs for other materials such as earth, sand, brick, or heavy concrete can be derived from the TVT for concrete by density scaling:

$$\text{TVT in material} = \text{TVT in concrete} \times \frac{\text{density of concrete}}{\text{density of material}}$$

Barite ($BaSO_4$) concrete, with a density of 3.0 to 4.5 g cm^{-3}, has been used for reducing the shielding thickness where space is limited. The primary barrier can be made partly of steel to save space where necessary. Lead is the material commonly employed in the entrance door. The neutron production at energies above 10 MV requires that the door has hydrogenous material incorporated for protection against these neutrons.

19.3.5 ARCHITECTURAL AND EQUIPMENT DATA

NCRP Report No. 49 (page 108) states that, prior to the design of a facility, it is necessary to have the following architectural and equipment information:[10]

(1) Architectural

a. Drawings of radiation rooms and adjacent area, ... including position of radiation source, doors, and windows.
b. Information about occupancy below, above, and adjacent to radiation rooms.
c. Type of proposed, or existing, construction of floors, ceilings, and wall.
d. For megavoltage therapy installations, including cobalt, vertical sections and plot plans.

(2) Equipment

a. Below 150 kV.
    1) Purpose: therapy, radiography, fluoroscopy, etc.
    2) kV and weekly workload, if known.
b. 150 kV and above, including gamma beam apparatus.
    1) kV, or type of gamma source.
    2) mA or R per min (in present usage, rad or cGy per minute) at 1 meter.
    3) Weekly workload, if known, expressed in mA min, or cGy at 1 m.
    4) Restrictions in beam orientations without and with beam interceptor, if any.
c. Possible future increases in workload and radiation energy, and modification in beam orientation.

19.3.6 WORKLOAD (W)

Workload (W) is a measure of the degree of use of a particular external-beam therapy machine and is evaluated in terms of the dose delivered by the useful beam at 1 m from the source for 1 week of operation. W is expressed in Gy m^2 week^{-1}. For non-pulsed X-ray equipment operating below 1 MV, the workload has also been expressed in terms of milliampere-minutes (mA min) used per week.

Example 19.1

It is planned to install an isocentric 4-MV X-ray machine. It is expected that an average time of 7 min for setup and 3 min for irradiation will be needed for each patient treated on the machine. The average daily dose per patient is estimated to be 2.5 cGy at the isocenter of the machine, located at 0.8 m from the source. The clinic expects to work 14 h every day for 5 working days per week. Estimate the workload.

Machine time to be used per patient = 7 min (for setup) + 3 min (for treatment) = 10 min

Patients to be treated per hour = 60 min/10 min = 6 patients/h

Daily patient load in a 14-h working day = 14 h/d × 6 patients/hour = 84 patients/d

2.5 Gy is delivered at 0.8 m treatment distance for every patient. There are 5 working days per week. Total dose delivered by the machine per week

$$= (2.5 \text{ Gy/patient at } 0.8 \text{ m}) \times (84 \text{ patients/day}) \times (5 \text{ days/week})$$
$$= 1050 \text{ Gy week}^{-1} \text{ at } 0.8 \text{ m}$$

We want to express the workload as normalized at 1 m from the source. This normalization is achieved by multiplication of the above value by $(0.8 \text{ m})^2$. Thus,

$$W = (1050 \text{ Gy/week}) \times (0.8 \text{ m})^2$$
$$= 672 \text{ Gy m}^2 \text{ week}^{-1}$$

19.3.7 USE FACTOR (U)

In general, a radiation therapy machine may have its beam pointed in several directions during its use. The walls, floor, and ceiling to which the beam can be directed are to be designed to shield the primary radiation beam from the source. They are referred to as primary protective barriers. The other walls or barriers, toward which the radiation beam is not directed, are designed to protect against the scatter and leakage radiations. These are called secondary protective barriers. The use factor (U) is a beam direction factor that gives the fraction of the workload W for which the beam has a particular orientation. U for different directions can be based on specific details regarding the anticipated use of the particular equipment that is planned to be installed. Table 19.3 presents the values of U as obtained from the references cited.[10,17-19]

TABLE 19.3
Use Factors (U) (i.e., Beam Direction Factors) for Primary Protective
Barriers for Therapy Installations

Ref.	Floor	Walls	Ceiling[a]
NCRP[10]	1	1/4	1/4
Johns and Cunningham[17]	0.6	0.1	0.3
Farrow[18]	0.625	0.13	0.115
Cobb and Bjarngard[19]	0.48	0.6	0.29

Note: Values given are for use in situations where no specific data for the particular facility are available.

[a] Design features of some radiotherapy equipment may prohibit directing the beam toward the ceiling.

19.3.8 OCCUPANCY FACTOR (T)

Shielding is designed to protect the possible occupants of an area, rather than to protect the area itself. The purpose for which the protected area is used can be such that it may not be realistic to assume that the area is occupied by any one individual for all of the time that the beam is on. For example, toilets, elevators, hallways, and patients' waiting rooms are occupied only occasionally by any one individual. The occupancy factor (T) is used in the shielding evaluations to take into account such facts. Any area used by a radiation worker should be considered an area with full occupancy, with T = 1. Table 19.4 gives the values of T from NCRP Report No. 49, for nonoccu-pationally exposed persons, in the planning of shielding.[10] These values can be used if no other occupancy data specific to the facility are available. Full-occupancy areas (T = 1) are work areas such as offices, laboratories, shops, patient wards, and nurses' stations. Areas of partial occupancy (T = 1/4) are corridors, rest rooms, unattended parking lots, etc. Areas of occasional occupancy (T = 1/16) are waiting rooms, stairways, toilets, janitors' closets, etc. In some jurisdictions, local laws may forbid the use of a value of T less than 1/4.

TABLE 19.4
Occupancy Factors

Occupancy	T	Area
Full	1	Work areas, offices, laboratories, shops, nursing station, control panel, occupied spaces in near-by buildings
Partial	1/4	Corridors, restrooms, elevators using operators, unattended parking lots
Occasional	1/16	Waiting rooms, toilets, stairways, unattended elevators, janitors' closets, outside areas used by pedestrians or vehicular traffic

From NCRP Report No. 49,[10] to be used when no data specific to the facility are available.

19.4 ESTIMATING THE ALLOWABLE BARRIER TRANSMISSION

19.4.1 PRIMARY SHIELDING BARRIER

Figure 19.1a illustrates a beam from a teletherapy source head directed toward a wall (#1) of the treatment room. This wall should be designed to reduce the exposure of the occupants on its other side to the primary beam. In barrier calculations, the dose reduction due to the inverse-square fall-off should also be allowed for. For this we need to estimate the distance, d_B, from the source to the occupant behind the barrier. The distance d_B is a sum of three distances: the distance, d_W, from the source to the wall, the thickness of the wall, t_W, and a possible distance of clearance between the wall and the occupant, as shown in Figure 19.1b. NCRP Report No. 49 suggests that it can be assumed that there is a 30-cm clearance between any occupant and the wall. Because the purpose in the calculation itself is to determine the value of t_W, assuming that t_W is zero is a possible conservative assumption in the estimation of d_B, unless a first-guess value of t_W is known from past experience. By the definitions of the workload (W), the use factor (U), and the occupancy factor (T), the equivalent dose received in 1 week by a person standing at distance d_B in the absence of any shielding will be

$$\frac{W\,U\,T}{\left(d_B\right)^2} \tag{19-1}$$

Some therapy heads that are mounted on a gantry for isocentric rotation may have a counter-weight that intercepts the beam after it exits the patient, as shown in Figure 19.1a. If there is such a beam interceptor (also called beam stopper), the fraction, F_{BS}, of radiation that is transmitted by the beam interceptor should be taken into account in the shielding calculations. NCRP Report No. 102 recommends that a beam interceptor should transmit not more than 0.1% of the useful beam (i.e., $F_{BS} < 0.001$) and cover up to a 30° angle of the central ray. If the equivalent dose to a person behind the wall should not exceed the weekly limit P, the maximum acceptable transmission, B_P, through the primary barrier can be derived from the equation

$$\frac{W\,U\,T}{\left(d_B\right)^2}F_{BS} \times B_P = P \tag{19-2}$$

i.e.,

$$B_P = \frac{P\left(d_B\right)^2}{W\,U\,T}\frac{1}{F_{BS}} \tag{19-3}$$

19.4.2 SECONDARY PROTECTIVE BARRIER

Where there is no primary barrier, a secondary barrier will be needed to provide protection against leakage and scattered radiations.

Leakage Radiation

For any machine, the manufacturers specify the leakage fluence at 1 m from the source as a fraction, F_L, of the useful primary beam fluence at 1 m from the source (see Section 19.3.3). If the distance between a person behind the barrier and the source position is d_B (see Figure 19.1b), the maximum acceptable barrier transmission, B_L, that protects against leakage radiation is obtainable from the relation

$$\frac{W\,U\,T}{\left(d_B\right)^2}F_L \times B_L = P \tag{19–4}$$

i.e.,

$$B_L = \frac{P\left(d_B\right)^2}{W\,U\,T}\frac{1}{F_L} \tag{19–5}$$

The use factor U is 1 for leakage radiation.

Scattered Radiation

The intensity of scattered radiation from the patient which reaches the barrier is related to the primary intensity at the patient position, the cross section of the beam (i.e., the volume irradiated), the angle of deflection of the scattered photons that reach the barrier, and the distance to the barrier. We define a scattering coefficient, α, as the ratio of the scattered dose for a beam of unit cross-sectional area (1 m^2) at a unit distance (1 m) away from the scatterer (i.e., the patient) to the primary dose delivered to the scatterer.

Examples of the values of α that can be used for shielding calculations are given in Table 19.5. The value of α changes with the energy of the primary beam and the angle θ of the scatter with respect to the direction of the primary. In general, a machine may have collimators that provide a maximum possible beam cross section of A_{pat} at its normal source-to-patient distance, d_{pat}. Because the workload, W, is specified at a distance of 1 m from the source, the primary dose to the scatterer (i.e., the patient) is $W/(d_{pat})^2$, with d_{pat} measured in meters. Because the values of α are for a beam of 1 m^2 cross section, for a beam of cross section A_{pat} (measured in square meters), the scattered dose at 1 m from the patient is

$$\frac{W}{\left(d_{pat}\right)^2}\left(\alpha\,A_{pat}\right) \tag{19–6}$$

The dose to a person behind the barrier will also be reduced because of the inverse-square fall-off of the scatter fluence over the distance d_B between the person and the scatterer. Hence, in general, the maximum acceptable barrier transmission, B_S, for the scattered radiation is related to P by the expression

$$\frac{W\,U\,T}{\left(d_{pat}\right)^2}F_S\,B_S = P \tag{19–7}$$

where F_S is the scatter factor given by

TABLE 19.5
Values of Scatter Coefficient α

Primary Beam	Scattering Angle θ[a]					
	30°	**45°**	**60°**	**90°**	**120°**	**135°**
^{137}Cs gamma rays	0.1625	0.125	0.1025	0.07	—	0.0475
^{60}Co gamma rays	0.15	0.09	0.0575	0.0225	—	0.015
4-MV X-rays	—	0.068	—	—	—	—
6-MV X-rays	0.175	0.045	0.0275	0.015	—	0.01

Note: α is the ratio of scattered dose at 1 m from the patient to the primary dose incident on the patient for a beam cross section of 1 m^2. Converted from data in NCRP Report No. 49,[10] which are for a beam of cross section 400 cm^2.

[a] $\theta = 0$ for forward scatter.

$$F_S = \frac{\alpha A_{pat}}{\left(d_B\right)^2} \tag{19–8}$$

Hence,

$$B_S = \frac{P\left(d_{pat}\right)^2}{WUT} \frac{1}{F_S} \tag{19–9}$$

All walls should have enough shielding to protect against 90° side scatter from the patient. The use factor U is 1 for 90° scatter. Sometimes, additional consideration will need to be given to photons scattered in a forward direction (at angles less than 90°) with respect to the incident beam. For example, this happens if the primary barrier of a side wall is designed to be just wide enough to cover the primary beam (as in Figure 19.1a). If so, the primary barrier may cover a 25° to 30° angle with respect to the central axis of the primary beam. Then the wall beyond the primary barrier should be designed to protect, not only against the leakage through the source housing and 90° scatter, but also against forward scatter from the patient that travels beyond the primary barrier when the beam is directed toward the wall.

Forward-scattered photons are of higher energy than 90° scatter and are more penetrating. Furthermore, the scatter coefficient, α, is greater for forward scatter. When one calculates the barrier thickness for protection against such forward scatter, adoption of a value of U of less than 1.0 can be meaningful. The value of U can be identical to that adopted for the calculation of the thickness of the adjacent primary barrier.

In the above analysis, we addressed scatter and leakage separately, although protection is needed against both simultaneously. To take this into account, the NCRP suggests that, after an independent calculation of the two barrier thicknesses, one should check the difference between them. If the difference exceeds one TVT, using the greater of the two thicknesses will be adequate. Otherwise, one HVT should be added to the greater thickness and adopted as the barrier thickness needed.

19.4.3 ENTRANCE DOOR BARRIER

Most radiotherapy rooms are designed to have a maze entrance. Some plans of maze designs are shown in Figure 19.2. The walls of the entrance path are designed to be such that leakage or scattered radiation from the isocenter cannot reach the door directly without undergoing scatter. A maze of proper design can reduce the lead shielding needed at the door. Multiple reflections through a maze with folds or turns is an effective means of reducing both the energy and the fluence of photons reaching the door. Protection against neutrons can also be achieved by making the maze entrance sufficiently long through several turns, if needed.

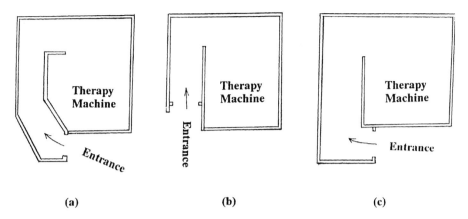

FIGURE 19.2   Three different designs of maze entrances to therapy rooms are shown in (a), (b), and (c).

The kinematics of Compton scattering of high-energy photons (see Section 7.5.3) is such that the maximum energy of photons scattered at 90° is 0.511 MeV. It is possible to show that, for 180° scatter, the scattered photon energy is 0.511/2 = 0.255 MeV, irrespective of the energy of the high-energy primary photon. This is also true when 180° scatter occurs as a consequence of two successive 90° scattering events. Hence, shielding data for 0.25 MeV can be used for shielding against a second scatter. However, for high-energy machines (operating far above the pair-production threshold of 1.02 MeV), there will be a significant number of annihilation photons of 0.511 MeV. Two or three scattering events at smaller angles in a single object can also result in a backscattered photon of energy higher than 0.511 MeV. In such cases, shielding data for 1-MV X-rays can be used.

In a treatment room having a single straight maze entrance (as shown in Figure 19.2b), the walls facing the entrance door to the treatment room can scatter the radiation scattered from the patient and the leakage from the source head toward the door. In principle, any scatterer can have a scatter factor of the form shown in Equation (19–8). If the wall that scatters is at a distance $d_{1,2}$ from the isocenter, the dose at the wall due to scatter from the patient is given by

$$\frac{W U T}{\left(d_{pat}\right)^{2}}\left(F_{S}\right)_{1}$$

where $\left(F_{S}\right)_{1}$ is the scatter factor for the first scatterer (i.e., the patient), and is given by

$$\left(F_{S}\right)_{1} = \frac{\alpha\, A_{pat}}{\left(d_{1,2}\right)^{2}} \tag{19–10}$$

If the wall is treated as a second scatterer having a scatter coefficient α_{2} and an area of irradiation A_{2}, the scatter factor, $\left(F_{S}\right)_{2}$, for the second scatterer is given by

$$\left(F_{S}\right)_{2} = \frac{\alpha_{2}\, A_{2}}{\left(d_{B}\right)^{2}} \tag{19–11}$$

where d_{B} is the distance between the second scatterer (i.e., the wall) and the entrance. Accordingly, we modify Equation (19–7) to obtain the following expression for the dose, $\left(D_{door}\right)_{S}$, received by a person at the door due to patient scatter:

$$\left(D_{door}\right)_S = \frac{W\,U\,T}{\left(d_{pat}\right)^2}\left(F_S\right)_1\left(F_S\right)_2 \tag{19–12}$$

For this dose to be reduced to the weekly limit P, the door should have shielding that attenuates the scatter by a factor $(B_{door})_S$, given by

$$\left(B_{door}\right)_S = \frac{P\left(d_{pat}\right)^2}{W\,U\,T}\frac{1}{\left(F_S\right)_1}\frac{1}{\left(F_S\right)_2} \tag{19–13}$$

The concept of Equations (19–12) and (19–13) can be extended to several successive scatterers. More complex methods of scatter evaluation by Monte Carlo and transport theoretical methods are possible,[20-22] but are not discussed here.

The factor $(F_S)_2$ is also applicable to the scattering of the leakage radiation by the wall toward the door. The dose at the door, $(D_{door})_L$, due to the wall scattering of the leakage radiation is

$$\left(D_{door}\right)_L = W\,U\,T\frac{F_L}{\left(d_{1,2}\right)^2}\left(F_S\right)_2 \tag{19–14}$$

For this dose to be reduced to the weekly limit P, the door should have shielding that attenuates this radiation by a factor $(B_{door})_L$, given by

$$\left(B_{door}\right)_L = \frac{P\left(d_{1,2}\right)^2}{W\,U\,T}\frac{1}{F_L}\frac{1}{\left(F_S\right)_2} \tag{19–15}$$

The total dose at the door, D_{door}, is given by the sum of $(D_{door})_S$ and $(D_{door})_L$. The door shielding should be adequate to give protection against both scattered and leakage radiations. After the door shielding is calculated separately for scattered and leakage radiations, the actual door thickness needed to protect against both of them can be arrived at based on the considerations discussed in Section 19.4.2.

19.4.4 ROOF PROTECTION AND SKYSHINE

The area above the ceiling of the treatment room may or may not be planned to be an occupied area. If there will be occupancy, the area of the roof struck by the primary beam should have sufficient thickness to function as a primary protective barrier, and the remaining part of the roof should offer protection against leakage and scattered radiation.

Even in situations where there is no occupancy directly above the ceiling, possible irradiation of occupants in upper stories of neighboring buildings should not be overlooked (see Figure 19.3). In addition to the possibility of direct irradiation, the radiation scattered by air, called skyshine or airshine, can pose a problem.[11,23-25] The skyshine can contribute a significant dose in areas behind the walls of the treatment room, if the ceiling offers only weather protection and no shielding. If a source delivers a dose rate, D_{1m}, at 1 m from it in air, and if the solid angle subtended at the source by the irradiated volume of air is Ω, an estimate of the dose rate from skyshine, $D_{skyshine}$, at a lateral distance, d_p (Figure 19.3), can be obtained from the following equation:[11]

$$D_{skyshine} = \frac{2.5\times10^{-2}\times D_{1m}\times\Omega^{1.3}}{\left(d_p\right)^2} \tag{19–16}$$

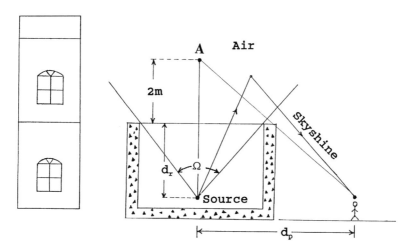

FIGURE 19.3 Diagram illustrating air scatter or skyshine. Ω is the solid angle subtended at the source by the aperture of the open roof.

For radiotherapy rooms, Ω is the solid angle subtended by the area of the roof irradiated. If a circular roof is irradiated, as shown in Figure 19.4, Ω is given by $2\pi(1 - \cos \phi)$, where ϕ is the polar angle of inclination between the center and the periphery of the roof. In practical situations, the irradiated area of the roof is likely to be close to a square. In such cases, it is possible to find an approximate value of Ω for skyshine calculations by replacing the square or rectangular area by an equivalent circular area. For scatter and leakage radiations, Ω is the value subtended by the entire ceiling. For the primary beam, Ω should be calculated for the largest primary beam cross section provided by the machine. D_{1m} can be substituted by $(WUT\ F_{BS})$, $(WUT\ F_L)$, and $(WUT\ \alpha\ A_{pat})/(d_{pat})^2$ for primary, leakage, and scatter components, respectively. NCRP Report No. 51 suggests that the acceptable transmission through the roof, $B_{skyshine}$, can be assessed from[11]

$$B_{skyshine} = \frac{P\left(d_r + 2\right)^2}{D_{skyshine}} = \frac{P\left(d_r + 2\right)^2 \left(d_p\right)^2}{2.5 \times 10^{-2} \times D_{1m} \times \Omega^{1.3}} \qquad (19\text{–}17)$$

where d_r is the height of the roof from the source in meters. (The term $(d_r + 2)^2$ is the square of the distance from the source to a point 2 m above the roof, as shown in Figure 19.3.)

Roof shielding of 1 to 2 TVT may often be needed for a therapy facility so that an unacceptable dose from skyshine is prevented.

19.5 HIGH-ENERGY X-RAYS AND NEUTRON PRODUCTION

19.5.1 NEUTRON SHIELDING AT THE DOOR

At low photon energies, photoneutron production is absent or negligible. At energies above 10 MV, production of photoneutrons increases.[11,12,15,26] The photoneutrons result from interaction of photons in materials in the source head, collimators, the patient, and also the materials in the room. From the point of view of dose to the patient, the neutron dose is insignificant compared to the photon dose.[15,27,28] For a dose of 1000 cGy delivered by photons, the neutron dose may be in the range of 0.06 to 0.1 cGy. However, for radiation safety of personnel, protection against neutrons cannot be ignored. For understanding the neutron problem, the reader is referred to the references cited above, in particular NCRP Report No. 79.[15]

Neutron fluence is reduced by slowing of neutrons through elastic scattering interactions with nuclei of the shielding material.[2,12,29,30] The slowing-down process is called moderation. In elastic scattering of neutrons with hydrogen nuclides, much energy is transferred to the hydrogen nuclides

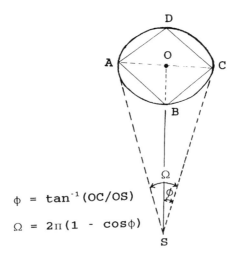

$$\phi = \tan^{-1}(OC/OS)$$

$$\Omega = 2\pi(1 - \cos\phi)$$

FIGURE 19.4 Solid angle subtended by the aperture of a circular roof at the source S. ϕ is the polar angle subtended by the circular periphery. Points A, B, C, and D on the circumference of the circle form the corners of a rectangular aperture.

(which recoil as protons). This large energy transfer happens because the mass of the hydrogen nucleus is almost the same as that of the impinging neutron. Collision of neutrons with heavy nuclides does not cause much loss of energy by the neutrons. Thus, heavy metals are poor neutron shields compared to hydrogenous materials. Water is a good moderator, and so are many plastic materials. The water content of concrete makes it an effective neutron attenuator.

NCRP Report No. 79[15] presents the following empirical expressions for concrete and polyethylene that relate the tenth-value thickness, TVT_N (in centimeters), for reduction of neutron dose equivalent around medical accelerators to the average neutron energy, E_n (in mega-electron volts):

$$TVT_N = \left(15.5 + 5.6\,\overline{E}_n\right) \text{ cm for concrete}$$

and

$$TVT_N = \left(6.2 + 3.4\,\overline{E}_n\right) \text{ cm for polyethylene}$$

NCRP Report No. 79 also states that the value of $\overline{E}_n$ would not exceed 1 MeV for medical accelerators. Thus, TVT_N would be less than 21 cm of concrete.

Normally, a therapy room that is shielded with concrete walls can also provide shielding against neutrons. However, neutrons can bounce off the walls and pass through the entrance way to reach the door. The area outside the door is a high-occupancy area. Furthermore, when the equivalent dose from neutrons is evaluated, the radiation weighting factors for neutrons (which are higher than those for X-rays) should not be overlooked. Therefore, the door needs to contain a sufficient thickness of a hydrogenous material (like polyethylene) to reduce the neutron dose to the occupants at the entrance. NCRP Report No. 79 states that the average energy of neutrons reaching the door is very low, in the neighborhood of 100 keV, and incorporation of 2 in. (5 cm) of polyethylene in the door would reduce the fast-neutron component by a factor of 10. Because neutrons that have slowed down considerably (called thermal neutrons) are captured by boron nuclides, polyethylene impregnated with boron offers advantage.

Approximate methods of estimating the neutron dose equivalent at the entrance to the room are reported in the literature.[15,31,32] In one method, which assumes a TVT_N for neutrons of 5 m in air, the equivalent dose, $(D_{door})_N$, from neutrons at the door is derived as

$$\left(D_{door}\right)_N = \frac{W\,F_N\,W_R}{\left(d_{maze}\right)^2\,10^{L/5}} \tag{19-18}$$

where F_N is the neutron dose at 1 m from the isocenter, expressed as a fraction of the dose delivered there by the useful photon beam; W_R is the radiation weighting factor for the neutrons; d_{maze} is the distance (in meters) from the isocenter to the near-end of the maze; and L is the length (in meters) of the central path through the maze from its room end to the entrance door. Equation (19–18) has been ascertained by experimental measurements to err on the safe side.[33]

Neutrons can also be produced in the room through photon reactions in objects, including primary barriers of steel.[34,35] The adequacy of protection against neutrons should be confirmed by radiation surveys during the inaugural operation of the therapy machine. X-ray dosimeters and survey instruments that may normally be available in a radiotherapy clinic are not adequate for neutron measurements. The neutron survey should be done with neutron-sensitive monitoring devices, such as boron trifluoride (BF_3) proportional counters, or by foil activation methods (see Section 5.4).[15,36-40]

19.5.2 NEUTRON CAPTURE GAMMA RAYS

Neutrons are captured (or absorbed) by many nuclides in reactions that release gamma rays. Such neutron capture gamma rays are emitted from walls, materials in the room, and the door. Capture gamma rays are penetrating. A prominent reaction is neutron capture in hydrogen that releases a 2.2-MeV photon. Capture of a neutron in boron releases a gamma photon of 0.478 MeV. There are other neutron capture reactions in concrete that can release gamma rays having even higher energies, of up to 10 MeV. (Several capture gammas may be emitted from a single neutron capture.) The lead shielding in the door should offer protection against both the scattered photons and the capture gamma rays. The capture gamma rays from hydrogenous material in the entrance door should be absorbed in a lead layer in the outer face of the door. The hydrogenous layers for neutron shielding can be sandwiched between lead sheets to provide structural balance to the door. The overall shielding at the door should offer protection against scattered photons, neutrons, and neutron capture gamma rays. A properly designed maze can reduce all of these components at the door.

19.5.3 INDUCED RADIOACTIVITY

Some of the nuclei resulting from a photoneutron reaction are radioactive.[15] Careful studies have shown that such photon-induced activity does not present a safety problem.[41] This is because the amount of activity induced, although detectable, is minimal and decays rapidly. Some radioactivity is induced in the patient also, resulting in a negligible additional dose to the patient.

19.6 AN EXAMPLE OF SHIELDING CALCULATIONS FOR A FACILITY

19.6.1 BASIC DATA AND ASSUMPTIONS

In the following sections, we evaluate the shielding requirements for an isocentric rotational 4-MV X-ray therapy machine. Unless specified otherwise, all shielding is provided by concrete of density 2.35 g cm^{-3}. The machine has no primary beam stopper, and patients are treated with the isocenter at 0.8 m from the source. It is capable of a maximum field size of 40 cm × 40 cm at the isocenter. The head leakage is 0.1% of the useful beam. The workload is anticipated to be 672 Gy m^2 week^{-1} (as derived in Example 19.1). The proposed floor layout of the department is shown in Figure 19.5. A corner location has been chosen. The building is a single-storied structure with no occupancy above.

Figure 19.6 shows the layout of the therapy room. The orientation of the gantry of the machine, the plane of rotation of the central axis of the beam, and the width of the beam are also shown.

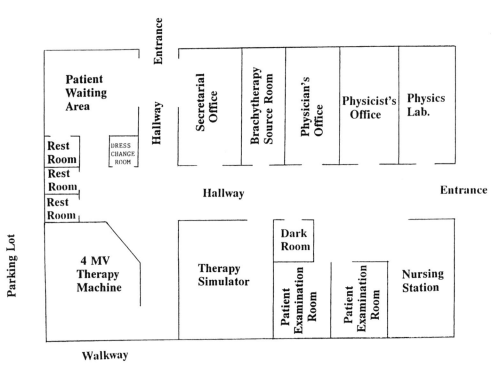

FIGURE 19.5 Sample floor plan of a radiotherapy department.

An entrance having a maze is used to ensure that neither primary nor secondary radiations from the machine or patient can directly reach the door. The photon fluence at the door is likely to be mostly due to the radiation scattered by the inside walls that face the door. Radiations scattered two or more times can be weak in both intensity and energy. Hence, the amount of shielding needed at the entrance door can be minimal. In this example, there is no need to be concerned about neutron shielding because no neutrons are produced at 4 MV energy.

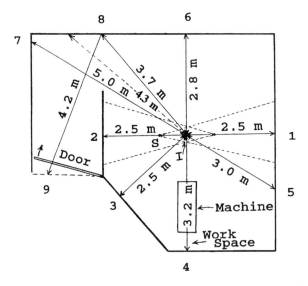

FIGURE 19.6 Floor layout for installation of an isocentric therapy machine. The isocenter of rotation is above point I, and the plane of rotation of the central axis of the beam includes points 1 and 2. Distances between various points are also shown. See worksheets at the end of this chapter.

In shielding evaluations, some assumptions are inevitable when exact layout details or pertinent data are not available. If, in a particular assumption, one errs on the safe side and overestimates the shielding, this is called a conservative assumption. On the contrary, cost-saving assumptions also can be made. We have tried to be conservative in carrying out the calculations for this facility. For example, where data for 4 MV are not available, we have used values available for either cobalt-60 or 6 MV, depending upon which of these results in a higher shielding estimate. The reader is advised to make a critical appraisal of our assumptions and to repeat these calculations independently.

19.6.2 SIDE WALLS

Figure 19.6 shows several locations, marked by numbers 1 to 9, where the barrier thicknesses should be estimated for providing adequate safety. A worksheet that can be used for estimating the shielding has been appended at the end of this chapter. The shielding needed at locations 1 to 8 has been calculated on this worksheet. All of the parameters have been assigned appropriate values based on Figure 19.6 and on the data provided in this chapter. The barriers at positions 1 and 2 are primary barriers. At positions 3 to 8, only secondary barriers are needed. For locations 3 and 5, an extra evaluation has been done giving special consideration to 45° forward scatter.

Sometimes a point, such as location 9 in Figure 19.6 that lies just outside the entrance door, may be subjected to different components. (Location 9 receives radiation from the patient that penetrates the wall, the scatter that comes through the maze and the door, and scatter from skyshine.) Although one can consider only one component at a time during the shielding evaluations, it is important to ensure that the sum of the components does not exceed the acceptable dose limit. In such instances, the required safety can usually be achieved by addition of 1 or 2 HVT for the largest of the separately derived thicknesses (as pointed out in Section 19.4.2).

If the beam is obliquely incident on a barrier, the thickness calculated is along a path that is inclined to the wall and aligned with the direction of the beam and is not perpendicular to the wall. However, because scattered photons produced in the wall can travel perpendicular to the wall and have smaller path lengths, this can result in overdosing. This is especially so if the angle of inclination is more than 45°. As a matter of precaution, NCRP Report No. 49 recommends that, if the beam obliquity is taken into account and the perpendicular thickness of the wall is reduced, one HVT be added to the wall thickness to ensure safety. Lines 28 to 31 in the worksheet are meant for adding a safety factor for conditions such as these.

19.6.3 ENTRANCE DOOR SHIELD

The door is designed to protect anyone who might be at location 9 of Figure 19.6, which can receive scatter from the walls facing the door. Although the area outside the door is a controlled area, we will use a minimal value of P of only 20 μSv, because of the consideration that the area has already been planned to receive 200 μSv week⁻¹ through wall transmission. We will use expressions (19–13) and (19–15) for assessing the shielding requirement for the door for scattered and leakage components separately.

For scattered radiation, we have

$$W = 672 \text{ Gy m}^2 \text{ week}^{-1}; \quad U = 1; \quad T = 1;$$

$$d_{pat} = 0.8 \text{ m}; \quad A_{pat} = 0.16 \text{ m}^2$$

From Table 19.5, for 90° scatter from the patient, for ^{60}Co we obtain $\alpha = 0.0225$. Distance from patient to wall $= d_{1,2} = 4.3$ m. Using Equation (19–10),

$$\left(F_s\right)_1 = \left(0.0225 \times 0.16 \text{ m}^2\right)/\left(4.3 \text{ m}\right)^2 = 1.947 \times 10^{-4}$$

The wall has a width of 1.5 m and a height of 3.0 m. Thus, the area of the wall contributing to scatter is

$$A_2 = 1.5 \text{ m} \times 3.0 \text{ m} = 4.5 \text{ m}^2$$

For the wall scatter coefficient we will use the value for ^{137}Cs (0.66 MeV) for 90° scatter from Table 19.5. Hence, $\alpha_2 = 0.07$. Distance from wall to door, $d_B = 4.2$ m. Substituting in Equation (19–11), we obtain

$$\left(F_S\right)_2 = \left(0.07 \times 4.5 \text{ m}^2\right)/\left(4.2 \text{ m}\right)^2 = 1.786 \times 10^{-2}$$

$$P = 20 \text{ } \mu\text{Gy week}^{-1} \quad \text{(See NCRP Report No. 116, p35).}[1]$$

Substituting in Equation (19–13) gives

$$\left(B_{door}\right)_S = \frac{20 \text{ } \mu\text{Gy week}^{-1} \left(0.8 \text{ m}\right)^2}{672 \text{ Gy week}^{-1} \text{ m}^2 \times 1.947 \times 10^{-4} \times 1.786 \times 10^{-2}}$$
$$= 5.478 \times 10^{-3}$$

$$\text{TVTs needed} = n = -\log_{10}\left(B_{door}\right)_S = 2.26$$

Adopting the (TVT$_e$) of 0.7 cm of lead for 90° scatter of ^{137}Cs photons from Table 19.2, we obtain

$$\text{Lead shielding needed} = 2.26 \times 0.7 \text{ cm} = 1.6 \text{ cm}$$

For leakage radiation, with $F_L = 0.001$ and $d_{1,2} = 4.3$ in Equation (19–15), we obtain

$$\left(B_{door}\right)_L = \frac{20 \text{ } \mu\text{Gy week}^{-1} \times \left(4.3 \text{ m}\right)^2}{672 \text{ Gy week}^{-1} \text{ m}^2 \times 0.001 \times 1.786 \times 10^{-2}}$$
$$= 3.08 \times 10^{-2}$$

$$\text{TVTs needed} = n = -\log_{10}\left(B_{door}\right)_L = 1.51$$

Adopting the (TVT$_e$) of 2.1 cm in lead for ^{137}Cs photons of 0.66 MeV, we obtain

$$\text{Lead shielding needed} = 1.51 \times 2.1 \text{ cm} = 3.2 \text{ cm}$$

Overall shielding for the door: we notice that the lead shielding needed for scatter and for leakage is, respectively, 1.6 cm and 3.2 cm. The difference between the two is $\approx$1.6 cm, which is more than the TVT of 0.7 cm that we have used for the scatter component. Hence, we can incorporate a thickness of 3.2 cm of lead in the door.

19.6.4 SKYSHINE SHIELDING

There is no occupancy above the roof in this example. However, protection of the surroundings against skyshine is required. We can use the concepts outlined in Section 19.4.4 and Equation (19–17) for the purpose of evaluating the shielding to be provided by the ceiling. First, we will address independently the shielding against (a) the primary beam directed upward, (b) the leakage radiation, and (c) scattered radiation.

(a) Shield against skyshine from primary beam

Let us consider that the primary beam has a maximum rectangular cross section of 0.4 m × 0.4 m at a distance of 0.8 m from the source. The radius of a circle of the same area is

$$\left[(0.4 \text{ m} \times 0.4 \text{ m})/\pi\right]^{1/2} = 0.226 \text{ m}$$

The polar angle subtended by the circle at the source

$$\phi = \tan^{-1}\left[0.226/0.8\right] = 15.77°$$

$$\text{Solid angle } \Omega = 2\pi(1 - \cos\phi) = 0.236 \text{ steradian}$$

$$\text{Distance of roof from source, } d_r = 2.5 \text{ m}$$

The machine rotates such that the source is at a height of 0.5 m from ground level when the beam is pointed upward. The diagram in Figure 19.7 connects a point **A** chosen to be at 2 m above the roof on the central axis of the beam, which is pointed upward, and a point **C** on the edge of the ceiling at 2.5 m distance, which is regarded to be the nearest point on the periphery of the roof from the central axis of the beam. We can consider that the points on the ground up to point **B** where line **AC** meets the ground are already protected by the side walls. Only beyond this distance does protection against skyshine have to be achieved by the shielding in the ceiling. Thus, the value of d_p for use in expression (19–17) is ascertained geometrically to be

$$d_p = (2 \text{ m}/2.5 \text{ m}) \times (0.5 \text{ m} + 2.5 \text{ m} + 2.0 \text{ m}) = 4.0 \text{ m}$$

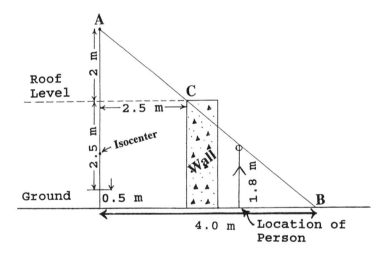

FIGURE 19.7 **B** is the nearest point at which scatter from point **A** can reach the ground unshielded by the side wall.

We will further assume that W = 672 Gy m^2 week^{-1}, F_{BS} = 1 for no primary-beam stopper, T = 1 for full occupancy, U = 1/2 for a primary beam pointed upward, D_{1m} = WUT F_{BS} = 336 Gy m^2 week^{-1}, and P = 20 μGy week^{-1} for an uncontrolled area. Thus, substituting in Equation (19–17), we obtain

$$B_{\text{skyshine}} = \frac{20 \text{ μGy week}^{-1} (2.5 + 2)^2 \times (4.0 \text{ m})^2}{2.5 \times 10^{-2} \times 336 \text{ Gy m}^2 \text{ week}^{-1} \times (0.236)^{1.3}}$$

$$= 5.04 \times 10^{-3}$$

The number of TVTs needed is

$$n = -\log_{10}\left(5.04 \times 10^{-3}\right) = 2.3$$

$$\left(TVT_e\right)_P = 29 \text{ cm} \quad (\text{from Table 19.1 for 4 MV})$$

Shielding needed = 2.3 × 29 cm = 67 cm. Thus, the part of the ceiling struck by the primary beam should have a thickness of 67 cm.

(b) Shield against skyshine from head-leakage radiation

For leakage radiation, the value of Ω should be based on the entire roof area. We will assume that the roof is approximately a 5 m × 6 m = 30 m² rectangular area, and that the source is 1 m below the roof. The radius of a circle having the same area is

$$\left[30 \text{ m}^2/\pi\right]^{1/2} = 3.1 \text{ m}$$

The polar angle formed by a circle of the above radius at a source 1 m below the roof is

$$\phi = \tan^{-1}\left[3.1/1\right] = 72°$$

The solid angle Ω is

$$\Omega = 2\pi\left(1 - \cos\phi\right) = 2\pi\left(1 - 0.309\right) = 4.34 \text{ steradians}$$

Furthermore,

$$W = 672 \text{ Gy m}^2 \text{ week}^{-1}; \quad F_L = 0.001; \quad T = 1; \quad U = 1;$$

$$D_{1m} = \left(WUT\right) \times F_L = 672 \text{ Gy m}^2 \text{ week}^{-1} \times 0.001$$

$$= 0.672 \text{ Gy cm}^2 \text{ week}^{-1}$$

$$d_p = 4 \text{ m}; \quad d_r = 1 \text{ m}; \quad P = 20 \text{ μSv week}^{-1};$$

$$B_{skyshine} = \frac{20 \text{ μSv week}^{-1} \times \left(1 \text{ m} + 2 \text{ m}\right)^2 \times \left(4 \text{ m}\right)^2}{2.5 \times 10^{-2} \times 0.672 \text{ Gy week}^{-1} \times 4.34^{1.3}}$$

$$= 2.54 \times 10^{-2}$$

Number of $(TVT_e)_L$ needed:

$$n = -\log_{10}\left(2.54 \times 10^{-2}\right) = 1.6$$

For a $(TVT_e)_L$ of 29 cm, the shielding needed for protection against skyshine from leakage radiation is

$$n \times \left(TVT_e\right)_L = 1.6 \times 29 \text{ cm} = 47 \text{ cm}$$

(c) Shield against skyshine from patient scatter

The scattered radiation comes from the patient, who is positioned at the isocenter of treatment. The distance of the isocenter below the roof is

$$\text{height of roof from ground} - \text{height of isocenter} = 3.0 \text{ m} - 1.3 \text{ m} = 1.7 \text{ m}$$

Thus, $d_r = 1.7$ m. The radius of a circle having the same area as the roof is 3.1 m (as calculated before). The polar angle subtended by such a circle at a point 1.7 m below it is

$$\tan^{-1}\left[3.1/1.7\right] = 61°$$

The solid angle Ω is

$$\Omega = 2\pi\left(1 - \cos\phi\right) = 2\pi\left(1 - 0.481\right) = 3.26 \text{ steradians}$$

Furthermore,

$$W = 672 \text{ Gy m}^2 \text{ week}^{-1}; \ U = 1; \ T = 1;$$

$$\alpha = 0.0225; \ A_{pat} = 0.16 \text{ m}^2; \ d_{pat} = 0.8 \text{ m};$$

$$P = 20 \ \mu\text{Sv week}^{-1}; \ d_p = 4 \text{ m}; \ d_r = 1.7 \text{ m};$$

$$D_{1m} = \left(WUT\right)\left(\alpha A_{pat}\right)/\left(d_{pat}\right)^2$$

$$= \left(672 \text{ Gy week}^{-1} \text{ m}^2 \times 0.0225 \times 0.16 \text{ m}^2\right)/\left(0.8 \text{ m}\right)^2$$

$$= 3.78 \text{ Gy m}^2 \text{ week}^{-1}$$

Substituting all of the above values in expression (19–17), we obtain

$$B_{skyshine} = \frac{20 \ \mu\text{Sv week}^{-1} \times \left(1.7 + 2\right)^2 \times \left(4.0 \text{ m}\right)^2}{2.5 \times 10^{-2} \times 3.78 \text{ Gy m}^2 \text{ week}^{-1} \times \left(3.26\right)^{1.3}}$$

$$= 9.97 \times 10^{-3}$$

The number of $(TVT_e)_S$ needed is

$$n = -\log_{10}\left(9.97 \times 10^{-3}\right) \approx 2.0$$

For $(TVT_e)_S = 17$ cm (from Table 19.2) for the first scattered radiation, the shielding needed for protection against the skyshine from scattered radiation component is

$$1.9 \times \left(TVT_e\right)_S \approx 2.0 \times 17 \text{ cm} = 34 \text{ cm}$$

The difference between the above value and the thickness of 47 cm which we calculated for protection against leakage radiation is less than the $(TVT_e)_S$ of 17 cm. Hence, we will add one $(HVT)_L = 9$ cm to 47 cm and adopt a thickness of 56 cm of concrete for the part of the ceiling that is not struck by the primary beam. Here, it is worthwhile to mention that the skyshine produced by multiple scattering is weaker in energy than the first scattered radiation from the patient, for which the $(HVT)_S$ that we used applies. Thus, the above evaluation is conservative.

Figures 19.8a, b, and c are cross-sectional views of the walls of the treatment room that we just planned.

19.7 OZONE PRODUCTION

Ozone and other noxious gases are produced by the interaction of ionizing radiation with air. Because X-ray beams interact less in air than do electron beams, the problem of ozone production is negligible during the use of X-ray beams. However, electron beam interaction with air can produce a considerable amount of ozone. This is particularly so when total-skin electron treatments are carried out with a large field cross section and a large treatment distance. The ozone should be cleared by provision of adequate ventilation to the room. Ozone is radiomimetic (i.e., mimics

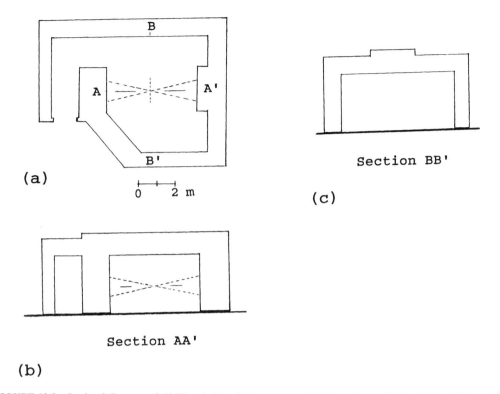

(a)

(c)

(b)

Section BB'

Section AA'

FIGURE 19.8 Sectional diagrams of shielding design of a therapy room. (a) A section parallel to the floor, (b) a section perpendicular to the maze and through the isocenter of the machine, and (c) a section parallel to the maze and through the isocenter.

radiation) in its adverse effects. The threshold for ozone effects is 0.1 parts per million. Nitric oxide and nitrogen dioxide are also produced by ionizing radiation and are harmful, but they have much higher thresholds than does ozone.[11] Kits marketed commercially are available for measurement of the concentration of these gases.

19.8 MISCELLANEOUS ASPECTS OF PLANNING A FACILITY

There should be sufficient overlap between the door and the side walls of a treatment room to prevent radiation leakage through gaps. If there is a gap between the door and the floor, radiation can be reflected by the floor and emerge outside the treatment room. Incorporation of layers of lead sheets below the door (i.e., under the floor) can reduce the reflection.

Provision should be made for passing cables into the room for physics measurements to be made on the beam. All of the conduits for wires and cables should preferably be incorporated in the secondary protective barriers. They should follow a slanted or curved course through the barrier to prevent passage of radiation through them to the outside.

There are various other aspects, in addition to the radiation shielding, to which attention should be paid in planning of an external-beam therapy facility.[10-12] Any radiotherapy room should be planned so as to provide a pleasing environment for patients and staff. The access to the room should be such that nonambulatory patients in stretchers can be moved in and out comfortably. In the access planning, one should also consider the need for moving in the therapy equipment during installation. The machine should be installed with sufficient space around it for servicing. The room should also have sufficient space for storage of treatment aids and accessories. There should be good ventilation for removal of the heat generated by the machine, to provide comfort for patients and staff, and to prevent accumulation of ozone. Air conditioners and ducts for ventilation should be located at heights of 8 feet or more. Air conditioners that vent to the outside should be covered by concrete baffles on the outside. Recesses in the walls for placement of localizing lasers can be planned in advance.

The door should be designed in such a way that a patient can open it from the inside of the room in an emergency. The doors are very heavy, especially those for use with high-energy beams. Electromechanical door opening and closing devices, which can also be operated manually in case of power failure, should be installed.

The control console should be placed in close proximity to the access door, so that the operator can readily control who enters the radiation room and when. The facility design should permit two-way oral communications between the patient in the treatment room and the operator at the control console outside.

Provisions for viewing the patient under treatment by the operating staff should be made. A closed-circuit television viewing system can be useful for this purpose. This system may be augmented by a system of viewing that utilizes a lead-glass window in the entrance door as well as a mirror.

Warning signs are a part of the access control system, and they should have a standard format. Unless otherwise specified by law or regulations, the format should include

1) Words that indicate the degree of hazard
2) A statement of the type of hazard
3) The standard radiation warning symbol
4) A brief statement of instructions for avoiding unwanted exposure

A light should be installed at the entrance to the room to indicate the "beam on" condition to persons outside the room. An electrical interlock must be installed on the door of the therapy room. The interlock shall be wired into the electrical circuit in such a manner that, when the door is opened for any reason, the generation of the radiation beam will automatically be terminated and irradiation can be resumed only by manual resetting of the controls, after the door is closed.

Radiation alarms that include a flashing light when the beam is "on" must be installed in the room to warn the staff about the "beam-on" condition. Systems that give an audible signal that can be heard prior to and during the generation of the beam should also be provided. Emergency switches for turning off the machine should be installed in the treatment room at different points within easy reach of the staff. The staff should be trained to observe the alarm and how to act if the alarm flashes or sounds. Radiation safety measures such as signs and interlocks are the subject of NCRP Report No. 88, entitled "Radiation Alarms and Access Control Systems."[42] Machines using radioisotope sources are equipped with manual mechanisms to restore the source to the "off" position. Staff should be educated about, and made familiar with, the tools and working of the mechanism of the particular machine. An emergency action procedure should be posted for the benefit of the staff.

Some accelerators use klystrons to provide microwave power. Klystrons operate with pulsed electron currents at voltages in the range of 100 to 250 kV and are sources of X-rays themselves. A shielding thickness of 1 to 2 in. of lead is needed for reducing the X-ray leakage from the klystrons to safe levels.[11] After installation, a radiation survey should be conducted around the klystrons. Wrapping films around them can reveal radiation leaking through gaps, if any, in the lead shielding. The film-wrap approach can also be used for checking the machine-head leakage.

The medical physicist on occasion needs to provide a protective-barrier report prior to the construction of a therapy facility. The report typically gives the architect the thicknesses of the protective walls. Most machine vendors may be able to provide a floor and shielding plan for their machines. During the construction phase before the concrete is poured, a careful check should be carried out on the general layout and the distances between the forms that hold the cement while it hardens. Samples of concrete should be obtained and checked for density during the construction phase, so that expensive corrections later on can be avoided. A close consultation between the architect, machine vendor, and a qualified physicist can result in a safe and well-planned facility.

All facilities should be surveyed and certified by a qualified physicist to be safe based on actual radiation levels measured around the installation. In some legal jurisdictions, a copy of the survey may need to be forwarded to the local authorities.

WORKSHEET FOR SHIELDING CALCULATION

Machine Model:_____; Energy:_____; W =_____ Gy m^2 week^{-1};
Beam Stopper Attenuation F_{BS} = _____; Leakage F_L = _____;

---

1. Position shielded

---

2. Controlled area?

---

3. Limit P (μGy week^{-1})

---

4. Factor U

---

5. Factor T

---

6. d_W (m)*

---

7. t_W (Anticipated) (m)

---

8. $d_B = (d_w + t_w + 0.3)$ (m)

---

9. $B_P = (P\ d_B{}^2)/(WUT\ F_{BS})$

---

10. $n = -\log_{10}(B_P)$

---

11. $(TVT_e)_P$ (cm)

---

12. $n \times (TVT_e)_P$ (cm)

---

13. $B_L = (P\ d_B{}^2)/(WUT\ F_L)$

---

14. $n = -\log_{10}(B_L)$

---

15. $(TVT_e)_L$ (cm)

---

16. $n \times (TVT_e)_L$ (cm)

---

17. d_{pat} (m)

---

18. A_{pat} (m^2)

---

19. Angle θ

---

20. α

---

21. $F_S = \alpha\ A_{pat}/(d_B)^2$

---

22. $B_S = P\ (d_{pat})^2/(WUT\ F_S)$

---

23. $n = -\log_{10}(B_S)$

---

24. $(TVT_e)_S$ (cm)

---

25. $n \times (TVT_e)_S$ (cm)

---

26. Larger of 16 or 25

---

27. $(HVT)_L$ for leakage (cm)

WORKSHEET FOR SHIELDING CALCULATION (Cont.)

----

28. Do 16 and 25
    differ <1 $(TVT)_S$?

----

29. If "yes" add 1 $(HVT)_L$

----

30. Any thickness added
    for extra safety

----

31. Recommended thickness (cm)

----

*   For primary-barrier calculations, the value of d_W is the sum of the source-to-isocenter distance and the isocenter-to-wall distance. For scatter and leakage barriers, the value is an average distance represented by the latter.

WORKSHEET FOR SHIELDING CALCULATION — EXAMPLE

Machine Model: <u>X-80</u>; Energy: <u>4 MV</u>; W = <u>672</u> Gy m^2 week^{-1};
Beam Stopper Attenuation F_{BS} = <u>1.0</u>; Leakage F_L = <u>0.001</u>;

	1	2	3	4
1. Position shielded	1	2	3	4
2. Controlled area?	No	Yes	Yes	Yes
3. Limit P (μGy week^{-1})	20	200	200	200
4. Factor U	1/4	1/4	1	1
5. Factor T	1/4	1	1	1
6. d_W (m)*	3.3	3.3	2.5	3.2
7. t_W (Anticipated) (m)	1.5	1.5	0.5	0.5
8. $d_B = (d_W + t_W + 0.3)$ (m)	5.1	5.1	3.3	4.0
9. $B_P = (P\ d_B{}^2)/(WUT\ F_{BS})$	1.24×10^{-5}	3.1×10^{-5}		
10. $n = -\log_{10}(B_P)$	4.91	4.51		
11. $(TVT_e)_P$ (cm)	29	29		
12. $n \times (TVT_e)_P$ (cm)	142	131		
13. $B_L = (P\ d_B{}^2)/(WUT\ F_L)$			3.24×10^{-3}	4.76×10^{-3}
14. $n = -\log_{10}(B_L)$			2.49	2.32
15. $(TVT_e)_L$ (cm)			29	29
16. $n \times (TVT_e)_L$ (cm)			72	67
17. d_{pat} (m)			0.8	0.8
18. A_{pat} (m^2)			0.16	0.16
19. Angle θ			90°	90°
20. α			0.0225	0.0225
21. $F_S = \alpha\ A_{pat}/(d_B)^2$			3.31×10^{-4}	2.25×10^{-4}
22. $B_S = P\ (d_{pat})^2/(WUT\ F_S)$			5.76×10^{-4}	8.47×10^{-4}
23. $n = -\log_{10}(B_S)$			3.24	3.07
24. $(TVT_e)_S$ (cm)			17	17
25. $n \times (TVT_e)_S$ (cm)			55	52
26. Larger of 16 or 25			72	67
27. $(HVT)_L$ for leakage (cm)			9	9
28. Do 16 and 25 differ <1 $(TVT)_S$?			No	Yes

WORKSHEET FOR SHIELDING CALCULATION — EXAMPLE (Cont.)

29. If "yes" add 1 $(HVT)_L$			—	9
30. Any thickness added for extra safety			—	—
31. Recommended thickness (cm)	142	131	72	76

* For primary-barrier calculations, the value of d_W is the sum of the source-to-isocenter distance and the isocenter-to-wall distance. For scatter and leakage barriers, the value is an average distance represented by the latter.

WORKSHEET FOR SHIELDING CALCULATION — EXAMPLE
(Contd.)

Machine Model: <u>X-80</u>; Energy: <u>4 MV</u>; W = <u>672</u> Gy m^2 week^{-1};
Beam Stopper Attenuation F_{BS} = <u>1.0</u>; Leakage F_L = <u>0.001</u>;

1. Position shielded	5	6	7	8
2. Controlled area?	No	No	Yes	No
3. Limit P (μGy week^{-1})	20	20	200	20
4. Factor U	1	1	1	1
5. Factor T	1/4	1/4	1	1/4
6. d_W (m)*	3.0	2.8	5.0	3.7
7. t_W (Anticipated) (m)	0.5	0.5	0.5	0.5
8. $d_B = (d_W + t_W + 0.3)$ (m)	3.8	3.6	5.8	4.5
9. $B_P = (P\ d_B{}^2)/(WUT\ F_{BS})$				
10. $n = -\log_{10}(B_P)$				
11. $(TVT_e)_P$ (cm)				
12. $n \times (TVT_e)_P$ (cm)				
13. $B_L = (P\ d_B{}^2)/(WUT\ F_L)$	1.72×10^{-3}	1.54×10^{3}	1.0×10^{-2}	2.41×10^{-3}
14. $n = -\log_{10}(B_L)$	2.76	2.81	2.0	2.62
15. $(TVT_e)_L$ (cm)	29	29	29	29
16. $n \times (TVT_e)_L$ (cm)	80	82	58	76
17. d_{pat} (m)	0.8	0.8	0.8	0.8
18. A_{pat} (m^2)	0.16	0.16	0.16	0.16
19. Angle θ	90°	90°	90°	90°
20. α	0.0225	0.0225	0.0225	0.0225
21. $F_S = \alpha\ A_{pat}/(d_B)^2$	2.49×10^{-4}	2.78×10^{-4}	1.07×10^{-4}	1.78×10^{-4}
22. $B_S = P\ (d_{pat})^2/(WUT\ F_S)$	3.06×10^{-4}	2.74×10^{-4}	1.78×10^{-3}	4.29×10^{-4}
23. $n = -\log_{10}(B_S)$	3.52	3.56	2.75	3.37
24. $(TVT_e)_S$ (cm)	17	17	17	17
25. $n \times (TVT_e)_S$ (cm)	60	61	47	57
26. Larger of 16 or 25	80	82	58	76
27. $(HVT)_L$ for leakage (cm)	9	9	9	9

28. Do 16 and 25 differ <1 $(TVT)_S$?	No	No	Yes	No
29. If "yes" add 1 $(HVT)_L$	—	—	9	—
30. Any thickness added for extra safety	—	—	—	—
31. Recommended thickness (cm)	80	82	67	76

* For primary-barrier calculations, the value of d_w is the sum of the source-to-isocenter distance and the isocenter-to-wall distance. For scatter and leakage barriers, the value is an average distance represented by the latter.

WORKSHEET FOR SHIELDING CALCULATION — EXAMPLE
(Contd.)

Machine Model: <u>X-80</u>; Energy: <u>4 MV</u>; W = <u>672</u> Gy m^2 week^{-1};
Beam Stopper Attenuation F_{BS} = <u>1.0</u>; Leakage F_L = <u>0.001</u>;

1. Position shielded	3*	5*
2. Controlled area?	Yes	No
3. Limit P (μGy week^{-1})	200	20
4. Factor U	1/4	1/4
5. Factor T	1	1
6. d_W (m)**	2.5	3.0
7. t_W (Anticipated) (m)	0.5	0.5
8. $d_B = (d_W + t_W + 0.3)$ (m)	3.3	3.8
9. $B_P = (P\, d_B{}^2)/(WUT\, F_{BS})$		
10. $n = -\log_{10}(B_P)$		
11. $(TVT_e)_P$ (cm)		
12. $n \times (TVT_e)_P$ (cm)		
13. $B_L = (P\, d_B{}^2)/(WUT\, F_L)$	3.24×10^{-3}	1.72×10^{-3}
14. $n = -\log_{10}(B_L)$	2.49	2.76
15. $(TVT_e)_L$ (cm)	29	29
16. $n \times (TVT_e)_L$ (cm)	72	80
17. d_{pat} (m)	0.8	0.8
18. A_{pat} (m^2)	0.16	0.16
19. Angle θ	45°	45°
20. α	0.068	0.068
21. $F_S = \alpha\, A_{pat}/(d_B)^2$	1.0×10^{-3}	7.42×10^{-4}
22. $B_S = P\, (d_{pat})^2/(WUT\, F_S)$	7.74×10^{-4}	1.03×10^{-4}
23. $n = -\log_{10}(B_S)$	3.11	3.99
24. $(TVT_e)_S$ (cm)	23	23 (6 MV data from Table 19.2)
25. $n \times (TVT_e)_S$ (cm)	72	92
26. Larger of 16 or 25	72	92
27. $(HVT)_L$ for leakage (cm)	9	9

28. Do 16 and 25 differ <1 (TVT)$_S$?	Yes	Yes
29. If "yes" add 1 (HVT)$_L$	9	9
30. Any thickness added for extra safety	—	—
31. Recommended thickness (cm)	81	101

* Repeat calculations for 45° scatter with U = 1/4. U = 1 for leakage.

** For primary-barrier calculations, the value of d_W is the sum of the source-to-isocenter distance and the isocenter-to-wall distance. For scatter and leakage barriers, the value is an average distance represented by the latter.

REFERENCES

1. National Council on Radiation Protection and Measurements, NCRP Report No. 116, Limitation of Exposure to Ionizing Radiation, National Council on Radiation Protection and Measurements, Bethesda, Maryland, 1987.
2. Dennis, J.A., On the recommendations of ICRP/90/G-01, Radiat. Res., Vol 123, p349-350, 1990.
3. Dennis, J.A., EURADOS-CENDOS discussion on ICRP draft recommendations, Health Phys., Vol 59, p936, 1990.
4. Cameron, J.R., Hormesis and high fliers: Radiation risk revisited, Letter, Phys. Today, Vol 45, p13, 14, and 94, 1992.
5. Yallow, R.S., Is radiation less harmful than BEIR-V reports (letter), Phys. Today, Vol 44, p13, 14, and 101, 1992.
6. Kocher, D.C., Perspective on historical development of radiation standards, Health Phys., Vol 61, p519-527, 1991.
7. National Council on Radiation Protection and Measurements, Recommendations on Limits for Exposure to Ionizing Radiation, NCRP Report No. 91, National Council on Radiation Protection and Measurements, Bethesda, Maryland, 1987.
8. International Commission on Radiation Protection, Recommendations of the ICRP, ICRP-60, Ann. ICRP, Vol 21, No. 1–3, Pergamon, Oxford, 1991.
9. National Council on Radiation Protection and Measurements, Implementation of Principles of As Low As Reasonably Achievable for Medical Personnel, NCRP Report No. 107, National Council on Radiation Protection and Measurements, Bethesda, Maryland, 1990.
10. National Council on Radiation Protection and Measurements, Structural Shielding Design and Evaluation for Medical Use of X-rays and Gamma Rays up to 10 MeV, NCRP Report No. 49, National Council on Radiation Protection and Measurements, Bethesda, Maryland, 1976.
11. National Council on Radiation Protection and Measurements, Radiation Protection Design Guidelines for 0.1–100 MeV Particle Accelerator Facilities, NCRP Report No. 51, National Council on Radiation Protection and Measurements, Bethesda, Maryland, 1977.
12. Swanson, W.P., Radiological Safety Aspects of the Operation of Electron Linear Accelerators, IAEA Technical Report Series No. 188, International Atomic Energy Agency, Vienna, 1979.
13. Mckenzie, A.L., Shaw, J.E., Stephenson, S.K., and Turner, P.C.R., Radiation Protection in Radiotherapy, IPSM Report No. 46, The Institute of Physical Sciences in Medicine, London, 1986.
14. International Commission on Radiological Protection, Protection Against Ionizing Radiation from External Sources Used in Medicine, ICRP Publication 33, Pergamon Press, Oxford, 1982.
15. National Council on Radiation Protection and Measurements, Neutron Contamination from Medical Electron Accelerators, NCRP Report No. 79, National Council on Radiation Protection and Measurements, Bethesda, Maryland, 1984.
16. National Council on Radiation Protection and Measurements, Medical X-ray, Electron Beam, and Gamma-ray Protection for Energies up to 50 MeV (Equipment Design, Performance, and Use), NCRP Report No. 102, National Council on Radiation Protection and Measurements, Bethesda, Maryland, 1989.
17. Johns, H.E., and Cunningham, J.R., Physics of Radiology, 4th Edition, p545, Charles C Thomas, Springfield, Illinois, 1983.
18. Farrow, N., The effect of linear accelerator use on primary barrier design, Phys. Med. Biol., Vol 30, p1151-1153, 1985.
19. Cobb, P.D., and Bjarngard, B.E., Use factors for medical linear accelerators, Health Phys., Vol 31, p463-465, 1976.
20. Bigg, P.J., Calculation of shielding door thicknesses for radiation therapy facilities using the ITS Monte Carlo program, Health Phys., Vol 61, p465-472, 1991.
21. Yuan-Chyuan Lo, Albedos for 4-, 10-, and 18-MV bremsstrahlung X-ray beams on concrete, iron, and lead — normally incident, Med. Phys., Vol 19, p659-666, 1992.
22. Jaeger, R.G. (Ed. in Chief), Radiation Attenuation Methods, Chapter 3, in Engineering Compendium on Radiation Shielding, Vol 1, Shielding Fundamentals and Methods, Springer-Verlag, Berlin, 1968.
23. Clarke, E.T., Photon fields near earth-air interface, p255, in Engineering Compendium on Radiation Shielding, Vol 1, Jaeger, R.G. (Ed. in Chief), Springer-Verlag, New York, 1968.
24. Jenkin, T.M., Accelerator boundary doses and skyshine, Health Phys., Vol 27, p251-257, 1974.
25. Borak, T.B., A simple approach for calculating gamma ray skyshine for reduced shielding applications, Health Phys., Vol 29, p423-425, 1975.
26. Heitler, W., The Quantum Theory of Radiation, 3rd Edition, Oxford University Press, London, 1954.
27. Nath, R., Epp, E.R., Swanson, W.P., and Bond, V., Neutrons from medical accelerators: An estimate of risk to the radiotherapy patient, Med. Phys., Vol 11, p231-241, 1984.
28. Hoffman, R.J., and Nath, R., On the sources of radiation exposure of technologists in a radiotherapy center with high energy X-ray accelerators, Health Phys., Vol 24, p525-526, 1973.
29. Jaeger, R.G. (Ed. in Chief), Section 8.2, Attenuation of neutrons, p497-530, in Engineering Compendium on Radiation Shielding, Vol 1, Springer Verlag, Heidelberg, 1968.
30. National Council on Radiation Protection and Measurements, Protection Against Neutron Radiation, NCRP Report No. 38, National Commission on Radiation Protection and Measurements, Washington, D.C., 1971.
31. Kersey, R.W., Estimation of neutron and gamma radiation doses in the entrance mazes of SL75-20 linear accelerator treatment rooms, Medicamundi, Vol 24, p151-155, 1979.

32. McCall, R.C., Jenkins, T.M., and Shore, R.A., Transport of accelerator produced neutrons in a concrete room, IEEE Trans. Nucl. Sci., Vol 26, p1593-1602, 1979.

33. McGinley, P.H., and Butker, E.K., Evaluation of neutron dose equivalent levels at the maze entrance of medical accelerator treatment rooms, Phys. Med. Biol., Vol 18, p279-282, 1991.

34. McGinley, P.H., Photoneutron production in the primary barriers of medical accelerator rooms, Phys. Med. Biol., Vol 34, p777-783, 1989.

35. McGinley, P.H., Long, K., and Kaplan, R., Production of photoneutrons in a lead shield by high-energy X-rays, Phys. Med. Biol., Vol 33, p975-980, 1988.

36. McGinley, P.H., Wood, M., Mills, M., and Rodriguez, R., Dose levels due to neutrons in the vicinity of high-energy medical accelerators, Med. Phys., Vol 3, p397-402, 1976.

37. Tosi, G., Torresin, A., Agosteo, S., Foglio Para, A., Sangiust, V., Zeni, L., and Silari, M., Neutron measurements around medical electron accelerators by active and passive techniques, Med. Phys., Vol 18, p54-60, 1991.

38. Agosteo, S., Foglio Para, A., and Maggioni, B., Neutron fluxes in radiotherapy rooms, Med. Phys., Vol 20, p407-414, 1993.

39. Sanchez, F., Madurga, G., and Arrans, R., Neutron measurements around an 18 MV linac, Radiother. Oncol., Vol 15, p259-265, 1989.

40. Bading, J.R., Zeitz, L., and Laughlin, J.S., Phosphorus activation neutron dosimetry and its application to an 18 MV radiotherapy accelerator, Med. Phys., Vol 9, p835-843, 1982.

41. Glasgow, G.P., Residual radioactivity in radiation therapy treatment aids irradiated on medical linear accelerators, in Radiotherapy Safety, Symposium Proceedings No. 4, American Association of Physicists in Medicine, New York, 1984.

42. National Council on Radiation Protection and Measurements, Radiation Alarms and Access Control Systems, NCRP Report No. 88, National Council on Radiation Protection and Measurements, Bethesda, Maryland, 1986.

ADDITIONAL READING

1. Chilton, A.B., Shultis, J.K., and Faw, R.E., Principles of Radiation Shielding, First Ed., Prentice-Hall, Englewood Cliffs, New Jersey, 1984.

2. Jaeger, R.G. (Ed. in Chief), Engineering Compendium on Radiation Shielding, Vol 1, Springer-Verlag, Heidelberg, 1968.

3. International Commission on Radiological Protection, Protection Against Ionizing Radiation from External Sources Used in Medicine, ICRP Publication 33, Pergamon Press, Oxford, 1982.

4. Mckenzie, A.L., Shaw, J.E., Stephenson, S.K., and Turner, P.C.R., Radiation Protection in Radiotherapy, IPSM Report No. 46, The Institute of Physical Sciences in Medicine, London, 1986.

5. National Council on Radiation Protection and Measurements, Neutron Contamination from Medical Electron Accelerators, NCRP Report No. 79, National Council on Radiation Protection and Measurements, Bethesda, Maryland, 1984.

6. Swanson, W.P., Radiological Safety Aspects of the Operation of Electron Linear Accelerators, IAEA Technical Report Series No. 188, International Atomic Energy Agency, Vienna, 1979.

7. National Council on Radiation Protection and Measurements, Structural Shielding Design and Evaluation for Medical Use of X-rays and Gamma Rays up to 10 MeV, NCRP Report No. 49, National Council on Radiation Protection and Measurements, Bethesda, Maryland, 1976.

8. National Council on Radiation Protection and Measurements, Radiation Protection Design Guidelines for 0.1–100 MeV Particle Accelerator Facilities, NCRP Report No. 51, National Council on Radiation Protection and Measurements, Bethesda, Maryland, 1977.

9. National Council on Radiation Protection and Measurements, Medical X-ray, Electron Beam, and Gamma-Ray Protection for Energies up to 50 MeV (Equipment Design, Performance, and Use), NCRP Report No. 102, National Council on Radiation Protection and Measurements, Bethesda, Maryland, 1989.

10. Thomadsen, B. (Ed.), Radiotherapy Safety, Proceedings of a Short Course at the University of Wisconsin, March 1982, American Association of Physicists in Medicine, American Institute of Physics, New York, 1984.

11. McGinley, P.H., Miner, M.S., and Mitchum, M.L., A method for calculating the dose due to capture gamma rays in accelerator mazes, Phys. Med. Biol., Vol 40, p1467-1473, 1995.

12. Mills, M.D., Almond, P.R., Boyer, A.L., Ochran, T.G., Madigan, W., Rich, T.A., and Dally, E.B., Shielding considerations for an operating room based intraoperative electron radiotherapy unit, Int. J. Rad. Oncol. Biol. Phys., Vol 18, p1215-1221, 1990.

13. Maitz, A.H., Dade Lunsford, L., Wu. A., Lindner, G., and Flickinger, J.C., Shielding requirements on-site loading and acceptance testing of the Leksell Gamma Knife, Int. J. Rad. Oncol. Biol. Phys., Vol 18, p469-476, 1990.

Chapter 20

RADIATION SAFETY IN BRACHYTHERAPY

20.1 INTRODUCTION

In brachytherapy, small sources that contain radioactive material within a capsule are used. The current methods of brachytherapy can be divided into low-dose-rate (LDR) and high-dose-rate (HDR) techniques,[1,2] which present different hazard control problems. LDR techniques have been practiced since the discovery of radium; HDR techniques have become possible in modern times because of the development and availability of artificially produced radioactive sources of very high specific activities. Whereas LDR brachytherapy is performed with sources of low activity, of the order of a few gigabecquerel, sources having activities of 100 GBq may be employed for HDR brachytherapy. Such high-activity sources used in HDR brachytherapy should be handled only with a remote afterloading device installed in a room specially planned to have sufficient space, distance from the source to personnel, and shielding. The HDR precautions are not unlike those adopted for teletherapy treatments, with remote-control devices, shielding, safety interlocks, and radiation alarms. For an understanding of the safety and quality control problems encountered in HDR remote-loading brachytherapy, the reader is referred to the American Association of Physicists in Medicine (AAPM) Report 41[3] and other publications[4,5] cited at the end of this chapter. Our discussion here mainly addresses the conventional LDR techniques, which are the subject of Report No. 40 from the National Council on Radiation Protection and Measurements (NCRP).[6]

It is interesting to compare external-beam therapy with LDR brachytherapy from a radiation safety point of view. In Chapter 19, which deals with external-beam therapy, much emphasis was placed on shielding evaluations, because control of the parameters of time and distance could not provide the needed levels of safety. In LDR brachytherapy, the sources are of much lower strengths than those of the sources used for external-beam therapy. Shielding is necessary for storage and transport of LDR sources. However, during their handling, loading, or removal, a sufficient level of safety can be achieved by use of distance and time. Shielding can be added for the purpose of ALARA (as low as reasonably achievable) at the time of source handling and patient treatment.

Whereas radioisotope sources having activities of the order of 100 TBq are needed for external-beam therapy, LDR brachytherapy sources have activities of the order of only gigabecquerel. Although an external therapy beam is dangerous because it can deliver a lethal dose in a very short time, the external-beam treatment is done with great care in a well-shielded therapy room with engineered safety features, remote "on" and "off" mechanisms, safety interlocks, etc. LDR brachytherapy sources can be used without such elaborate built-in safety mechanisms. However, the potential for overexposure from them should not be underestimated. Many incidents of high radiation exposures have resulted because of careless handling of LDR brachytherapy sources. In this chapter, we discuss the radiation hazard control in LDR brachytherapy.

20.2 ROLE OF TIME AND AFTERLOADING

As a general safety rule, one should work with any radiation source only for the minimum time one needs for its loading or removal. Since the early 1960s, afterloading techniques in brachytherapy have contributed to much reduction in the time spent in the handling of sources and hence in the radiation exposure to personnel.[7-10] This was not so in the first decades of the practice of brachytherapy, when the radioactive sources were loaded into applicators (i.e., source carriers or guide tubes) at the very beginning of the procedure. These applicators were then inserted in the tissues or body cavities of patients. The disadvantage of such a method was that it involved handling of radiation sources even during inserting and positioning of the applicators. The practice of using applicators with sources already loaded has been abandoned. Instead, empty applicators are first inserted and manipulated until they are in the correct configuration in the patient. It is only after ensuring that they have been properly placed with respect to the tumor or anatomic structures in the body that the radioactive sources are loaded into the applicators. Hence, the sources are said to be "afterloaded," and the technique is called "afterloading" technique.

Afterloading methods can be manual or remote. In manual afterloading, the sources are mounted at the tip of a long handle. The sources, which are held by hand at the inactive end of the long handle, are inserted into the applicators. In remote afterloading, a sophisticated remote-handling apparatus steers the sources into and out of the applicators by an electromechanical or pneumatic mechanism which has a timer to control the duration of treatment. Remote-loading techniques have been used for both LDR and HDR treatments.

20.3 ROLE OF DISTANCE

When radioactive sources are handled, it is necessary to maintain a safe distance between the body and the sources. Handling them at too short a distance can result in an unacceptably high dose. As an example, let us compare two possibilities. First, let us say that a worker takes 5 min (300 sec) to pick up and load a brachytherapy source into a catheter by using forceps of 15 cm length. Alternatively, another worker picks up the source with his finger tips and does the loading quickly, in just 1 sec. In the latter instance, the fingers are on the surface of the metallic capsule of the source, and the surface may be only 0.5 mm from the radioactive material in the source. We know that the dose is directly proportional to the time of irradiation, but is inversely proportional to the square of the distance. If we take into account the differences in the times and distances in the two situations, the dose received by the finger tips in the second case will be more than that in the first case by a ratio given by

$$\frac{(15\text{ cm})^2}{(300\text{ sec})} \times \frac{1\text{ sec}}{(0.05\text{ cm})^2} = 300$$

In other words, it will take as long as 25 h (i.e., 300×5 min) for the worker who used the 15-cm forceps to be subjected to the high dose received by the other worker who touched the source capsule. Thus, distance is a very effective parameter for reducing the radiation dose. Especially in brachytherapy, speed of execution cannot substitute for the benefit of distance and inverse-square dose fall-off. At close distances, a very high dose can be received in fractions of seconds.

Sources should never be touched. All source manipulations should be done with forceps or tongs at least 15 cm in length. It is worthwhile for workers to practice the use of forceps or any remote handling procedure with nonradioactive "dummy" sources, to develop timing efficiency for handling the actual radiation sources.

20.4 ROLE OF SHIELDING

Shielding is essential for the safe storage and transport of brachytherapy sources. Shielding can be employed, as well, for the purpose of ALARA, to add to the advantages already contributed by control of distance and time. A movable shield placed by the bedside of the patient can reduce the dose levels in the hallways and adjacent rooms.

The physical characteristics and shielding data for several radioisotope sources used in brachytherapy are given in Table 17.1 in Chapter 17. ^{137}Cs and ^{192}Ir have been preferred over ^{226}Ra, ^{60}Co, and ^{182}Ta for temporary implants, because of the more efficient shielding of their radiation by lead. The merits of newer sources such as ^{241}Am, ^{145}Sm, and ^{169}Yb have also been considered for potential use in the future. The very low energy of the photons emitted by these sources (and also by ^{125}I and ^{103}Pd for permanent implants) makes effective shielding possible even by 0.5 mm of lead.

20.5 MONITORING INSTRUMENTS

Radiation survey meters of the ionization and GM (Geiger-Mueller) counter types should be readily available in the department. The former should be capable of measuring air-kerma rates from 10 μGy h^{-1} to 1 Gy h^{-1} (i.e., exposure rates from approximately 1 mR h^{-1} to 100 R h^{-1}). The latter should have enough sensitivity to measure levels of 0.1 μGy h^{-1} (i.e., 0.01 mR h^{-1}), comparable to the background. The survey meters should be calibrated periodically by an authorized calibration laboratory providing traceability of the readings to the national and international standards. The meters should be checked often with a test source so that their correct performance is ensured.

20.6 SOURCE STORAGE AND PREPARATION

Brachytherapy sources must be stored in a safe having 3 to 4 TVL of lead shielding (Figure 20.1). The storage safe may have many drawers with holes or recesses for placement of the sources. Each source should have an identification label, engraved mark, or color code that can readily be seen. A fixed magnifying glass should be installed as an aid for reading the identification. Hand-held magnifiers may contribute to unnecessary exposure. Sources can be categorized or grouped in terms of their type, radioisotope content, or strength and stored in separate drawers for quick retrieval for use. The storage safe is to be placed behind an L-shaped block offering 2 to 4 TVL of lead shielding with a lead-glass visor (Figure 20.1). The worker should stand in front of the L-block so that the body is well shielded during retrieval of the sources from the safe and preparation for loading. Forceps and tongs should be provided for ready use. A well-type lead container should be available besides the lead block for temporary storage during the selection and preparation of sources for afterloading. Threading through the eyelet of any source should be done after the source is inserted in a hole in a lead block, so that most of its radioactive length is blocked, with only the eyelet portion protruding outside the shield.

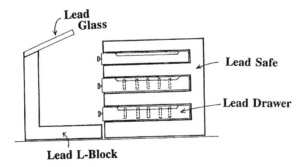

FIGURE 20.1 A lead safe designed with drawers and slots for placement of encapsulated brachytherapy sources. An L-shaped lead block with a lead glass visor is located in front of the safe.

Beta sources, such as ^{90}Sr-^{90}Y, are to be handled behind a shield of a low-Z transparent plastic material such as acrylic. Lead is not a good β-ray shield because the interaction of β radiation with lead produces bremsstrahlung. Beta sources are usually mounted on the tip of a rod (Figure 20.2) that has a plastic shield mounted behind the source. Ophthalmic β applicators may deliver a dose of 100 Gy on their surface in only a few seconds. The source should always be held in such a way that the plastic shield intervenes between the source and the operator. Fingers should not be placed too close to the surface of the source. The source applicator should be stored in a specially designed plastic container having a sufficient thickness of plastic to absorb the β radiation (Figure 20.2b). The applicator should be taken out of its box only for the short time needed for use. All preparation of the patient should be done in advance. The duration of irradiation may be very short, lasting just a few seconds. It is worthwhile to establish a method of timing by using a stopwatch to control

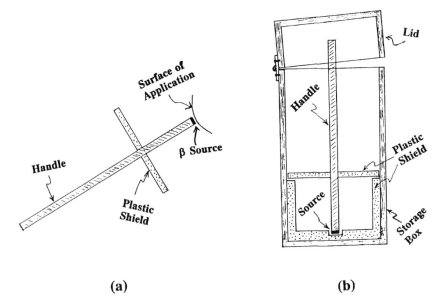

(a)   **(b)**

FIGURE 20.2   (a) Typical appearance of an ^{90}Sr β-ray eye applicator with the source at the tip of a rod and a plastic shield mounted behind the source. (b) The applicator is stored in a plastic box.

the period of treatment exactly. The procedure should be practiced so that it will be accurate and safe when being used on a patient.

The radiation levels in the source storage room should be surveyed frequently to ensure that no source is left outside the storage safe. Survey meters should be readily available in the source room for locating any misplaced, dropped, or lost source. The room where the sources are stored should be locked, and access should be allowed only to authorized personnel.

20.7 SOURCE INVENTORY

A record of the brachytherapy sources available in the department and of their actual locations should be maintained. A misplaced or lost brachytherapy source can become a radiation hazard to the public. The removal of any source from storage, its insertion in a patient, its removal from the patient after completion of treatment, and its return to storage should all be recorded in a log book. Records of receipt, storage, use, and return of rental sources should likewise be maintained.

The use of flexible radioactive wires (of ^{192}Ir, ^{182}Ta, or ^{198}Au) can create special problems.[11] A single long wire may be acquired and cut into the desired lengths for use; thus, the total number of sources to be tracked can change. Proper record-keeping of how a particular long wire is used and disposed of is necessary for control of the radiation hazard. Cut pieces of radioactive wires should be traced and accounted for to prevent loss.

20.8 SOURCE WIPE TESTS

A basic precaution required with the use of radioactive materials is to prevent any spread of radioactive contamination. The possibility for such a spread is minimal with brachytherapy sources, provided the sources are always handled in such a way as not to threaten the integrity of the encapsulation.[12,13] Sources should not be heated or subjected to steam for sterilization, because that would damage the capsule. Only chemical sterilization should be used. All brachytherapy sources should be checked periodically for any leakage of radioactivity resulting from cracking or rupture of the capsule. Wiping the surface of a source capsule with cotton swabs and counting the wipes for any radioactive emission by a high-sensitivity counter can reveal any breach in the capsule.

Radium sources are particularly hazardous and should be tested frequently for radon leakage.[14] In radium sources, there is pressure build-up due to both α particles (which are gaseous helium ions) and the radium decay product of radon gas. Leakage of radon from radium sources with defective encapsulation can become a major radiation hazard, because the diffusing radon can contribute to the deposition of its radioactive daughter products on walls, surfaces, and floors throughout a department. Many radium sources used in the past have been phased out and replaced by the safer non-radium substitutes.

The tools used for cutting radioactive wires are likely to become contaminated, albeit with a low probability. Hence it is advisable to keep these tools isolated from others. Wipe tests on them can reveal any contamination, which may require a clean-up.

20.9 SOURCE TRANSPORT

Radioactive sources are transported from the source storage facility to the patient room for loading into the patient. A lead-shielded transport container that can be rolled on wheels is useful for this purpose (Figure 20.3). A transport container specifically designed to carry the afterloading inserts for the particular applicators in use at a given clinic can be obtained commercially.

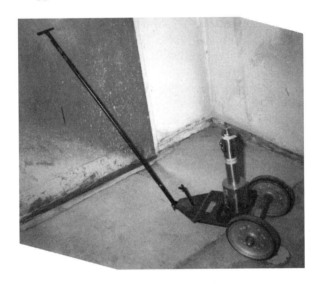

FIGURE 20.3   A lead-walled cart for transporting brachytherapy sources between the source storage area and the patient room.

Shipping of radioactive sources to other institutions or receipt or return of sources from or to source vendors should be done in containers that have sufficient shielding. The dose rates on the surface of these containers can be reduced further by the use of internal spacers which increase the distance of the container surface from the sources. In most jurisdictions, there are regulations concerning the transport of radioactive materials. These usually require signing of shipping certificates indicating the type of source (needles, wires, sealed, unsealed, etc.), the radioisotope, the amount of activity, and the radiation levels on the surface and at 1 m from the shipping container, and they require labeling of the container with radioactivity warning signs.

20.10 SAFETY OF NURSES AND VISITORS DURING TREATMENT

LDR brachytherapy is a procedure that can extend over several days. Proper care is necessary for avoiding unnecessary irradiation of auxiliary medical staff, particularly nurses, attending the patient, and also exposure of visitors.[15] Preferably, a private room should be made available. This is a regulatory requirement in some jurisdictions. A corner room should be selected where possible, so that traffic is minimal. The location of the patient's bed in the room should be such that irradiation of other patients, staff, and visitors is minimized. After the sources are inserted in the patient, the radiation levels at different points in the room and adjacent areas should be surveyed and noted. Efforts should be made to ensure that the radiation levels in areas to which the public may have access are minimal. Air-kerma rates of less than 2 μGy h^{-1} can usually be achieved in the hallways and at the door by proper selection of the position of the bed in the room and the choice of the room itself. Any chair in the room where a visitor may sit can be moved to a location with a low radiation level, preferably less than 2 mR h^{-1} (which corresponds approximately to 17 μGy h^{-1} air-kerma rate). The visiting time may be restricted to less than an hour.

The dose rate at the bedside and at 1 m from the patient should be recorded. The nursing staff should be advised to keep a distance of at least 2 m from the patient if possible without compromising nursing care. A maximum duration for nursing at the bedside of the patient can be indicated as guidance to the nurses. This can be based on the projected number of radioactive patients whom a nurse may attend in a year during her rotation in the clinic, and on the ALARA policy of the institution. If nursing for an extended period is warranted, the (afterloaded) sources may be removed temporarily and placed in the lead transport container, which may be left in the room until the end of treatment.

Figure 20.4 shows the different warning signs that can be posted. These include a warning sign for the entrance door to the patient's room (Figure 20.4a) indicating the radioisotope and the activity in use. Other signs in Figure 20.4 mark the patient's chart to alert the nurses (Figure 20.4b and c) about either temporary or permanent radioactive implants. Bedside lead shields can be acquired and used for ALARA.[16,17] The patient should wear a wrist band indicating that he or she is radioactive. Nurses should be educated and informed about radiation safety principles so that they understand how to work with radiation, rather than fearing the radiation.[18] They should be made familiar with the appearance of the sources, applicators, and warning signs.

20.11 PROCEDURE AFTER TREATMENT

At the end of treatment, all sources should be removed from the patient except in the case of permanent implants (as discussed in Section 20.12). A procedure for safe removal of sources should be established in the institution for minimum exposure to personnel. The removal technique should not cause physical damage to the sources. It is also important to have a method that will definitely succeed in removing the sources. There have been instances of afterloaded sources left lodged in patient tissues after an attempt at removal. The patient's body should be surveyed to ensure that all radiation sources have been removed prior to his or her discharge from the hospital. The room should be surveyed for radiation levels so that any left-over or dropped source is detected. All trash from the room should be surveyed for radiation emission prior to disposal. Only after it has been ascertained that all sources have been recovered for return to storage can the safety signs be removed. Without much delay, the removed sources should be taken back for inventory and storage.

20.12 PERMANENT IMPLANTS

Radiation sources of ^{222}Rn, ^{198}Au, ^{125}I, and ^{103}Pd have been used for permanent implants. In the U.S., the use of ^{222}Rn is a thing of the past. ^{125}I, and ^{103}Pd, have lower radiation energies than does ^{198}Au, and hence they are more efficiently shielded by lead. Furthermore, compared to ^{198}Au, they have longer mean lives, giving a longer irradiation period. This results in a lower strength of sources at the time of implantation for the delivery of any desired dose. Even during hospitalization, the patient's self-shielding is greater for ^{125}I and ^{103}Pd than for ^{198}Au.[19] Overall, ^{125}I and ^{103}Pd are preferable to ^{198}Au from the point of view of the radiation safety of hospital personnel.

For permanent implants, the same precautions as for removable implants should be taken while the patient is hospitalized. Local regulations should be observed in deciding on the appropriate

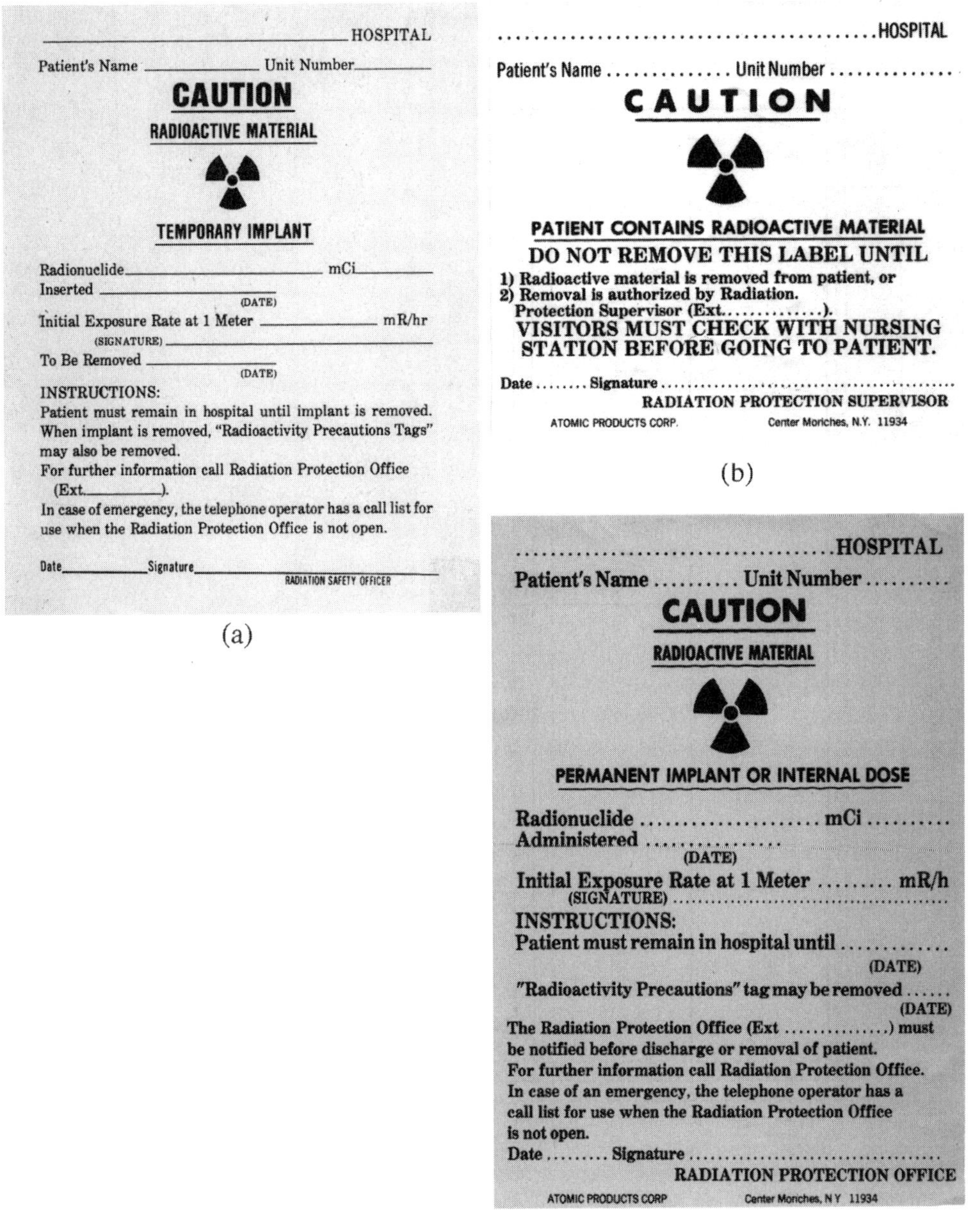

FIGURE 20.4 Radiation warning signs (a) for labeling the entrance door of the patient treatment room, (b) for labeling the patient's treatment chart for a temporary implant, and (c) for labeling the patient's treatment chart for a permanent implant.

time for the discharge of these patients. One guideline requires that the radioactivity in a patient with a permanent implant should reach less than 1.11 Gbq (30 mCi) for the patient to be discharged from the hospital.[6] According to another guideline, the radiation level at 1 m from the patient should be less than 50 μSv h^{-1} (5 mrem h^{-1}) for discharge.[20]

Radioactive seeds may be expelled in urine or other body excretions, especially in the case of permanent prostate implants. The urine should be checked for the presence of radioactive seeds. Any source, if found, should be segregated and taken to the storage room. The source either can be stored for decay over a period of 10 half-lives or can be returned to the source vendor for disposal.

After discharge, a patient with a permanent implant should be advised to follow certain precautions to reduce the irradiation of other members of the household. The patient may be asked to maintain a distance of 1 m from others as much as possible. Particular care should be taken to avoid exposure of pregnant women and persons below the age of 18 years. The patient's relatives should be properly educated and informed and should not be driven to panic. The hazards should not be overrated because, unlike the staff in the hospital, the patient's relatives are not frequently close to patients implanted with radiation sources.

If a patient containing radioactive materials dies in the hospital, the volume of tissue implanted can be excised and isolated to be left to decay. This precaution can also be taken if the body is autopsied.

20.13 PERSONNEL MONITORING

In addition to the use of chest monitors, the use of wrist and finger radiation monitoring badges is helpful and desirable for those who handle brachytherapy sources. The doses recorded by these monitors can alert the radiation safety officer to the possible need to improve the source-handling procedures.

20.14 CONCLUSION

The use of brachytherapy sources need not be feared if care is exercised. A proper understanding of the importance of the role of distance in improving radiation safety is very important. Sources should never be touched for saving time or for obtaining quick results in a panic situation. Preloading techniques should be replaced by afterloading methods.

REFERENCES

1. Martinez, A.A., Orton, C.G., and Mould, R.F. (Eds.), Brachytherapy HDR and LDR, Proceedings of Remote Afterloading: State of the Art Conference, Nucletron Corporation, Columbia, Maryland, 1990.
2. Joslin, C.A.F., Brachytherapy: A clinical dilemma, Int. J. Radiat. Oncol. Biol. Phys., Vol 19, p801-802, 1990.
3. American Association of Physicists in Medicine, Remote Afterloading Technology, AAPM Report No. 41, American Association of Physicists in Medicine, American Insitute of Physics, New York, 1993.
4. IEC, Particular Requirements for the Safety of Remote Controlled Automatically Driven Gamma-ray Afterloading Equipment, International Standard IEC 601, Medical Electrical Equipment, Part 2, Bureau de la Commission Electrotechnique Internationale, Geneva, 1989.
5. Almond, P.R., Remote Afterloading, p601-619, in AAPM Monograph No. 9, Advances in Radiotherapy Treatment Planning, Wright, A.E., and Boyer, A.L. (Eds.), American Association of Physicists in Medicine, New York, 1983.
6. National Council on Radiation Protection and Measurements, Protection Against Radiation from Brachytherapy Sources, NCRP Report No. 40, National Council on Radiation Protection and Measurements, Washington, D.C., 1972.
7. Paine, C.H., Modern afterloading methods for interstitial radiotherapy, Clin. Radiol., Vol 23, p263-272, 1972.
8. Henschke, U.K., Hilaris, B.S., and Mahan, G.D., Afterloading in interstitial and intracavitary radiation therapy, Am. J. Roentgenol., Vol 90, p386-395, 1963.
9. Suit, H.D., Moore, E.B., Fletcher, G.H., and Worsnop, R., Modification of Fletcher ovoid system for afterloading, using standardized radium tubes (milligram and microgram), Radiology, Vol 81, p126-131, 1963.
10. Horowitz, H., Kereiakes, J.G., Bahr, G.K., Cluxton, S.E., and Barrett, C.M., An afterloading system utilizing cesium-137 for the treatment of carcinoma of the cervix, Am. J. Roentgenol., Vol 91, p176-191, 1964.
11. Arnott, S.J., Law, J., Ash, D. et al., Problems associated with iridium-192 wire implants, Clin. Radiol., Vol 36, p283-285, 1985.
12. International Organisation for Standardisation (ISO), Sealed Radioactive Sources — Leak Test Methods, Technical Report 4862, Geneva, Switzerland, 1979.
13. British Standards Institution, Sealed Radioactive Sources, BS5288, British Standards Institute, London, 1976.

14. Wood, V.A. (Ed.), A collection of radium leak test articles, U.S. Public Health Service Publication, MORP 68-1, U.S. Government Printing Office, Washington, D.C., 1968.

15. National Council on Radiation Protection and Measurements, Precautions in the Management of Patients Who Have Received Therapeutic Amounts of Radionuclides, NCRP Report No. 37, National Council on Radiation Protection and Measurements, Washington, D.C., 1970.

16. Thomadsen, B., van de Geijn, J., Buchler, D., and Paliwal, B., Fortification of existing rooms for brachytherapy patients, Health Phys., Vol 45, p607-615, 1983.

17. Gitterman, M., and Webster, E.W., Shielding hospital rooms for brachytherapy patients: Design, regulatory and cost/benefit factors, Health Phys., Vol 46, p617-625, 1984.

18. Sedham, L.N., and Yanni, M.I., Radiation therapy and nurses' fears of radiation exposure, Cancer Nursing, Vol 8, p129-134, 1985.

19. Dawes, T.J.O.K., and Aird, E.G.A., Preliminary experience with ^{125}I seeds in Newcastle upon Tyne, Clin. Radiol., Vol 36, p359-364, 1985.

20. United States Nuclear Regulatory Commission, Rules and Regulations, Code of Federal Regulation, Energy, Part 10, Paragraph 35.75, p532, Revised Jan 01,1994, U.S. Government Printing Office, Washington, D.C.

ADDITIONAL READING

1. American Association of Physicists in Medicine, Advances in Radiation Oncology Physics, Dosimetry, Treatment Planning, and Brachytherapy, American Association of Physicists in Medicine Monograph No. 19, American Institute of Physics, New York, 1993.

2. Institute of Physical Sciences, Report 46, Chapter 3, Brachytherapy, in Radiation Protection in Radiotherapy, Mckenzie, A.L., Shaw, J.E., Stephenson, S.K., and Turner, R.C.R. (Eds.), Institute of Physical Sciences in Medicine, London, 1986.

3. Institute of Physical Sciences in Medicine, Report 45, Dosimetry and Clinical Uses of Afterloading Systems, Alderson, A.R. (Ed.), Institute of Physical Sciences in Medicine, London, 1986.

4. American Association of Physicists in Medicine, Symposium Proceedings No. 4, Radiotherapy Safety, Thomadsen, B. (Ed.), American Institute of Physics, New York, 1982.

5. American Association of Physicists in Medicine, Recent Advances in Brachytherapy Physics, Shearer, D.A. (Ed.), American Insitute of Physics, New York, 1981.

6. International Atomic Energy Agency, Physical Aspects of Radioisotope Brachytherapy, IAEA Technical Report Series No. 75, International Atomic Energy Agency, Vienna, 1967.

SUBJECT INDEX
VOLUME I

A

AAPM, 134
Abbreviations, 190–191
Absorption
    of bone, 208–211
    of energy
        and dose, 119–120
        local, 66, 73–74
    mass-energy absorption coefficient, 210, 225–231
    photoelectric, 62–66, 75
    of photons, 59–60, 78
Accelerating tube, 103, 104
Acceleration of electrons, 81, 85, 93, 103
Accelerators
    direct-voltage electrostatic, 103–105
    electron, 93
    induction, 103
    linear, 103, 105–112
    particle, 103–115
Accredited dosimetry calibration laboratory (ADCL), 130, 135
Acronyms, 190–191
ADCL, 130, 135
Air
    electron mass stopping powers in, 215–216
    mass attenuation coefficients, 226
    mass energy absorption coefficients, 226
    mass energy transfer coefficients, 226
Air dose, 122, 124–125
Air kerma, 123–127
    relationship to dose, 125–127
    relationship to exposure, 124, 125
Air-kerma rate constant, 137–140
Air output factor, See Normalized air output factor
Air output rate, calibrated, See Calibrated air output rate
Air-tissue interface, 94
Alpha decay, 26, 27, 28
Alpha particles, 1, 25, 56, 149
    collision and, 49–52
    in particle accelerators, 113
Alpha track, 49
Alternating current (AC), 85, 111, 112
Aluminum
    covalent bonds of, 12, 15
    electron mass stopping powers in, 221
    mass attenuation coefficients, 228
    mass energy absorption coefficients, 228
    mass energy transfer coefficients, 228
Aluminum filter, 90
Aluminum oxide, covalent bonds of, 12, 15
American Association of Physicists in Medicine (AAPM), 134
Ammonia, covalent bonds of, 12, 15
Angular distribution, of scattered photons, 68, 69
Angular emission of photoelectrons, 66, 68, 69

Anode
    in Coolidge X-ray tube, 82, 85, 86
    rotating, 84
Anthracene, 149
Antimatter, 18
Antineutrino, 28
Antiparticles, 16, 18, 28
Antiprotons, 18
Antiquarks, 17, 18
Appendices, 215–231
Applied potential, the role of, 143–144
Atomic attenuation coefficient, 61, See also Attenuation coefficient
Atomic level, 7–9
Atomic mass, 4, 11, 61, 70
Atomic mass unit (amu), 11
Atomic number, 4, 6, 11, 27
    effective, 75–76, 202
    photoelectric interaction and, 65
    photon energy and, 72–73, 74
    radioactive decay and, See Decay schemes
    vs. Compton cross section, 70, 74
Atomic orbits, 4, 7–9, 11, 12, 14–15
Atomic physics, historical background, 3
Atomic shells, 7–10, 12, 30, 31–32, 90
Atoms
    formation of, 3–7
    physical characteristics of, 3–4
Attenuation coefficient, 59–62
    atomic, 61
    for bone, 209
    electronic, 61–62
    linear, 60–61
    mass, 61, 65, 225–231
    for mixtures and compounds, 75–76
Attractive force, 16, 17, 25
Auger electron, 10
    emission from electron capture, 30
    emission from photoelectric effect, 63, 66
Avogadro's number, 11–12, 61, 70
Axis of beam, 155, 156
    central-axis dose profile, 157–159
    off-central axis points, 200–201
Azimuthal quantum number, 7

B

Back-pointing device, 100, 101
Back-scatter factor (BSF), 165, See also Peak scatter factor
Barium-137, 94
Baryons, 16, 17, 18, 19
Batho's method, 204–206, 207–208
Beam
    cross section of, 110, 155, 156
    dose delivered by a, 136–137

electron, 49
external-beam therapy (teletherapy), 93–101
and filter material, 90
flatness of, 200
hardening of the, 90, 91
light beam localizer, 96, 99
need for calibration of the, 131
photon, 59
quality, 157
    half-value thickness and, 90–91
    peak scatter factors and, 165
shape, 95, See also Field size; Geometric penumbra
useful, 83–84
Beam geometry, 76–78, 96–98, 155–157
Becquerel unit, 37
Benzene, 153
Beryllium, 4
Beta decay, 25, 27–28
    beta-minus decay, 28–29
    beta-plus decay, 29–30
Beta particles, 25–30, 143, 149
Betatron, 103, 110–112
Binding energy, 3, 9, 26, 63
BIPM, 130
Bismuth-210, 29
Blocked fields, 193, 194
Blood, radiation of, 1
Body constituents, effective atomic number (Z) for, 75
Body inhomogeneities, correction for, 202–208
Bonds, types of molecular, 12, 14–15
Bone
    attenuation and absorption in, 208–211
    depth-dose profiles, 211
    effective atomic number and density, 75, 202–203
    electron mass stopping powers in, 217
    mass attenuation coefficients, 227
    mass energy absorption coefficients, 210, 227
    mass energy transfer coefficients, 227
Bosons, 16
Boson vectors, 16
Bottom quarks, 17, 18
Bound electrons, 66
Bound state of atoms, 12, 14
Brachytherapy, 93, 94
Bragg-Gray cavity, ideal, 133–134
Bragg ionization curve, 51–52
Bremsstrahlung, 52–55, 74, 81, 124, See also X-rays
    angular distribution, 53
    energy distribution, 74
    production of, in Coolidge X-ray tube, 82
Broad-beam geometry, 76–77, See also Beam geometry
Build-up caps, 129, 131, 132, 135
Build-up factor, 77–78, 135
Bureau International des Poids et des Mesures (BIPM), 130

C

Calcium
    mass attenuation coefficients, 229
    mass energy absorption coefficients, 229
    mass energy transfer coefficients, 229

Calcium fluoride, electron mass stopping powers in, 222
Calibrated air output rate (CAOR), 173–174
    derivation of dose rate and, 175–176
    effective rectangular field and, 194, 195
    off-central axis points and, 200, 201
    PDD and, 178, 182, 184
Calibrated peak output rate (CPOR), 173–174
    derivation of dose rate and, 175–177
    effective rectangular field and, 194–195, 196
    PDD and, 184, 186
Calibration
    of beams, need for, 131
    of a film, 147
Calibration factor, 130–131, 135
Calorimetry, 153
Capacitance, 144
Capacitors, 103–104
Carbon
    electron mass stopping powers in, 220
    isotopes of, 11
    mass attenuation coefficients, 225
    mass energy absorption coefficients, 225
    mass energy transfer coefficients, 225
    as standard for atomic masses, 11
Cathode, 81–82
Cavity chambers, 128–130, 133–137
Central-axis dose profile, 157–159
Ceric sulphate, 153
Cesium-137, 34, 94, 139–140
Chamber, walled, in a medium, 13, 134–135
Characteristic curve, 148
Charge
    of electrons, 10, 71–73
    of elementary particles, See Charged particles
    relationship to exposure, 124
Charged-particle equilibrium (CPE), 120–121, 123, 131
Charged particles, 15, 16, See also Alpha particles; Beta particles; Gamma particles
    collision loss, 49–52, 133
    moving, 52
    radiative loss, 52–56
Charmed quarks, 17, 18
Chemical bonds, 12, 14–15
Chemical dosimeters, 152–153
Clinical linear accelerator, 108–110
Clinical physicist, 1, 2
Cobalt-59, 46–47
Cobalt-60, 28–29, 39–40, 48
    beam, calibration of, 131, 135
    bone and depth-dose profile, 209, 211
    dose
        to tissue in air for, 131–132
        in water for, 132–133
    dose rate, to tissue in air, 161
    effect of field radius on TAR and SAR, 197
    energy released in disintegration, 140
    machines, 95–98
    output factors for, 174
    percent depth doses for, 167–169
    tissue-air ratios for, 164

Cobalt-61, 48
Cockcroft-Walton voltage multiplier, 103–104
Coherent Thompson scattering, 7, 59, 62
Cold cathode tubes, 81
Collimator, 95, 96, 109
Collision loss, 49–52, 133
Collision stopping power, 215–223
Colors of quarks, 17, 18
Compounds, attenuation coefficient for, 75–76
Compton cross section, 68–70
Compton effect, 68, See also Compton scattering, incoherent
Compton scattering, incoherent, 59, 66–70, 74, 75, 159, 160
Condenser chamber, 144–145
Conservation law of electric charge, 26
Conservation law of lepton number, 26
Conservation law of mass-energy, 4, 66–67
Conservation law of momentum, 66
Conservation law of nucleon number, 26
Convolution approach, 209
Coolidge X-ray tubes, 81–88
Copper
    mass attenuation coefficients, 229
    mass energy absorption coefficients, 229
    mass energy transfer coefficients, 229
Copper filter, 90
Corpuscular radiation, 1
Cosmic rays, 18
Coulomb, 10
Coulomb field, 52
Covalent bonds, 12, 14, 15
Crookes' tubes, 81
Cross section
    of beam, 110, 155, 156
    Compton, 68–70
    of pair production, 72
    photoelectric, 66
Crystals, 150–151
CT numbers, 210
CT scans, 209–210
Curie unit, 37
Curvature of surface, 200
Cyclotron, 103, 112–113
Cylindrical cavity chamber, 129, 132, 145

D

Dalton, 3
Daughter nuclides, 41–45
Daughter product build-up and decay, 41–42
Day's method, 199–200
Decay chains, 41–45
Decay constant, 39, 40, 41
Decay schemes, 26–27, 28, 29, 30, 31, 32
Deflector, 113
Delivery period, for uniform dose, 93
Delta rays, 56
Densitometer, 147
Density
    of body constituents, 202
    ionization, 51–52, 56

of the lung, 208
of the medium, 61
optical, 147, 148
Depletion layer, 150
Depth, 161–162
    beam quality and, 158
    calculation of dose in the, 159
    effective, 203–204
    ratio of kerma to dose at, 122–123
    treatment, 155, 156
    water-equivalent, 204
Depth-dose, 165–166, 175, 177, 193, 211; percent, See Percent depth dose
Deuterium, 5, 7, 113
Deuterons, in particle accelerators, 113
Diagnostic radiology, 84, 85, 148–149
Diameter, of radiotherapy dose, 93
Diaphragms
    adjustable, 98
    collimating, 97, 98, 99, 159, 160
    in ionization chambers, 127, 128
    within wave guides, 107
Dielectric-filled waveguide, 107, 108
Diminution of photon flux, 59–60
Diodes, semiconductor, 85–86, 150
Dirac's theory of the electron, 71, 72
Direct current (DC), 108
Direct-voltage electrostatic accelerators, 103–105
Disintegration, 93, 139–140
Dissipation of energy, 82
Dose, 119–120
    accumulation of, 98
    air, 122, 124–125
    build-up of, by secondary electron release, 97–98, 120, 121–122
    calculation of
        in the depth, 159
        parameters, 161–162
    definition, 1
    delivery period, 93
    determination of, 133
    distance from the source and, 93, 137, 138, 155, 156
    electron beams, delivered by, 136–137
    energy transfer and, 59, 139, 225–231
    gathering depth-dose data, 175
    kerma profiles and, 121–123
    measuring by thermoluminescent dosimeters, 151–152
    in medium, 125–127
    percent depth dose, 165–166
    relationship to kerma, 119, 121, 122–123
    relationship to air kerma and exposure, 125–127
    skin, 90, 94, 158–159
    to spinal cord, 184
    of therapeutic X-rays, 85
    to tissue in air, 131–132, 159–160, 161
    typical uniform, 93
    in water, 132–133
    to water, 137
Dose output
    calibrated, See Calibrated air output rate; Calibrated peak output rate

factors, 173–174
Dose profile, central-axis, 157–159
Dose rate
    absolute, 131, 159
    methods of deriving, 175–177
    at off-center axis points, 201
Dosimeters, 117
    chemical, 152–153
    ferrous sulfate, 152–153
    film as an inaccurate calibrator, 147–148
    Fricke, 152–153
    thermoluminescent, 150–152
Dosimetry, 117
    additional corrections and special situations,
        193–211
    basic ratios and factors for, 155–191
Down quarks, 17, 18
Drift-tube waveguide, 107, 108
Duration, of treatment, 84, 177
Dynodes, 150

E

Effective atomic number (Z), 75–76, 202
Effective depth, 203–204
Effective field size, 204
Effective rectangular field, 193–196
Einstein, Albert, 3, 23, 63
Einstein's theory of relativity, 3, 23, 67
Electric charge, 4, 10, 15, 16
Electric field, 21, 22, 72, 103
    in ionization chambers, 127
    in linear accelerators, 105, 115
Electricity, and magnetism, 21
Electric potential, 7.143–144, 150
Electromagnetic force, 16
Electromagnetic radiation, 1, 9, 10, 21–24
Electrometer, 129, 135, 143, 144
Electron beam, 49
Electron capture, 30–31, 52
Electron contamination dose, 97–98, 159
Electronic attenuation coefficient, 61–62
Electron leptons, 16, 17, 18
Electron-neutrino leptons, 16, 17
Electron-positron annihilation, 72
Electrons, 1, 3, 4
    acceleration of, 81, 85, 93, 103
    Auger, See Auger electrons
    binding energies of, 9
    charge of, 10, 71–73
    emission composed of, 81, See also X-rays
    emissions from, 62
    free vs. bound, 66
    "holes," 150
    orbits, See Orbits of electrons
    recoil, 67, 68, 70, 75
    secondary, 9, 97–98, 120, 121–122
        as addition to skin dose, 97–98
        from ionization chamber wall, 134, 136
    shells, 4, 7–11, 12, 30, 31–32, 90
    tracks of, 50, 121–122
Electron scattering, 49–51

Electron volt, 10–11, 103, 107
Electrostatic accelerators, 103–105
Elementary particles, 15–19, See also Charged particles;
        Fluence
    forces between, 18
    research in, 18
    wave-like behavior of, 24
Elements
    binding energies of atomic orbital electrons, 9
    definition, 4
    formation of, 3–7
    list of, 6
    periodic table, 12, 13
Energy, 3
    absorption of local, 66, 73–74
    amount absorbed and dose, 119–120
    binding, 3, 9, 26, 63
    bremsstrahlung, 54–55, 74
    continuous, of beta particles, 28, 29
    of dissipation, 82
    and electron scattering, 50
    electron volt and, 10, 103, 107
    in ionization detectors, 143–144
    law of conservation, 4
    of nucleons, 26
    of photons, 23, 62–66, 70, 72–73, 138, 210
    potential, 7, 143–144, 150
    propagation of, 21–24
    of quarks, 18
Energy distribution, 74
Energy fluence, 117–118
Energy fluence rate, 118
Energy states, 7–8
Energy transfer, 119, 139; mass energy transfer coefficient,
        225–231
Equilibrium, secondary electron, 120–121
Equivalent squares and circles, 177–178, 179
"Ether," 23
EV, 10–11, 103, 107
Excitation, 1, 9–10; and nuclide stability, 5
Exclusion principle, Pauli's, 7
Exposure, 123–124
    duration of, 84, 177
    measurement of, 127–131
    relationship to air kerma, 124, 125
    relationship to dose, 125–127
Exposure calibration factor, 130–131, 135
Exposure rate, calculation of, 139
External-beam therapy (teletherapy), 93–101
Extrapolation chamber, 146
Eyler's exponential constant, 38

F

Fall-off, inverse-square, 160–161
Ferrous sulfate dosimeter, 152–153
Field localizer, 96, 99
Field size
    of beam, 155, 156, 161–162
    and derivation of dose rate, 175–177
    effective, 204
    effective rectangular, 193–196

electron contamination and, 159
  equivalent squares and circles, 177–178, 179
  irregularly-shaped, with shields, 193, 194
Field width, effective, 189–190, 204
Filament tube, 81–88
Film, 146–149
  as an inaccurate calibrator, 147–148
  calibration of a, 147
  diagnostic, 148–149
  high-energy port, 149
  response curves, 147–148
Filter
  aluminum, 90
  copper, 90
  material of, and beam, 90
  thickness of, 84
  Thoreaus, 90
  in X-ray tube, 82, 84, 88, 90
Fixed-SAD technique, 156, 162, 176
Fixed-SSD technique, 156, 162, 165–166, 175 176
Flavors of quarks, 17, 18
Fluence, 117, 118, 120, 122, 131
  in ionization chambers, 127, 134–135
  primary and scatter, 76–77
  secondary electron, 120
Fluence rate, 118
Fluorine, ionic bonds of, 12, 14
Fluoroscopy, diagnostic, 85
Focal spot, 83, 84–85
Foil, electron-scattering, 109, 110
Free-air ionization chamber, 127–128
Free electrons, 66
Frequency of waves, 21–24
Fricke dosimeter, 152–153
Full-wave rectification, 86–88

G

Gamma particles, 23, 25, 31–33, 149
Gamma ray energy, 31–32
Gas-discharge X-ray tube, 81, 82
Gas multiplication, 143
Geiger-Mueller (GM) counter regions, 143, 144
General Electric Company, 81
Geometric penumbra, 96–98
Germanium, 150
Glossary, 190–191
Gluons, 16, 17, 18
Gold-198, 32, 33
Gravitational field, 10, 11
Gravitational force, 16
Gray unit, definition, 119
Grids, 148–149
Guard plates, 127, 128
G value, 153

H

Hadrons, 16, 17, 18, 19
Half-life, 26, 38, 39–40
  neutron activation and, 46
  of photonuclear reaction products, 78

of radiotherapy isotopes, 94
Half-value thickness (HVT), 61, 90–91, 157
Half-wave rectification, 85–86
H & D curve, 148
Heat, 9, 21–22
Heat generation
  avoidance of overheating, 84–85
  in Coolidge X-ray tubes, 82–83, 84
Heavy ions, 1
Heel effect, 84
Helium, 4, 113
  alpha decay, 26, 27
  binding energies of, 9
  during fusion, 35
  isotopes of, 5
High-neutron-flux reactor, 93
High-voltage supply and rectification, 85–88
Historical background
  of atomic physics, 3
  of radiation physics, iii
Homogeneity index, 91
Hot-cathode tubes, 81–82
Hydrogen, 4, 5
  covalent bonds of, 12, 14, 15
  during fusion, 35
  isotopes of, 5, 7, 113
  mass attenuation coefficients, 225
  mass energy absorption coefficients, 225
  mass energy transfer coefficients, 225
Hydrogen bomb, 34
Hydrogen bonds, 12, 14–15
Hyperons, 18

I

ICRU, 117
In-air output, See Calibrated air output rate
Incoherent Compton scattering, 59, 66–70, 74, 75, 159, 160
Induced nuclear transformations, 35
Induction accelerators, 103
Infrared radiation, 23
Inhomogeneities, lung and bone, 202–208
Inhomogeneity correction factor, 202–208
  comparison of, obtained by different methods, 206–208
  discontinuity of, across an interface, 205
Intensifying screens, 148–149
Intensity, 77–78, 90
Internal conversion, 26, 31–32
International Commission on Radiation Units and Measurements (ICRU), 117
International Union of Pure and Applied Physics, 11
Inverse-square factor, 160, 162, 176
Inverse-square fall-off, 160–161
Iodine-125, 31, 40
Iodine-131, 29, 30
Ionic bonds, 12, 14
Ionization, 1, 9 10
Ionization chambers
  cavity, 128–130, 133–137
  free-air, 127–128

in a medium, 133, 134–135
Ionization density, 51–52, 56
Ionization detectors, 143–146
Ions, heavy, 1
Iridium-191, 48
Iridium-192, 94
Iris-loaded waveguide, 107, 108
Irradiation parameters, 161–162
Isobars, 5
Isocentrically mounted system, 109
Isomeric state, 32
Isomeric transition, 5, 26, 32–33
Isotones, 5
Isotopes
    decay of
        corrections for dose, 93
        a single, 37–41, See also Disintegration
    definition, 5
    for radiotherapy, 93–94
    sources of, 93–94, 137, 138
    stable, 5
    unstable, 5

J

Joule, 10, 83

K

Kerma
    air, 123–127
    air-kerma rate constant, 137–140
    definition, 119
    mass and, 119
    ratio of, to dose at depth, 122–123
    relationship to dose, 119, 121, 122–123
    water, 123
Kerma profiles, dose and, 121–123
Kinetic energy
    of Compton recoil electrons, 67, 68, 70, 75
    of photoelectrons, 66
K shell, 7–10, 12, 30, 31–32
    characteristic X-rays, 90
    in photoelectric effect, 63, 64

L

Lateral electronic equilibrium, 208
Laws of conservation, See individual conservation laws
Lead
    collision and radiative loss in, 53
    electron mass stopping powers in, 223
    mass attenuation coefficients, 231; vs. photon energy for,
        65
    mass energy absorption coefficients, 231
    mass energy transfer coefficients, 230
    for source shielding, 95
    types of photon interactions, 75
Leptons, 16, 17, 18
LET, 56
Light
    transmitted, intensity of, 147

velocity of, 3
visible, 23
Light beam localizer, 96, 99
Light waves, 21–22
Linear accelerators (linacs), 103, 105–110, 115
Linear attenuation coefficient, 60–61
Linear density of ionization, 56
Linear energy transfer (LET), 56
Line focus, 83
Lithium, 4, 5
    binding energies of, 9
    ionic bonds of, 12, 14
Lithium fluoride, 12, 14; electron mass stopping powers in,
        222
Loaded waveguides, 107, 108
Local energy, 66, 73–74
Lorentz force, 103
L shell, 7–10, 12, 30, 31–32, 90
Lung
    density
        and effective atomic number, 202–203
        and lateral electronic equilibrium and, 208
    phantom geometry of, 203

M

Magnetic field, 21, 22, 25, 26; in particle accelerators, 109,
        110, 112, 114
Magnetic peeler, 111
Magnetic quantum number, 7
Magnetism, and electricity, 21
Mass
    atomic, 4, 11, 61, 70
    Avogadro's number, 11–12, 61
    dose and, 119–120
    of elementary particles, 15
    of gas in Bragg-Gray cavity, 133
    kerma and, 119
    molecular, 11
    of quarks, 18, 24
Mass attenuation coefficient, 61, 65; for various materials,
        225–231
Mass defect, 25–26
Mass-energy absorption coefficient, 210, 225–231,
        See also Absorption
Mass-energy conversion, 24
Mass energy transfer coefficient, 225–231, See also
        Energy transfer
Mass-equivalent thickness, 61
Mass number, 5, 27
Mass unit, atomic, 11
Mean free path, 61
Mean life, 15, 19, 38, 40–41
Mercury, 32
Mesons, 1, 16, 17, 18, 19
Methyl methacrylate
    mass attenuation coefficients, 227
    mass energy absorption coefficients, 227
    mass energy transfer coefficients, 227
Microtron, 103, 114–115
Microwave technology, 23, 115
Mixtures, attenuation coefficient for, 75–76

Modeling, 203, 209
Molecular bonds, 12, 14–15
Molecular mass, 11
Molybdenum-99, 33, 44–45
Monitor unit, 184
Monitor units per degree of arc, 190
Monte Carlo techniques, 203, 209
M shell, 7–10, 30, 90
Muon-neutrino leptons, 16, 17, 18
Muscle
    electron mass stopping powers in, 218
    mass attenuation coefficients, 227
    mass energy absorption coefficients, 227
    mass energy transfer coefficients, 227

N

Narrow-beam geometry, 76, See also Beam geometry
National Council on Radiation Protection and Measures, 117
Negative muon leptons, 16, 17
Negative tau leptons, 16, 17
Negatron, 28, 71; -positron pair production, 59, 71–73, 74, 75
Neon, 4, 9
Neutrinos, 16, 30–31
Neutron, 1, 3
    atomic structure and, 4–5
    charge, 4
    decay of, 28
    in particle accelerators, 113
    physical characteristics, 4
    -proton balance, 27–38
    quarks in, 17
    and stability of isotopes, 5
Neutron activation, 45–48
Neutron flux, 47
Nickel, from cobalt-60 decay, 28–29
Nitrogen
    covalent bonds of, 12, 15
    isotopes of, 5
    mass attenuation coefficients, 225
    mass energy absorption coefficients, 225
    mass energy transfer coefficients, 225
Normalized air output factor (NOAF), 174
    derivation of dose rate and, 175–176
    effective rectangular field and, 194, 195
    off-central axis points and, 200
    PDD and, 178, 183
Normalized peak output factor (NPOF), 173–174
    derivation of dose rate and, 175–177
    effective rectangular field and, 194–195, 196
    PDD and, 184, 186
Normalized peak scatter factor (NPSF), 165, 174
NPOF, See Normalized peak output factor
NPSF, 165, 174
"n-type" semiconductor material, 150, 151
Nuclear decay scheme, See Decay schemes
Nuclear fission, 26, 33–34
Nuclear force, 16
Nuclear fusion, 26, 34–35

Nuclear reaction, 35
Nuclear reactors, 34, 45
Nuclear transitions, 25–35
    induced, 35
    of technetium-99m, 32–33, 44–45
Nucleons, 25
Nucleus, 4–5, 25–35
Nuclide, 26, 28

O

Off-center ratios in air, 200–201
Off-central axis points, 200–201
Optical density, 147, 148
Optical distance indicator (ODI), 98–100
Orbits of electrons, 4, 7–11, 12, 31–32, 90
    bonds and, 12, 14–15
    collision loss and, 51
Oscillator
    microwave, 108
    radio frequency, 105, 106
Outcome, 1, 2
Outer space, and elementary particle research, 18
Output
    in-air, See Calibrated air output rate; Normalized air output factor
    peak, See Calibrated peak output rate; Normalized peak output factor
    voltage of, 85
Overheating of X-ray tube, 82–85
Oxalic acid, 153
Oxygen
    covalent bonds of, 12, 14, 15
    isotopes of, 5
    mass attenuation coefficients, 226
    mass energy absorption coefficients, 226
    mass energy transfer coefficients, 226

P

Pair production, 59, 71–73, 74, 75
    cross section, 72
    negatron-positron, 71–73
    threshold energy, 71–72
    yield, 72–73
Pancake cavity chamber, 129, 146
Parallel-plate cavity chamber, 129, 146
Parameters, 161–162
Particles, See Charged particles; Elementary particles; Fluence
Patient support, 98, 99
Pauli's exclusion principle, 7
Peak output, See Calibrated peak output rate; Normalized peak output factor
Peak scatter factor (PSF), 163, 170, 177
    derivation of dose rate, 175–176
    effective rectangular field and, 194, 195
    inhomogeneity correction factor and, 206
    normalized, 165, 174
    output factors and, 174
    PDD and, 178, 180, 181–184, 186, 187
Peeler (betatron), 111

Penumbra
    geometric, 96–98
    transmission, 98
Percent depth dose (PDD), 165–166, 178
    converting for one SSD to another, 180–190
    relationship to TAR and TMR, 178, 180
Periodic table of elements, 4, 12, 13
Phantom materials, 75, 155, 162, 205; tissue-phantom ratio,
    170, 173
Phase stability, 106–107, 115
Phosphorous-32, 113
Photoelectric absorption, 59, 62–66
Photoelectric cross section, 66
Photoelectric effect, 63–65, 74
Photoelectric interaction, 65–66
Photoelectrons, 9, 63
    angular emission of, 66, 68, 69
    kinetic energy of, 66
Photographic film detector, 146–149
Photographic process, 146–147, See also Film
Photomultiplier, 150
Photon field, 16
Photon fluence, 120–121
Photon flux, 59–60
Photons, See also Electromagnetic radiation; Gamma
    particles
    the electromagnetic spectrum and, 23–24
    interactions of, 59–78
    wavelength of, 24
Photonuclear reaction, 59, 78
Physicist
    clinical, 1
    cooperation between, and physician, 1–2
Physics, historical background of atomic, 3
Pions, 18
Planck's constant, 23
Plasma state of matter, 34
Plastic
    in parallel-plate chambers, 146
    use in cavity ionization chambers, 128–129
    as water-substitute in dose assessment, 137
Polonium, 25
Polyethylene
    electron mass stopping powers in, 218
    mass attenuation coefficients, 228
    mass energy absorption coefficients, 228
    mass energy transfer coefficients, 228
Polymethyl methacrylate, electron mass stopping powers
    in, 218
Polystyrene
    electron mass stopping powers in, 220
    mass attenuation coefficients, 228
    mass energy absorption coefficients, 228
    mass energy transfer coefficients, 228
Port films, 149
Positioning, of patient, 98, 99
Positrons, 28, 29–30; negatron-positron pair production,
    71–73, 74, 75
Power supply, 108, 109; three-phase, 87
Pressure
    in gas-discharge X-ray tubes, 81
    normal (NTP), 124

Pressure correction factor, 130
Primary-air ratio (PAR), 196, 197, 198, 199
Proportional counter region, 143, 144
Protons, 1, 3
    beta-plus decay and, 29–30
    charge, 4
    collision loss and, 51
    during electron capture, 30–31
    in particle accelerators, 113
    physical characteristics, 4
    quarks in, 17
Prout, 3
"p-type" semiconductor material, 150, 151

Q

Quanta, and the electromagnetic spectrum,
    23–24
Quantum chromodynamics, 16
Quantum electrodynamics, 16
Quantum mechanics, 7
Quantum number, 7
Quarks, 16–19, 25

R

Radiation chemical yield, 153
Radiation dose, See Dose
Radiation dosimetry, See Dosimetry
Radiation field, 117, See also Field size
Radiation therapy. *See* Radiotherapy
Radiation units and measurements, 117–140
Radiative loss, 52–56
Radiative stopping power, 215–223
Radioactive decay, 26–34
    calculations, 37–48
    chains, 41–45
Radioactivity, discovery of natural, 25
Radio frequency (RF) oscillator, 105, 106
Radiography, See Diagnostic radiology
Radioisotopes, See Isotopes
Radiotherapy
    brachytherapy, 93, 94
    cobalt-60 machines for, 95–98
    definition of, 1
    equipment for, 93–101
    film used in, 146–149
    historical background, 43
    radioisotopes for, 93–94
    teletherapy, 93–101
Radio waves, 21–22
Radium, 25
Radium-226, 94
    alpha decay to radon, 27, 28
    decay chain of, 42
    secular equilibrium of, 43–44
Radium-E, 42
Radon, contamination by, 44
Radon-222, 27, 28, 43
Rad unit, 126
Reactors
    high-neutron-flux, 93

nuclear, 34, 45
Rectangular field, effective, 193–196
Rectification, 85–88
    full-wave, 86–88
    half-wave, 85–86
    self-, 85, 86
Reference state, 7
Relativity, 3, 23, 67
Resistors, 103, 104
Resolution of image, 83
Resonance accelerators, 103, 105–112
Rest energy of quarks, 18, 19
Roentgen rays, 81, See also X-rays
Roentgen unit, 126
Rotating anode, 84
Rubidium-37, 34

S

SAD, 155, 156, 162, 176
Saturation activity, 47, 48
Scatter
    angular distribution of, 67, 68, 69
    in blocked fields, 193, 194
    coherent Thompson, 59, 62, 75
    during dose to tissue in air, 159–160
    electron, 49–51
    incoherent Compton, 59, 66–70, 74, 75, 159, 160
    percent by collimator, 161
    use of grid to minimize, 148–149
Scatter-air ratio (SAR), 196–197, 198, 199, See also
        Tissue-air ratio
Scatter build-up factor, 77–78, 135
Scatter factor, peak, See Peak scatter factor
Scatter-radius integration, 197–199
Scintillation detector, 149–150
Secondary emissions, 9, 97–98, 117, 120, 121–122; from
        ionization chamber wall, 134, 136
Secular equilibrium, 43–44
Self-rectified circuit, 85, 86
Semiconductor diodes, 85–86, 150
Shells, See Electrons, shells
Shielding blocks, 193, 194
Silicon, 150
    electron mass stopping powers in, 221
    mass attenuation coefficients, 229
    mass energy absorption coefficients, 229
    mass energy transfer coefficients, 229
Silver bromide emulsions, 24, 146–147
Skin dose, 90, 94, 158–159
Sodium, binding energies of, 9
Sodium-22, 31
Source capsule, 96
Source head, 93, 95, 98, 109
Source of isotopes, 93–94, 137, 138
Source on-off mechanism, 95, 96
Source-to-axis distance (SAD), 155, 156; fixed, technique,
        156, 162, 176
Source-to-skin distance (SSD), 93, 97, 155, 156, 163, 196
    converting PDD from one to another, 180–190
    fixed, technique, 156, 162, 165–166, 175–176
    optical distance indicator, 98–100

Special theory of relativity, 3, 23, 67
Spectrometer, 149, 150
Spin, of elementary particles, 15
Spin quantum number, 7
SSD, See Source-to-skin distance
Stability
    of elementary particles, 15–16
    of isotopes, 5, 6
    phase, 106–107, 115
Stable isotopes, 5
Stable nuclide, definition, 26
Standard International (SI) System, 119
Standards, radiation unit calibration, 130–131
Standard temperature and pressure (STP), 130,
        133
Standing wave, 107–108
Standing wave linear accelerator, 107–108
Stem effect, 145
Stopping power, 51, 52, 53, 215–223
Strange quarks, 17, 18
Strong force, 16, 17, 25
Support of patient, 98, 99
Surface curvature, 200

T

TAR, See Tissue-air ratio
Target, See also Thickness of medium
    body inhomogeneities, correction for, 202–208
    heat generation and, 83
    modification of field for odd-shaped, 193, 194
    off-central axis points, 200–201
    of photonuclear reaction products, 78
    surface curvature of, 200
Tau-neutrino leptons, 16, 17, 18
Technetium generator, 44–45
Technetium-99m, 32–33
Teflon, electron mass stopping powers in, 218
Teletherapy, 93–101
Temperature
    normal (NTP), 124
    -pressure correction factor, 130
Thallium-activated sodium iodide, 149
Therapeutic radiology, X-ray, 84, 88
Thermionic emission, 9, 81
Thermoluminescence, 150–151
Thermoluminescent dosimeters (TLDs), 150–152
Thermonuclear bomb, 34
Thickness of filter, 84
Thickness of medium, 60, 61, 62, 69
    fractional transmission and, 77
    half-value, 61, 90–91, 157
    of ionization chamber wall, 134–135
    scatter build-up factor and, 77, 135
    for source shielding, 95
Thimble cavity chamber, 129, 145
Thompson scattering, 59, 62, 75
Thoreaus filter, 90
Three-phase transformers, 87–88
Threshold energy
    for negatron-positron pair production, 71–72
    for photonuclear reactions, 78

Tin
    mass attenuation coefficients, 230
    mass energy absorption coefficients, 230
    mass energy transfer coefficients, 230
Tissue
    dose to, in air, 131–132, 159–160, 161
    effective atomic number and density of, 202
    electron mass stopping powers in, 217
    mass-energy absorption coefficient, 210
    soft
        behavior of water as analogy for, 123
        effective atomic number (Z) for, 75
    substitute materials for, 75
Tissue-air interface, 94
Tissue-air ratio (TAR), 163, 176, 177, See also Scatter-air
       ratio
    for cobalt-60, 164
    in Day's method, 199
    in effective rectangular field, 194, 195
    inhomogeneity correction factor and, 204–208
    off-central axis points and, 201
    relationship to PDD, 178, 180
    in scatter-air ratio correction, 196, 197
    in scatter-radius integration, 198, 199
    TMR and, 166, 170
    for unblocked field, 199
Tissue maximum ratio (TMR), 166, 170, 176, 177
    for arc, 189–190
    derivation of dose rate and, 176, 177
    effective rectangular field and, 193, 195, 196,
       198
    relationship to PDD, 178, 180, 184–190
    for X-rays, 172
Tissue-phantom ratio, 170, 173
TLD reader, 151–152
TMR, See Tissue maximum ratio
Top quarks, 17, 18
Transformers, 85, 86, 87–88, 89
Transient equilibrium, 44–45
Transmission penumbra, 98
Transuranic element, 5
Traveling-wave linear accelerator, 107–108
Treatment duration, 84, 177
Treatment (source) head, 93, 95, 98, 109
Triplet production, 72
Tritium, 5, 7
Tube current, 84
Tube potential, 84
Tungsten, 81
    electron mass stopping powers in, 223
    for source shielding, 95

U

Ultraviolet radiation, 23
Units and measurements, 117–140
Unstable isotopes, 5
Unstable nuclide, 5
Up quarks, 17, 18
Uranium
    radioactivity of, 25
    for source shielding, 95

Uranium-235, 34
Uranium-238, 94

V

Vacuum tube, 85–86
Van de Graaff electrostatic generator, 104–105
Vector bosons, 16
Velocity
    of electromagnetic waves, 21, 23, 24, 106–107
    of light, 3, 67, 107
    of particles, 106, 107, 111
Volt, electron, 10–11, 103, 107
Voltage
    of alternating current, 85
    in condenser chamber, 144, 145
    Coolidge tube operating, 87
    high-voltage supply and rectification, 85–88
    in ionization detectors, 143
Voltage multiplier, 103–104
Volume integration, 209

W

Water
    collision and radiative loss in, 53
    covalent bonds of, 12, 14
    dose in, 132–133
    dose to, 137
    electron mass stopping powers in, 215–216
    hydrogen bonds of, 14
    mass attenuation coefficients, 226; vs. photon energy for,
      65
    mass energy absorption coefficients, 210, 226
    mass energy transfer coefficients, 226
    secondary electron tracks through, 121–122
    types of photon interactions, 75
Water kerma, 123
Wave guides, 107, 108, 109
Wavelength, 21–24; shift in, during Compton scattering,
    67
Wave propagation, 21–22
Weak force, 16, 25
Weight
    of components in mixtures and compounds, 75
    definition, 11
W value, 124–125, 153

X

Xenon-131, 29, 30
X-ray circuit, 88, 89
X-ray machines, 81–91, 108–110,
      See also Accelerators
X-rays, 1, 10, 23, See also Bremsstrahlung
    bone and depth-dose profile for, 209, 211
    in electromagnetic spectrum, 23
    emission of
        from electron capture, 30
        from photoelectric effect, 63, 66
    historical background, 81
    image sharpness, 83

intensifying screens to enhance effect of, 148–149
output factors for, 174
percent depth doses for, 170, 171
spectra and quality of, 88, 90–91
tissue maximum ratio for, 172
X-ray tubes
Coolidge, 81–88

gas-discharge, 81, 82
self-rectified, 85–88

Z

Z, See Effective atomic number
Zinc sulfide, 149

AUTHOR INDEX
VOLUME I

A

Ahnesjo, A., 213
Almond, P.R., 141
Anderson, D.W., 55, 57, 78
Arnott, N., iii
Ashkin, J., 50, 53, 57
Attix, F.H., 51, 57, 78, 140, 141, 153, 210, 212, 215, 225

B

Batho, H.F., 204, 205, 207, 212
Battista, J.J., 212, 213
Becquerel, H., 25
Bergen, M.J., 215
Berkley, L.H., 212
Bernard, M., 212
Bethe, H., 50, 53, 57
Bichsel, H., 51
Bilelajew, A.F., 212
Bjarngard, B.E., 212
Bourland, J.D., 213
Boyer, A.L., 57, 213
Bragg, W., 51, 52
Brahme, A., 212
Buffa, A., 141
Burlin, T.E., 141

C

Cassell, K.J., 213
Chaney, E.L., 212, 213
Chen, X.G., 211
Chin, L.M., 212
Chui, C.S., 213
Clarkson, J.R., 197, 212
Cockcroft, J.D., 103, 104
Compton, A.H., 66 –70, 74, 75
Constantinou, C., 79
Coolidge, W., 81, 82
Crookes, W., 81
Cundiff, J.H., 212
Cullip, T.J., 212
Cunningham, J.R., 54, 191, 204, 212
Curie, M., 25, 43, 94
Curie, P., 25

D

Das, I.J., 212
Day, M.J., 199, 212
Deasy, J., 211
de Broglie, L., 24
Desobry, G.E., 57
Dirac, P.A.M., 71, 72
Distasio, J., 115

Driffield, V.C., 148
Duane, W., iii
Dunscombe, P.B., 212
Dutreix, A., 141
Dutreix, J., 141, 212

E

Eichmiller, F.C., 212
Einstein, A., 3, 63
Eklof, A., 212
El Khatib, E., 212
Evans, R.D., 78, 225
Evans, R.E., 57
Eyler, L., 38

F

Failla, G., 212
Farahani, M., 212
Fermi, E., 57
Fleischman, R.C., 141
Fricke, H., 152
Ford, J.C., 115
Fox, R.A., 212

G

Gabriel, T.A., 212
Galileo, G., iii
Galvin, J.M., 211
Goetsch, S., 141
Golden, R., 170, 172
Gross, W., 212

H

Hanson, A.O., 57
Hanson, W.F., 141, 212
Henkelman, R.M., 213
Hettinger, G., 141
Hobday, P.A., 213
Holmes, T., 211
Holt, J.G., 141
Horton, J.L., 212
Hubbell, J.H., 78, 225
Humphries, L.J., 141
Hurter, F., 148

I

Israel, H.I., 19, 78

J

Johns, H.E., 54, 191

K

Kallman, P., 212
Karzmark, C.J., 115, 116
Kase, K.R., 206, 212
Kereiakes, J.G., 115
Khan, F.M., 141, 212
Kijewski, P.K., 212
Kinsella, T., 211
Klein, E.E., 212
Kramers, H.A., 57
Kubo, H., 141
Kulenkampff, H., 57
Kutcher, G., 141

L

Lanzl, L.H., 116, 140, 141
Lerner, R.G., 19
Lidowski, L., 213
Lind, B., 212
Loevinger, R., 140, 141
Lyman, E.M., 57

M

Mackie, T.R., 211, 212, 213
Malone, D.E., 213
Massey, J.B., 191
Mauceri, T., 206, 212
McLaughlin, W.C., 212
Meigoni, A.S., 212
Mendelleev, D., 12
Mijnheer, B.J., 212
Mohan, R., 213
Mok, E.C., 213
Morin, R.L., 212

N

Nath, R., 141
Nieminen, J.M., 212
Nunan, C.S., 115
Nizin, P.S., 212

O

O'Connor, J.E., 213
Orear, J., 57
Orton, C.G., 212

P

Paliwal, B., 211
Parker, R.P., 212, 213
Perry, D.J., 141
Peterson, M., 170, 172
Petterson, C., 141
Petti, P.L., 212
Price, W.J., 153

Q

Qian, G.-X., 212

R

Rashid, H., 212
Reckwerdt, P., 211
Rice, R.K., 212
Roentgen, W.C., 81
Roesch, W.C., 51, 52, 153, 210, 225
Rogers, D.W.O., 141, 212
Rozenfeld, M., 57, 141
Russ, S., iii
Rutherford, 25

S

Saxner, M., 213
Schluter, R.A., 57
Schmidt, G.C., 25
Schiff, L.I., 57
Scott, M.B., 57
Scrimger, J.W., 212, 213
Seltzer, S.M., 215
Shalek, R.J., 141
Shultz, R.J., 141
Siddon, R.L., 213
Silverman, R., 115
Smith, R.M., 211
Sontag, M.R., 204, 212
Soole, B.W., 57
Spencer, L.V., 141
Spiers, F.W., 212
Stedeford, B., 141
Storm, E., 19, 57, 78
Swerdloff, S., 211
Suntharalingham, N., 141
Svenson, G.K., 212
Svensson, H., 141

T

Tanabe, E., 115
Thomas, S.J., 212
Thoreaus, 90
Tochilin, E., 78, 153, 212
Trepp, A., 213
Trigg, G.L., 19

V

van de Geijn, J., 212
Van de Graaff, R.J., 104, 105

W

Walton, E.T., 103, 104
Weatherburn, H., 141

Webb, S., 212
Werner, B.L., 212
White, D.R., 79
Wingate, C.L., 212
Wong, J.W., 213
Wright, K.A., 141
Wyckoff, H.O., 140

Y

Yang, J., 211

Z

Zhu, Y., 213

SUBJECT INDEX
VOLUME II

A

AAPM, 95–97, 195; TG-21 protocol, 65
Absolute activity, 88
Absolute-risk model, 152–153
Absorbed dose from radiation leakage,
163
Accelerator, 35, 55, 60, 162
Acceptable weekly equivalent dose limits,
162
Access control, 162, 183, 198, 199–200, See also
Door shielding
Activity units, 88, 90
Acute radiation syndrome, 143–144
Additive-risk projection model, 152
Adjacent sites treatment, 46–52, 79
Afterloading techniques, 88, 127, 135, 137,
195–196
Air conditioning, 182
Air-kerma rate constant for radium, 90
Air-kerma rate yield, 88, 90–91
Air-kerma strength, 90
Air-kerma yield of treatment, 92
    linear source, 102–103
    planar implant dosage tables, 117, 119
    planar molds, Manchester system, 121
    single-plane implant, 114, 122
    volume implant dosage table, 118, 123;
        Quimby system, 115
Air kerma to water dose conversion, 94
Airshine, 172
ALARA standards, 143, 155, 161, 195
Alarms, 183, 195
Alpha particles
    pressure build-up, 199
    radiation weighting factor, 148
Aluminum shielding, 70
American Association of Physicists in Medicine
    (AAPM), 65, 95–97, 195
Americium, 86, 196
Angular scattering, 59–60
Anatomic landmarks, 44
Animal experiments, 150
Annihilation photons, 171
Annual maximum dose limits, 155–157, 162
Annular zones, 13–14, 35
Apparent activity, 88
Architectural data, 166
Arc therapy, 77–79
Armpits, 75
"As low as reasonably achievable" (ALARA), 143,
    155, 161, 195
Atomic transitions, 85
Atomic weapons testing, 154
Attenuation, 98–99
    encapsulating material, 98

in water, 93
Autopsies, 202

B

Background radiation, 154
Backscattered electrons, 69–70
Backscattered photons, 171
Barite, 165
Barium contrast medium, 35
Basic dose rate, 113–114, 132
Beam angles, 50–52; wedge angle, 17, 18
Beam edge superposition, 48
Beam-flattening filters, 2, 4, 7, 55
Beam interceptor, 168
Beam-limiting diaphragms, 2–6
"Beam on" indicator, 183
Beam's-eye projection, 46
Bedside shields, 200
Beryllium-7, 154
Beta sources for brachytherapy, 85, 86; storage and
        handling, 197
Bilateral arcs, 26, 34
Biological damage, 143–144, 146
Biological effectiveness, 145–146
Bladder, 135, 137
Bodily excretions, 201
Body inhomogeneities, 72–74; contour shape correction,
        10–12
Body thickness, 21–26, 38
Bolusing, 22, 24
Bone, electron scattering in, 73–74
Boron-based shielding, 174
Boron trifluoride proportional counters, 175
Brachytherapy, 85–139, 195
    AAPM/ICGW approach, 95–97
    dosimetry, See Dosimetry, brachytherapy sources
    implanting procedure, 127
    interstitial application, 87–88
    intracavitary insertions, 88, 134–139
    low-dose-rate and high-dose-rate, 195
    multiple source array, 105–111
    permanent implants, 88, 134–139
    planar implant dosage table, 117, 119
    planning and implementing, 125–133
    radiation safety, 195–202
        afterloading techniques, 88, 127, 137, 195–196
        handling time, 196
        monitoring, 197, 202
        nurses and visitors, 199–200
        permanent implants, 200–202
        post-treatment procedures, 200
        shielding, 196
        source distance and, 196
        source wipe tests, 198–199
    radionuclide sources, 85, 86

inventory, 198
  procurement, 127
  radiographic localization, 127–130
  storage and handling, 196–200
  strength, 88–93, 125–126, 134
simple line source treatment, 103–104
single-plane implant, 87, 114, 120–121, 122
surface applications, 85, 119–120
systems, 111–118
  Manchester (Paterson and Parker), 115–117,
    119–125, 136–137
  Memorial Hospital (New York), 114–115
  Paris, 113–114, 132
  pitfalls of mixing approaches, 117–118
  Quimby, 112
temporary implants, 88
two-plane implants, 88, 107–109, 121–122
volume implants, 88, 107, 110, 112, 113, 115, 118,
    122–125
Breast irradiation, 26, 29, 125
Bremsstrahlung, 55, 56, 57, 61
Bronchial applications, 88, 100, 103
"Building blocks," 104, 105
Build-up, dose, See Dose build-up; Secondary electrons
Build-up zone, 13–14

C

Cable conduits, 182
Cadaver handling procedures, 202
Calibrated peak output rate (CPOR), 66
Cancers, 144, 150, 151, 155; lifetime risk projection,
    151–153
Capsule, 85
  effective attenuation coefficient, 98
  linear, 97–99
  metallic, 85, 89
Carbon-14, 154
Carcinogenic effect, 144, 150, 151–153
Catheters, 88, 127, 130
Centerline peripheral dose (CPD), 114
Central-axis dose profile, 21–22, 24, 26, 57, 61, 63–64
Cervical radiotherapy, 136–139
Cesium, 86, 95, 101, 102, 118, 170; shielding
    considerations, 196
Characteristic X-rays, 85
Chest irradiation, 24, 26, 29
Chest monitors, 157, 202
Childhood cancers, 144
Chromosomal aberrations, 146, 147
Circular areas, source strength distribution, 124
Closed-circuit television, 183
Cloud chamber, 63, 65
Cobalt-60, 4, 5, 86
  combined-beam dose distributions, 16
  gamma ray scatter coefficient, 170
  isodose curves for linear source, 101
  isodose distributions for common techniques, 26–34
  shielding considerations, 196
  water perturbation correction, 95, 118
Coefficient of equivalent thickness (CET), 74
Cold spots, 35, 50, 73, 79

Collimator, 4, 56, 66, 70; for intraoperative radiotherapy, 76
Collision energy loss, 174
Colpostats, 135–136
Communication system, 183
Compensating filters, 26, 29
Compton-scattering, 4, 171
Computed tomography (CT), 1, 43–46, 74
Computer-assisted dosimetry, 7, 13, 127, 132
Concrete shielding materials, 164–165, 174, 175
Congenital defects, 144
Contour shape corrections, 10–12
Contrast medium, 35
Control console, 183
Controlled-access areas, 162, 183, 199–200
Copper shielding, 70
Core, volume implant, 122
Cosmic radiation, 154
Crossed ends, 107, 121
Cumulative radiation dose, 156, 162
Curved surfaces, 10–12; electron arc therapy, 77
Cylindrical mold, 111

D

Density scaling, 165
Dental compound, 85
Depth-dose curves, 57, 60–62; electron arcs, 79
Depth-dose profile, central-axis, 21–22, 24, 26, 57, 61,
    63–64
Deterministic radiation effects, 144, 155
Diagnostic X-ray source, 35
Diaphragms, 2–6
Disposal of sources, 201–202
Distance
  effective SSD, 11, 70–71
  fixed SSD, 9, 65
  inverse-square fall-off, 56, 74, 100, 168, 169
  radiation safety considerations, 161, 168, 196
Distribution rules
  for implants, 119–125
    single-plane, 120–121
    two-plane, 121–122
    volume, 122–125
  surface applications, 119–120
    circular areas, 119, 124
    irregularly shaped areas, 120
    rectangular areas, 120
Door controls, 183
Door shielding, 166, 170–175, 177–178, 182, 183
Dosage tables
  linear sources, 102, 103
  planar implant, 117, 119
  planar mold, 121
  single-plane implant, 114, 122
  volume implant, 115, 118, 123
Dose
  basic rate, 113–114, 132
  normal tissue tolerance, 7, 39
  scatter, 4, See also Scattered radiation
  surface, 58–60, See also Dose build-up; Skin dose
  therapeutic, 151
  water, 93–97, 100–101

Dose and dose rate effectiveness factor (DDREF), 153
Dose building blocks, 104, 105
Dose build-up, See also Secondary electrons
   contour shape and, 10
   electron angular scattering, 59–60
   electron beams, secondary electron component, 58
   obliquity influence, 12–13
Dose distribution
   comparison of X-rays and electron beams, 74
   correction for contour shape, 10–12
   electron beam, See Electron beam dose distribution
   fixed-SSD technique, 9
   implanted systems, See Brachytherapy
   isocentric technique, 9
   isodose curves and surfaces, 1, See also Isodose curves
   for linear source, 97–102
   Manchester (Paterson and Parker) distribution rules, 119–125
   photon beam, See Photon beam dose distribution
   wedge filters and, 14–21
   zones, 13–14
Dose equivalent (H), 146, 147
Dose evaluation for radiation protection, 144–150
   effective dose, 149–150
   equivalent dose, 147–149
   microscopic energy deposition, 145
   quality factor and dose equivalent, 146–147
   radiation weighting factors, 147–149
   relative biological effectiveness, 145–146
   tissue weighting factors, 149
Dose output, electron beams, 65–67
Dose rate constant λ, 96
Dose-response projection, 151
Dose uncertainty, 151
Dose uniformity, 14, 38, See also Hot spots
   brachytherapy multiple source distribution, 105
   wedge filters and, 17, 22
Dose-volume plots, 40
Dosimetry, brachytherapy sources, 88
   AAPM/ICGW empirical approach, 95–97
   brachytherapy planning, 132–133
   linear sources, 97–102
     in air, 97–100
     dose distributions, 101
     in water, 100–101
   point source in water, 93–97
   radioactive seed implants, 95–97
Dosimetry, computer applications, 7, 13, 127, 132
Dumb-bell-type loading, 135
Dummy sources, 127, 130, 137, 196

E

Effective attenuation coefficient, 98
Effective dose, 149–150
   cumulative limits, 156
   occupational limits, 156
Effective SSD, 11, 70–71
Effective water-equivalent depth, 74
Elastic scattering, 173
Electromagnetic steering, 55
Electron, secondary, See Secondary electrons

Electron arc therapy, 77–79
Electron backscattering, 69–70
Electron beam angular scattering, 59–60
Electron beam dose distribution, 55–61
   adjacent fields, 79
   agreement of light and radiation fields, 71–72
   combined photon treatment, 79
   comparison with kilovoltage X-ray beams, 74
   depth-dose, 57, 60–62
     field size and, 62
     oblique incidence and, 63–64
   effective SSD, 70–71
   factors influencing, 56
   inhomogeneities and, 72–74
   intraoperative radiotherapy, 76–77
   machine-dependence, 61
   machine to patient, 55–56
   pencil beam, 55, 63
   selective shielding, 68
   surface dose build-up, 58–60
   total-skin treatment, 75–76, 181
Electron beam field shaping, 68
Electron beam field size, 62, 66
Electron beam leakage limits, 163
Electron beam output factors, 65–67
Electron beam radiation safety, See External-beam radiation safety
Electron beam range of penetration, 56, 60
Electron beam trimmers, 56, 66, 70
Electron-electron scattering, 55
Electron energy
   depth vs. dose distribution, 61
   penetrating power, 56
   scattering loss, 55
   shielding back-scattering properties and, 70
   surface dose and, 60, 62
Electron fluence
   angular deflection effects, 59–60
   electron arc therapy, 78
   electron beam dose build-up, 58–59
   inhomogeneities and, 72
   inverse-square fall-off, 56
   pencil beam, 55
   scatter, and beam-flattening filter, 7
   shielding-associated augmentation, 68
   tissue compensating filter and, 26
Electron-nuclear scattering, 55
Electron transport, 55
Elongation correction factors, 125
Embryo exposure limits, 156
Emergency action procedure, 183
Encapsulated sources, 85, 97–99
   effective attenuation coefficient, 98
   point source in water, 93
Endocurie therapy, 85
Energy straggling, 61
Entrance door shielding, 166, 170–175, 177–178, 182, 183
Entrance maze, 170–171, 175, 176
Entrance zone, 13–14, 35; wedge hot spots, 17, 21
Epidemiologic data, 143, 150, 151
Equally weighted parallel opposed beams, 21
Equivalent dose, 147–149

natural background radiation, 154
  neutron, 174
Esophagus treatment, 35–40, 88, 100
Excess cancers, 144, 150, 151
Exit dose, 74
Exit zone, 13–14, 35
External-beam radiation safety, 161–184, See also
      Shielding
  allowable barrier transmission, 168–173
  architectural and equipment data, 166
  comparison with brachytherapy, 195
  distance, 168
  entrance door barrier, 166, 170–172
  facility design and planning, 182–184
  gas production, 181–182
  leakage levels, 162–164
  neutron capture gamma rays, 175
  occupancy factor, 167–168
  patient monitoring, 183
  use factor, 167
  warning signs and indicators, 183
  weekly equivalent dose units, 162
  workload, 166
Eye
  lens opacification, 144
  recommended annual dose limits, 156–158
  shielding, 75

F

Facility design, 161, 166, 182–184, See also External-beam
      radiation safety; Shielding
  sample floor plan, 176
Fast neutrons, 174
Fatal accident risk, 155–156
Feathering, 50
Feet, 75; recommended annual dose limits, 156–158
Fetus exposure limits, 156
Field length, 7–8
Field shaping
  agreement of photon vs. electron field, 72
  CT for, 44–46
  electron beams, 68
Field size, 62, 66
Field width, 7–8
Film badges, 157
Filters
  beam-flattening, 2, 4, 7, 55
  tissue-compensating, 26, 29
  wedge, 2, 14–21
Finger badges, 157, 202
Fission neutrons, 146
Fixed source-to-skin distance (SSD), 9, 65
Flattening filter, 2, 4, 7, 55
Floor plans, 176
Fluence
  neutron, 173
  scatter, 7, 169
  electron, See Electron fluence
Fluoroscopic monitoring, 35
Focal spots, megavoltage X-ray machine, 4
Foil, electron beam scattering, 55

Foil activation methods, 175
Forceps, 196
Four-field box, 24, 38
Four-field-obliques, 26, 31
Full 360 degree rotation, 26, 32

G

Gamma radiation
  acute dose, 144
  brachytherapy, 85
  neutron capture, 162, 175
  radiation weighting factor, 148–149
  relative biological effectiveness, 146
  scatter coefficient, 170
  sealed sources leakage limits, 164
Gantry rotation, 9
Gas formation and leakage, 85, 181–182, 199
Geiger-Mueller (GM) counter, 197
Genetic effects, 144
Geometric edges, of photon beams, 2, 4
Given dose, 9
Gold-198, 86, 198
  implant applications, 134, 200
  water perturbation correction, 95, 118
Gonads, 149
Gynecologic applications, 134–139

H

Half-life, 134
Half-value thickness, 164
Hands, recommended annual dose limits, 156–158
Harmful effects of radiation, 143–144
Hazard warning signs, 183, 199, 200, 201
Heyman packing, 139
High-dose-rate brachytherapy, 195
Hinge angle, 17
Hot spots, 35
  adjacent electron fields, 79
  electron beam inhomogeneities, 73
  feathering and, 50
  wedge fields, 17, 21
Hydrogen-3, 154
Hydrogen nuclides, 173–174
Hydrogenous materials, 174, 175

I

ICRP standards and guidelines, 143, 153, 155–158,
      161
ICWG dosimetry approach, 95–97, 101–102
Implants, 87–88, 127, 130, See also Brachytherapy
  Manchester distribution rules, 119–125
  permanent, 88, 115, 134–139, 200–202
  removable, 88
  single-plane, 87, 114, 120–122
  temporary, 88
  volume, See Volume implants
Induced radioactivity, 175
Infinite limit approximation, 74
Integral dose σ, 40–42

International Atomic Energy Agency, 143
International Commission on Radiation Protection (ICRP), 143, 153, 155–158, 161
Interstitial Collaborative Working Group (ICWG) dosimetry approach, 95–97, 101–102
Intracavitary insertions, 88, 134–139
Intraluminal therapy, 88
Intraoperative radiotherapy (IORT), 76–77
Intrauterine irradiation, 88, 136–139
Inventory, 198
Inverse-square fall-off, 56, 74, 100, 168, 169
Iodine-125, 86, 94, 95, 115, 118; implant applications, 115, 134, 196, 200
Ionization chamber, 89–90, 157
Ionization current, 89
Iridium, 86, 89, 95, 113, 118, 119, 125, 196, 198
Irradiation duration, 91–93
Isocenter identification, 42
Isocentric radiotherapy facility layout, 176
Isocentric rotation, 9, 168
Isodose curves, 1
    adjacent sites treatment, 49, 79
    brachytherapy planning, 132–133
    cobalt-60 beam, 4, 5
    correction for contour shape, 10–12
    isocentric situations, 9
    linear sources, 101
    low-energy X-rays, 2–4
    megavoltage X-rays, 4–7
    multiple source array, 105–111
    obliquely incident electron beams, 64
    Paris approach, 113
    single-beam, 1–7
    vaginal cylinder, 135
    wedge angles, 17
Isodose shift correction method, 11
Isodose shift factors, 11
Isodose surfaces, 1; point source in water, 94

J

Japanese atomic bomb survivors, 150

K

Kerma rate, 90–91, See also Air-kerma yield of treatment
Klystrons, 183

L

Lateral subcutaneous dose, 23–24
$LD_{50/30}$, 144
Lead shielding, 68, 165, 166, 170–171, 175, 196, 197, 200, See also Shielding
Leakage radiation, 2, 4
    absorbed dose, 163
    entrance door shielding, 178
    maximum barrier transmission, 169
    recommended limits, 162–164
    secondary protective barrier, 169
    sealed sources, 85

skyshine protection, 180
Lethal dose, 144
Lifetime risk projection, 151–153, 155–156
Light-beam localizer, 52
Linear energy transfer (LET), 145; quality factor, 146–147
Linear-quadratic model, 151
Linear sources, 85, 97–102
    dose building blocks, 105
    source strength, 91, 98
Low-dose-rate (LDR) brachytherapy, 195
Lucite scatterer, 75
Lung, 38, 40, 46
Lymph nodes, 62, 136
Lung dose, 38, 40

M

Magnification factors, 130
Manchester system, 115–117, 119–125, 136–137
Mass stopping power, 74
Maximum acceptable transmission, 168
Maximum weekly dose, 162
Mayneord index, 40
Maze entrance, 170–171, 175, 176
Medical radiation exposures, 154
Memorial Hospital system, 114–115
Mental retardation, 144
Metallic capsules, 85, 89
Microscopic energy deposition, 145
Milliampere-minutes, 166
Milligram hour of treatment, 91–92
Milligram radium equivalent, 89
Minimum peripheral dose (MPD), 112, 114
Missing tissue problem, 10
Moderation, 173
Monitoring
    badges, 157, 202
    brachytherapy source safety, 197, 202
    instruments, 157, 197, 202
    of patients under treatment, 183
    of personnel radiation exposure, 157, 202
    radiotherapy simulation, 35
Multiple photon beams, 7–13
Multiple source arrays, 105–111
Multiplicative-risk projection model, 152–153
Mutations, 144, 146
Nitric oxide, 182

N

National Council on Radiation Protection and Measurements (NCRP), 143, 153, 155–158, 161–164, 168, 177, 195
Natural background radiation, 154
Neck, 24, 62
Net minimum dose (NMD), 116, 125
Neutron capture gamma rays, 162, 175
Neutron collision energy loss, 174
Neutron equivalent dose, 174
Neutron quality factors 147
Neutron radiation weighting factors, 148–149
Neutron relative biological effectiveness, 146

Neutron shielding, 173–175
Neutron survey instruments, 175
New York (Memorial Hospital) system, 114–115
Nitrogen dioxide, 182
Non-pulsed X-ray equipment, 166
Normalization depth, 9
Normalized peak output factors (NPOF), 66
Normal tissue dose tolerance, 7, 137
Nuclear reactor, 148, 154
Nuclear transitions, 85
Nuclear weapons testing, 154
Nylon ribbons, 115, 125–126
Nylon tube, 104, 130, 135
Nurse safety, 199–200

O

Oblique beams, 13–16, 26, 30–31, 43; total-skin electron
    treatment, 75
Obliquity
    dose build-up effects, 12–13
    electron depth dose and, 63–64
Occupancy factor (T), 167–168
Occupational effective dose limits, 156
Oncogenic transformation, 146
Organ weighting factor, 162
Orthogonal beams, 50–52
Orthogonal planar views, 105, 106
Orthogonal radiographic localization, 129–131
Orthogonal reconstruction, 130
Output factors, non-square electron fields,
    67
Ozone, 181–182

P

Palladium, 86, 94, 95, 118, 134, 196, 200
Paracervical triangle, 136
Parallel opposed beams, 21–27
    adjacent sites treatment, 49–50
    single beam matching, 50
    three-field techniques, 17, 21
Paris system, 113–114, 132
Partial isodose shift correction, 11
Paterson and Parker (Manchester) system, 115–117,
    119–125, 136–137
Patient education, 202
Patient monitoring, 183
Patient positioning, 9, 42, 43
    electron arc therapy, 77
    total-skin electron treatment, 75
Patient scatter, 162, 169, 170, 171
PDD, See Percentage depth dose
Peak output rate
    calibrated, 66
    electron arc therapy, 78
    electron beams, 70
    normalized, 66
Pencil beam, 55, 63
Penumbra, 2
    cobalt-60 beam, 4
    fall-of dose, 48

low-energy X-ray, 4
megavoltage X-rays, 4, 7
producers, 79
zone, 13–14, 35
Percentage depth dose (PDD), 74
    contour shape corrections, 10–12
    fixed-SSD technique, 9
    isocentric technique, 9
Peripheral dose, minimum (MPD), 112, 114
Peripheral sources, 105, 107, 123
Permanent implants, 88, 115, 134–139,
    200–202
Personnel monitoring, 157, 202
Phosphorus-32, 86
Photographic film, 68, 157
Photon backscattering, 171
Photon beam dose distribution, 1–52, See also
    X-ray beams
    adjacent sites treatment, 46–52
    agreement of light and radiation field, 71–72
    bilateral arcs, 26, 34
    combined beams, 7–13
    combined electron treatment, 79
    contour shape corrections, 10–12
    esophagus treatment example, 35–40
    four-field box, 21
    four-field-obliques, 26, 31
    full 360 degree rotation, 26, 32
    geometric edges, 2, 4
    isodose curves, 1
    parallel opposed beams, 21–27, 49–50
    posterior skip arc, 26, 33
    single-beam, 1–7
    three-field box, 21
    three-field-obliques, 26, 30
    wedge filters and, 14–21
    zones, 2, 13–14
Photon beam radiation safety, See External-beam
    radiation safety
Photon-induced activity, 175
Planar implant distribution rules, 120–122,
    125
Planar implant dosage table, 117, 119
Plaster-of-paris cast, 37–38
Platinum capsules, 85, 89
Pocket ionization chambers, 157
Point A, 136–137
Point B, 136–137
Point-source in water approximations, 93–97
Polyethylene shielding, 174
Port film, 35, 46, 47
Posterior skip arc, 26, 33
Potassium-40, 154
Power failure, 183
Practical range, 61
Pregnant women's exposure, 156, 202
Preloading, 88, 195–196
Primary electrons, 61
Primary protective barriers, 167, 168
Prostate implants, 201
Protective-barrier report, 183
Pseudo-arc technique, 79

Public radiation exposure limits, 155, 157–158, 162, 200

Q

Quality factor (Q), 146–147
Quimby system, 12

R

Radiation alarms, 183, 195
Radiation components, 85, 162
Radiation dose uncertainty, 151
Radiation harmful effects, 143–144
Radiation intensity profile, 2
Radiation leakage, See Leakage radiation
Radiation protection, See Safety standards; Shielding
Radiation risk assessment, 143, See also Safety standards
  absolute-risk and relative-risk models, 152–153
  ICRP nominal probability coefficients, 153
  uncertainties in, 150–153
    dose and dose rate effectiveness factor (DDREF), 153
    dose-response projection, 151
    lifetime risk projection, 151–153
    radiation dose, 151
    sample size, 150–151
Radiation Safety Committee (RSC), 157
Radiation safety officer (RSO), 157
Radiation safety standards, See Safety standards
Radiation survey meters, 197
Radiation weighting factors, 147–149, 162
Radiation worker, annual maximum dose limits, 155–157
Radioactive seeds, 85, 94, 104, See also Brachytherapy
  distribution rules, 121
  dummy sources, 130
  excretion, 201
  initial source strength, 134
  ribbons, 115, 125–126
  spherical volume, 107
Radioactive sources, See Radionuclide sources
Radioactive wires, 100, 103, 198–199; Paris approach, 113
Radioactivity units, for brachytherapy sources, 88–93
Radioactivity warning signs, 183, 199, 200, 201
Radiographic localization of brachytherapy sources, 127
Radiomimetic gas, 181
Radionuclide sources, 85, 86, See also specific radionuclides
  afterloading, 88, 127, 137, 195–196
  for brachytherapy, 195
  caution for using radium tables, 118
  cosmic ray-produced, 154
  dumb-bell-type loading, 135
  inventory, 198
  permanent implants, 200
  post-treatment procedures, 200
  preloading, 88, 195–196
  procurement, 127
  storage and handling, 196–199
  strength, 88–90, 125–126, See also Source strength
    time product, 91–93
  water perturbation corrections, 95, 118
  wipe tests, 198–199

Radiotherapy, intraoperative electron, 76–77
Radiotherapy simulator, 35, 127, 129
Radium, 85, 86, 88, 89
  caution for using tables, 118
  exposure rate constant, 89–90, 92
  needles, 85, 88
  safety considerations, 199
  shielding considerations, 196
  water perturbation correction, 95, 118
Radium-equivalent mass, 88, 89–90
Radon, 85, 86, 199; implant applications, 134, 200
Range straggling, 60
Ratio-of-TAR correction method, 11
Record-keeping, 198
Rectal radiosensitivity, 135, 137
Reentrant ionization chamber, 89–90
Reference dose rate, 112, 121
Relative biological effectiveness (RBE), 145–146
Relative-risk models, 152–153
rem, 146
Remote handling procedures, 88, 196
Remote "on" and "off" controls, 195
Removable implants, 88
Rind, volume implant, 122
Risk assessment, See Radiation risk assessment
Risk-benefit philosophy, 154–155
Roentgen equivalent man (rem), 146
Roof irradiation and protection, 172–173, 178–181
Ruthenium, 86

S

Safety interlocks, 185
Safety standards, 143, 161–184, 195–202
  architectural and equipment data, 166
  brachytherapy, 195–202, See also under Brachytherapy
  distance effects, 162, 196
  dose evaluation, 144–150
  external-beam, 161–184, See also External-beam radiation safety; Shielding
  facility design, 182–184
  general public, 155, 157–158
  handling time considerations, 195
  limits for adult workers, 155–156
  limits for pregnant workers, 156
  limits for workers under age 18, 156–157
  natural background radiation and, 154
  nurses and visitors, 199–200
  personnel monitoring and, 157
  post-treatment procedures, 200
  risk-benefit philosophy, 154–155
  shielding and, See Shielding
  source storage and handling, 196, 197–198
  time considerations, 161
Samarium, 86, 95, 196
Sample size considerations, 150–151
Scatter dose, 4
Scattered radiation, 2
  electrons
    angular deflections, 59–60
    back-scattering, 69–70
    effect of inhomogeneities, 72–74

electron-nuclear and electron-electron, 55
  pencil beam, 63
entrance door, 170–172, 177–178
flattening filter and, 7
lead shielding, 68
low-energy X-ray, 4
maximum barrier transmission, 169–170
neutrons, 173
point source in water model, 93, 94
secondary protective barrier, 169
skyshine, 172–173, 180–181
Scatter fluence, and beam-flattening filter, 7
Scattering coefficient α, 169, 170
Scattering foils, 55, 61
Sealed sources, 85
Seed implants, See Radioactive seeds
Selective shielding, 68–70, 75
Secondary electrons, 22, 56, 61, 58
  bolusing, 22, 24
  contour shape correction, 10
  megavoltage X-ray, 4
  obliquity effects on build-up, 12–13
  tissue compensating filter and, 26
Secondary protective barriers, 164, 167, 169–170
Seed implants, See also Brachytherapy
  AAPM/ICGW dosimetry approach, 95–97
  dose building blocks, 104
  point source in water dosimetry approximation, 94
Sex ratio alterations, 144
Shielding, 162, See also specific materials
  agreement of photon vs. electron fields, 72
  ALARA goals, 195
  assumptions, 177
  bedside, 200
  brachytherapy sources, 196, 197
  comparison of X-rays and electron beams, 74
  data, 164
  electron backscattering, 69–70
  electron beams, 68–70
  entrance door, 177–178, 182, 183
  example calculations, 175–181
  for external-beam therapy vs. brachytherapy, 195
  hydrogenous materials, 174, 175
  internal, 69–70
  materials, 164–166
  neutron capture, 175
  primary barriers, 167, 168
  protective-barrier report, 183
  recommended leakage levels, 162–164
  roof protection and skyshine, 172–173, 178–181
  secondary barriers, 167, 169–170
  selective, 68–70; total-skin electron treatment, 75
  side walls, 177
  use and occupancy factors, 167–168
  worksheet for calculations, 185–192
Shipping, 199
Side walls, 177
Sievart's integral, 99
Signs, 183, 199, 200, 201
Simulator, 35, 42–43, 127, 129
Single-field stereoradiography, 128
Single-plane implant, 87

air-kerma yield, 114
Manchester system distribution rules, 120–121, 122
orthogonal view, 105, 106
Skin dose, 60, 62
  bolusing effects, 22
  contour shape and, 10
  recommended annual dose limits, 156–158
  total-skin electron treatment, 75
Skin erythema, 144, 145
Skin gap, adjacent sites treatment, 48, 50
Skyshine, 172–173, 178–181
Sodium-22, 154
Soft-tissue necrosis, 145
Somatic effects, 144
Source, radionuclide, See Radionuclide sources
Source disposal, 201–202
Source inventory, 198
Source strength, 88–91, 125–126
  brachytherapy multiple source distribution, 105
  linear sources, 91
  permanent implants, 134
  specification
    by activity, 88, 90
    by air-kerma rate, 88, 90–91
    by radium-equivalent mass, 88, 89–90
    by water-kerma rate, 91
  time product, 91–93
  traceable, 88
Source-to-skin distance (SSD)
  effective, 11, 70–71
  fixed, 9, 65
Source wipe tests, 198–199
Spherical volume seed implant, 107
Spinal cord, 36, 38, 39–40, 43, 100
Steel, 165
Stereo radiography, 128
Sterilization, 198
Stillbirths, 144
Stochastic radiation effects, 144, 153, 155
Storage of radioisotope sources, 196
Strontium, 86
Superficial lesions, 68
Surface applications, Manchester distribution rules,
    119–120
Surgical openings, 76
Survey instruments, 197; for neutrons, 175

T

Tangentially opposing beams, 26
Tantalum, 86, 196, 198
Target volume, 1
  field width and field length, 8
  integral dose, 40–42
  localization, 35–36
  Paris approach, 113
  single-plane implant, 87
Target zone, 13–14
Temporary implants, 88
Tenth-value thickness (TVT), 164, 165, 174
Terrestrial emissions, 154
Therapeutic dose, 151

Therapy simulator, 35, 42–43, 129
Thermal neutrons, 148, 174
Thermoluminescent dosimeters, 157
Three-dimensional display, 1, 7
Three-field box, 21
Three-field-obliques, 26, 30
Three-field techniques, using wedges, 17, 21
360 degree rotation, 26, 32
Time considerations for radiation safety, 161, 195
Timing of treatments, 197–198
Tissue-air ratio (TAR), 9
Tissue-compensating filters, 26, 29
Tissue-equivalent bolus, 10, 22, 24
Tissue weighting factors, 149
Tolerance doses, 7, 39, 137
Tongue implants, 121
Total-skin electron treatment, 75–76, 181
Transverse contour, 7–8, 36
Treatment planning, See also Dose distribution; specific
    radiotherapies
    adjacent sites treatment, 46–52, 79
    brachytherapy, 111–118, 125–133
    caution for using radium tables, 118
    comparative evaluation of plans, 38–42
    computerized systems, 7
    CT data, 43–46
    dose-volume plots, 40
    electron beam, 62
    simple line source, 103–104
    therapy simulator, 35, 42–43
    2D model, 7–8
    zones for, 13–14
Trimmers, for electron beams, 56, 66, 70
Tritium, 154
Tube shift radiographic localization, 128
Tumor induction, 146
Two-plane implants, 88, 107–109; Manchester system,
    121–122
Two-plane separation factors, 124
Two-way communication system, 183

U

Uncertainties, in radiation risk assessment, 150–153
Unequally weighted parallel opposed beams, 22
Use factor (U), 167, 170
Urinary excretions, 201
U.S. National Cancer Institute, 95
Uterine applications, 88, 136–139

V

Vaginal insertions, 88, 134–136
Ventilation, 181–182
Visitor safety, 199–200
Vocal cord, 35

Volume implants, 88, 107, 110
    dosage table, 118
    elongation correction factors, 125
    Manchester system, 122–125
    New York system, 115
    Paris approach, 113
    Quimby system, 112, 115
Volume source array, 105

W

Wall scatter, 162, 167, 176, 177
Warning signs, 183, 199, 200, 201
Water
    kerma rate yield, 91
    linear source dosimetry, 100–101
    point source dosimetry, 93–97
Water-equivalent depth, effective, 74
Water-equivalent medium, 72
Water perturbation correction (WPC), 92–94, 100
Wax, 24, 85
Wedge angles, 17
Wedged oblique pair, 17
Wedge filters, 2, 14–21
Weekly equivalent dose units (P), 162
Weighting factors for radiation types, 147–149
Weighting factors for tissue types, 149
Wipe tests, 198–199
Wire conduits, 182
Workload (W), 166, 169
Worksheet for shielding calculation, 185–192
WPC (Water perturbation correction), 92–98, 100
Wrist badges, 157, 202

X

X-ray beams, See also Photon beam dose distribution
    allowable leakage limits, 163
    combined-beam dose distributions, 15
    comparison with electron beams, 74
    equipment workload, 166
    isodose curves
        low-energy beam, 2–4
        megavoltage beams, 4–7
    radiation weighting factor, 148
    scatter coefficients, 170
    shielding back scattering, 70, 164
    isodose distributions for common techniques,
        26–34
    therapy simulator, 35
X-ray dosimeters, 175
X-rays, and brachytherapy, 85

Y

Ytterbium, 86, 95, 196

AUTHOR INDEX
VOLUME II

A

Abe, M., 53, 83
Abrams, D., 52
Abrath, F.G., 82
Agarwal, S.K., 54, 83, 159
Ager, P.J., 54
Agosteo, S., 194
Aird, E.G.A., 141, 203
Al-Beteri, A.A., 81
Albert, R.E., 159
Alderson, A.R., 203
Almond, P.R., 82, 83, 84, 139, 194, 202
Amdur, R.J., 82
Anderson, J.A., 83
Anderson, L.L., 119, 140, 141
Andreo, P., 81
Arbari, A., 82
Armstrong, D.J., 54
Arnott, S.J., 202
Aron, B.S., 53
Arrans, R., 194
Asbell, S.O., 82
Ash, D., 140, 202
Attix, F.H., 82
Augenstein, L.G., 158
Auxier, J.A., 159

B

Bading, J.R., 194
Bagne, F., 83
Bahr, G.K., 202
Barest, G., 52
Barish, R.J., 159
Barrett, C.M., 202
Barrick, M.K., 159
Batho, H.F., 140
Bautro, N., 53
Beauvais, H., 54
Benner, S., 141
Bernard, M., 81, 82
Berstein, I.A., 82
Bethe, H.A., 81
Bhaduri, D., 83
Bielajew, A.F., 82
Biggs, P.J., 81, 82, 83, 193
Binder, W., 53
Bjarngard, B.E., 54, 82, 193
Bloch, P., 54
Bomford, C.K., 54
Bond, V., 159, 193
Boone, M.L.M., 82
Borak, T.B., 193
Born, C.G., 82, 83, 84
Bova, F.J., 82

Boyer, A.L., 82, 83, 139, 194, 202
Brady, L.W., 141
Brady, N.L., 82
Brahme, A., 81
Breitman, K.E., 140
Brenner, M., 82
Brewster, L.J., 52
Buchler, D., 203
Bunger, B.M., 159
Burkoritz, A., 54
Burns, D.J., 53
Burns, F., 159
Burns, J.E., 53
Busch, M., 140
Bush, R.S., 53
Butker, E.K., 194

C

Cameron, J.R., 193
Casebow, M.P., 141
Castro, V., 140
Ceve, P., 140
Chahbazian, D.J., 140, 141
Chaney, E.C., 52
Chassagne, D.J., 140, 141
Chen, G.T.Y., 54
Chilton, A.B., 194
Choi, M.C., 82, 83
Chui, C.S., 52
Chung-Bin, A., 159
Clarke, E.T., 193
Cluxton, S.E., 202
Cobb, P.D., 193
Cohen, M., 53, 54
Cole, A., 141
Constable, W.C., 54
Cook, J.R., 159
Cook, R., 83
Cox, J.D., 141
Crouch, E.A.C., 159
Cundiff, J.H., 82, 140
Cunningham, J.R., 54, 81, 139, 193
Cytacki, E., 141

D

Dade Lundsford, L., 194
Dally, E.B., 194
Davis, L.W., 54
Dawes, P.J.D.K., 54
Dawes, T.J.O.K., 203
Deibel, F.C., 81, 82
Delclos, L., 139, 141
Dennis, J.A., 193
Deutsch, M., 54

Ding, I.Y., 140
Dixon, R.L., 81
Dobblebower, R.R., 83
Doppke, K.P., 53, 82
Doss, L.L., 141
Duerkes, R.J., 82
Dunscombe, P.B., 83
Dupont, J.C., 54
Dutreix, A., 140, 141
Dutreix, J., 82, 141

E

Earl, J.D., 54
Early, L., 83
Ekstrand, K.E., 81
Ellett, W.H., 159
Ellis, F., 53
Elson, H.R., 82, 83, 84
Epp, E.R., 83, 193
Ewald, L.M., 82

F

Farrow, N., 193
Feber, B.S., 139
Feldman, A., 82
Fenster, A., 53
Fletcher, G., 139, 141, 202
Flickinger, J.C., 194
Foglio Para, A., 194
Frank, H., 82
Frass, B.A., 53, 54, 83
Freeman, C.R., 83
Freidel, H.L., 139
Fuchs, H., 53
Fuks, Z., 52
Fullerton, G.D., 83, 139

G

Gagnon, W.F., 53, 82
Garcia, D.M., 82
Garner, A., 83
George, F., III, 140, 141
Gerbi, B.J., 82
Giarattano, J.C., 82
Gibb, R., 139
Gibbs, F.A., 83
Gillin, M.T., 54, 141
Gitterman, M., 203
Glasgow, G.P., 82, 83, 141, 194
Glasser, O., 114, 115
Glatstein, E., 54, 83
Goitein, M., 52
Goldson, A.L., 83
Gregg, E.C., 53
Gromadzki, E.C., 140
Guerra, J., 83

H

Hale, J., 54
Hall, E.J., 53, 159
Hamberger, A.D., 141
Harder, D., 81
Harrison, L.B., 141
Heitler, W., 81, 193
Hendrickson, F.R., 54
Henschke, U.K., 139, 140, 202
Heyman, J., 141
Hilaris, B.S., 119, 139, 140, 141, 202
Hoffman, R.J., 193
Hogstrom, K.R., 81, 82, 83
Holoday, E.J.
Holodney, E. I., 117, 118, 140
Holt, J.G., 81
Hopfan, S., 54
Horowitz, H., 202
Horton, W.L., 53
Howellis, R., 140
Huda, W., 81
Hughes, H.A., 53
Huizenga, H., 81
Hunter, R.D., 82

I

Ishihara, H., 53
Iyer, P.S., 140

J

Jackson, S.M., 82
Jackson, W., 53
Jacky, J., 53
Jaeger, R.G., 193, 194
Jamshedi, A., 82
Jardine, J.H., 82
Jayaraman, S., 54, 58, 84, 140, 159
Jenkins, T.M., 54, 193, 194
Jette, D., 81
Johns, H.E., 53, 193
Johnson, P.M., 54
Jones, C.H., 141
Jones, D.E.A., 54
Joslin, C.A.F., 141, 202
Jungar, H., 82

K

Kagan, A.R., 141
Kalbaugh, K.J., 82
Kalend, A., 83
Kan, P.T., 140
Kao, M., 81
Kaplan, R., 194
Karcher, K.H., 53
Karjalainen, P., 82
Karzmark, C.J., 54, 83
Kazusa, C., 53
Keller, R.J., 140

Kepka, A., 54
Kereiakes, J.G., 82, 83, 84, 202
Kersey, R.W., 193
Khan, F.M., 53, 54, 81, 82, 83, 139
Khan, F.R., 141
Kim, T.H., 54
Kirsher, S.M., 83
Kirsner, S.M., 81
Klein, E.C., 53
Klevenhagen, S.C., 82, 84, 141
Kline, R.W., 54, 141
Koch, R.F., 141
Kocher, D.C., 158, 193
Kondo, S., 159
Krishnaswamy, V., 102, 140
Krispel, F., 83
Krohmer, J.S., 139
Kuan, H.M., 140
Kubo, Y., 53
Kuchnir, F.J., 82
Kurup, R.G., 81, 83
Kutcher, G.J., 52
Kwan, D., 141

L

Lam, K.S., 83
Lam, W.C., 83
Lambert, G.D., 82
Land, C.E., 159
Lanzl, L.H., 81, 140, 159
Laughlin, J.S., 52, 82, 114, 117, 118, 140, 194
Law, J., 202
Lax, I., 81
Leung, P.M.K., 53, 54
Levett, D.D., 83
Leavitt, D.D., 83
Levitt, S.H., 53, 82
Levitt, S.L., 139, 141
Leybovich, L.B., 83
Lichter, A.S., 53
Lightfoot, D.A., 82
Lillicrap, S.C., 54
Lindner, G., 194
Ling, C.C., 140
Ling, C.L., 53, 83
Lo, Y.-C., 193
Lommartzsch, P.K., 139
Long, K., 194
Lovett, R.D., 82
Lushbaugh, C.C., 158
Luxton, G., 140

M

Mabuchi, K., 158
Madigan, W., 194
Madurga, G., 194
Maggioni, B., 194
Maitz, A.H., 194
Mahan, G.D., 139, 202
Malaker, K., 83

Mandour, M.A., 81
Marinello, G., 140, 141
Mark, A., 52
Marks, R.D., 54
Markus, B., 81
Martin, C.L., 139
Martin, J.A., 139
Martin, S.J., 54
Martinez, A.A., 202
Mason, R., 158
Massey, J.B., 139
Mayneord, W.V., 40, 54
McCall, R.C., 82, 194
McCullough, E.C., 54, 83
McGinley, P.H., 194
Mckenzie, A.L., 81, 193, 194, 203
McKenzie, M.R., 83
McLellan, J., 81
McParland, B.J., 81, 82
McShan, D.L., 53
Meigooni, A.S., 140
Meisberger, L.L., 140
Meli, J.A., 140
Mendenhall, W.M., 82
Meredith, W.J., 103, 121, 122, 123, 140, 141
Meyer, J.L., 84
Michaelis, H.B., 83
Mills, M., 194
Mills, M.D., 81, 82, 194
Milton, R., 159
Miner, M.S., 194
Mira, J.G., 83
Mitchum, M.L., 194
Moeller, J.H., 83
Mohan, R., 52
Mok, E.C., 83
Mole, R.H., 158
Moliere, G., 81
Moore, E.B., 202
Moore, V.C., 53, 82
Moos, W.S., 140
Morawska-Kaczynska, M., 81
Morin, R.L., 139
Morton, R.J., 53
Mosher, C., 53
Mould, R.F., 202
Moyers, M.F., 81
Munro, P., 53
Murphy, D.J., 141

N

Nagata. Y., 53
Nath, R., 139, 140, 193
Neal, J.V., 158
Neblett, D.L., 141
Nelson, C.E., 83
Nisar, S., 139
Nishida, T., 53
Nori, D., 140, 141
Novack, D.H., 53, 83
Novins, K., 53

O

O'Neill, M.J., 83
Ocharn, G., 83
Ochran, T.G., 194
Ohta, H., 53
Olch, A., 141
Oliver, R., 53
Orton, C.G., 53, 202
Osian, A.D., 140

P

Page, V., 83
Pagnamenta, A., 81
Paine, C.H., 139, 140, 202
Paliwal, B., 81, 83, 84
Papiez, E., 83
Papiez, L., 81
Parker, H.M., 115, 119, 122, 125, 126, 140
Parsons, J.T., 82
Paterson, R., 115, 119, 122, 125, 126, 140
Paul, J.M., 141
Peacock, L.M., 83
Perez, C.A., 82, 141
Perry, D.J., 81
Peters, V.G., 82
Peterson, M.D., 53
Petti, P.L., 81
Pfalzner, P.F., 54
Philip, P.C., 141
Pierquin, B., 140, 141
Pillai, K., 53
Pizer, S.M., 53
Pla, C., 83
Pla, M., 83
Pochin, E.E., 159
Podgorsak, E.B., 83
Pohlit, W., 82
Pollari, H., 52
Potish, R.A., 139
Purdy, J.A., 53, 82
Purdy, J.M., 82
Puthawala, A.A., 141

Q

Quillin, R.M., 53
Quimby, E.H., 112, 113, 114, 115, 116, 139, 140

R

Raeside, D.E., 81
Rafkel, S., 83
Rao, P.S., 53
Rao, U.V.G., 140
Rawlinson, J.A., 53
Reft, C.S., 82
Reid, A., 54
Reuterwall, O., 141
Rich, T., 83, 194
Ritter, F.W.A., 140

Robins, J., 54
Rodgers, C.C., 53
Rodriguez, R., 194
Rogers, D.W.O., 82
Ron, E., 158
Rose, M.E., 81
Rosenman, J., 53
Rosenwald, J.C., 54
Ross, C.K., 82
Rossiter, M.J., 141
Rowell, H., 52
Rozenfeld, M., 54, 81
Rust, D.C., 54
Rustgi, S.N., 140
Rutledge, F.N., 141
Rytilla, A., 82

S

Sabbas, A.M., 81
Sabnis, S., 140
Sanchez, F., 194
Sandison, G.A., 81
Sangiust, V., 194
Saunders, J.E., 82
Saylor, W.L., 53
Scappicchio, M., 53
Schuer, T.H., 140
Scott, W.T., 53, 81
Sear, R., 53
Sedham, L.N., 203
Seibert, J.B., 53
Sewchand, W., 53, 54, 82
Shalek, R.J., 140, 141
Shapiro, S.J., 82
Sharma, S.H., 139, 141
Shaw, J.E., 193, 194, 203
Shearer, D.A., 141
Shearer, D.R., 203
Sherer, E., 159
Sherouse, G.W., 53
Shiu, A.S., 81, 83
Shohoji, T., 159
Shore, R.E., 159, 194
Shrott, K.R., 82
Shultis, J.K., 194
Siddon, R.L., 54
Sievert, R.M., 99, 140
Silari, M., 194
Siler, W.M., 117, 118, 140
Sill, J., 82
Simpson, L., 54
Sinclair, W.K., 139, 159
Skinner, A.L., 53
Slayton, R., 54
Smith, L.P., 81
Soleimani-Meigooni, A., 81
Souhami, L., 83
Stephenson, S.K., 193, 194, 203
Sternick, E.S., 81, 83, 140
Stewart, J.R., 83
Storchi, P.R.M., 81

Stovall, M., 140
Streffer, C., 159
Suit, H.D., 202
Supe, S.J., 139
Svensson, G.K., 54
Swanson, W.P., 193, 194
Syed, N., 139, 141

T

Takahashi, M., 53
Tapley, N., 82, 83, 141
Tepper, J.E., 52, 53, 54, 83, 141
Taylor, L., 114, 115
Thomadsen, B., 194, 203
Thomas, C.I., 139
Thompson, D., 158
Todd, M., 141
Tonnesen, G.L., 54
Torresin, A., 194
Tosi, G., 194
Tranter, F.W., 53
Trott, N.G., 139, 141, 159
Tsien, K.C., 53, 54
Turner, R.C.R., 193, 194, 203

U

Ulin, K., 81
Upton, A.C., 159

V

Van Dyk, J., 54
van de Geijn, J.A., 53, 83, 203
Veath, J.M., 84, 139

W

Wagner, L.K., 119, 140
Walker, S., 81
Wambersie, A., 141

Wang, C.C., 53
Wang, S., 83
Weatherwax, J.L., 114, 115
Weaver, J., 83
Weaver, K.A., 140
Webster, E.W., 53, 203
Welsh, A.D., 141
Werner, B.L., 81, 82
Wharton, J.T., 141
Wiles, J., 52
Wilkinson, J.M., 141
Williams, P.C., 82
Williamson, J.F., 54, 139, 140, 141
Wilson, J.F., 140, 141
Wilson, R., 159
Wollin, M., 141
Woo, M.K., 81
Wood, M., 194
Wood, V.A., 139, 203
Woods, M.J., 141
Worsnop, R., 202
Wright, A.E., 82, 139, 202
Wright, D.J., 54
Wright, S.J., 141
Wu, A., 83, 140, 194

Y

Yallow, R.S., 193
Yamaoka, N., 53
Yanni, M.I., 203
Young, D.J., 54
Young, M.E.J., 140

Z

Zeitz, L., 194
Zelle, M., 158
Zeni, L., 194
Zinreich, E., 83
Zwicker, R.D., 83, 140